Health and Safety Communication

Health and Safety Communication: A Practical Guide Forward is an easy introduction to the principles and practice of health and safety communications, providing all you need to know to design and implement communications efforts on a wide range of health and safety topics and issues. Whether you're a student grappling with a health communications course or a professional wishing to learn how to communicate health and safety messages effectively to a range of audiences using a variety of communications media, *Health and Safety Communication* is all you'll need.

This book incorporates two broad sections: the grounding and the applications. The model articulates a planning approach for designing, implementing and reviewing a range of communications approaches. The applications segment specifies numerous approaches, including workshops, print materials, campaigns, the media, public speaking and social media that can be used to convey what the health and safety specialist wants the audience to "know, feel and do" as a result of engagement with the communications approach. *Health and Safety Communication* blends sound foundations with practical strategies for health and safety communication so that messages can be communicated more effectively; after all, for changes to occur, the message must be received and respected.

Unique features of this book include a wide range of approaches and strategies, with numerous examples and tips provided throughout. "Messages from the field" incorporate examples and samples from over 30 individuals and organizations, offering their insights and suggestions. The applied approach of this definitive guide is designed to enhance the competence and confidence of those currently in health or safety arenas, as well as those seeking to incorporate health or safety messages in other settings such as businesses or communities.

David S. Anderson is Professor Emeritus of Education and Human Development at George Mason University, USA.

Richard E. Miller is Associate Professor at George Mason University, USA.

"It is a pleasure and very easy to recommend the new book by experts Drs. Anderson and Miller. As a physician, often asked to comment on health and science, or appear on national TV, I have been doing much of what they suggest. However, I have been a national expert helping to communicate science for at least 40 years. Their book masterfully summarizes a logical approach to becoming an understandable expert without such experience or intensive media training. Starting with the audience and moving to why do such an interview in the first place, the reader must grapple with their own motivations and intention. Moving on to what behavior changes, how to change and communicate and continuously improve your technique and message after each encounter. These 'Steps' become chapters and everything is explained clearly, without jargon and with very useful examples. This is a great and easy to use 'how to' and 'why' book by experts in health, communications and behavior change."

Mark S. Gold, M.D., DFASAM, DLFAPA, Chairman, Scientific Advisory Boards, RiverMend Health, Distinguished Professor

Donald R. Dizney Eminent Scholar and Chairman, Professor (Adjunct), Washington University School of Medicine, Department of Psychiatry, USA

Health and Safety Communication

A Practical Guide Forward

**David S. Anderson and
Richard E. Miller**

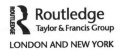
Routledge
Taylor & Francis Group

LONDON AND NEW YORK

First published 2017
by Routledge
2 Park Square, Milton Park, Abingdon, Oxon OX14 4RN

and by Routledge
711 Third Avenue, New York, NY 10017

Routledge is an imprint of the Taylor & Francis Group, an informa business

British Library Cataloguing in Publication Data
A catalogue record for this book is available from the British Library

Library of Congress Cataloging in Publication Data
A catalog record for this book has been requested

ISBN: 978-1-138-64742-8 (hbk)
ISBN: 978-1-138-64744-2 (pbk)
ISBN: 978-1-315-62704-5 (ebk)

Typeset in Bembo
by GreenGate Publishing Services, Tonbridge, Kent

Contents

11   Workshops   205

12   Social media   229

Figures and tables

Figures

Tables

About the authors

David S. Anderson Ph.D. is Professor Emeritus of Education and Human Development at George Mason University, where he served from 1987 to 2016. He was Professor and Director of the Center for the Advancement of Public Health, taught undergraduate and graduate courses, and directed over 180 national, state and local externally funded projects. He has served on several national, state and local advisory boards and has provided extensive keynote addresses, seminars and workshops. His areas of specialization include health promotion, communication and education, drug/alcohol abuse prevention, strategic planning and mobilization, and needs assessment and evaluation.

His strategic planning work emphasizes youth and young adults, school and community leaders, program planners and policy makers. He serves in a translational role with research, needs assessment and evaluation approaches appropriate for practitioners, policy makers, academics and scientists. Recent publications include *Wellness Issues for Higher Education* (2015) and *Further Wellness Issues for Higher Education* (2016); research includes the College Alcohol Survey (1979–2015), Wellness Assessment for Higher Education Preparation Programs and Understanding Teen Drinking Cultures in America. He developed *COMPASS: A Roadmap to Healthy Living* and *COMPASS Roadmap: Destination Health*.

Earlier in his career, he served as a college administrator, with positions as Director of Residence Life at Ohio University, Director of Residential Life at Radford University and Residence Hall Director at The Ohio State University. He received his Bachelor of Science Degree from Duke University, his Master of Arts Degree from The Ohio State University and his Ph.D. from Virginia Polytechnic Institute and State University.

Richard E. Miller Ed.D. is Associate Professor of health education at George Mason University. He has been a program specialist affiliated with the Center for the Advancement of Public Health at the University. Prior to his current faculty position, he was manager of health promotion at the Xerox Corporation and manager of occupational health at the University of Rochester's Medical Center. He has published widely in several peer-refereed journals in health education and promotion, employee assistance, occupational health and traffic safety. Currently he specializes in preparing driver education instructors and in that capacity he boasts of having driver-licensed over 3,000 high school students.

Preface

The world is fraught with thousands of health and safety issues that warrant attention. Whether it is the quality of water, immunization, emerging diseases, aggressive driving, obesity, fire safety, intellectual challenges or drug addiction, the opportunity to make a difference is omnipresent. Some of these issues have greater needs in some areas of the world than in others; and some of these issues are more pronounced among some groups or populations than in others. Whatever the issue or setting, whatever the audience or approach, opportunities exist to make changes in positive directions.

Thankfully, progress has been made, on so many fronts, to reduce the harm or concern associated with so many health and safety issues. And, thankfully, many dedicated professionals and concerned individuals, groups, organizations and agencies have the knowledge and skill to create change. However, while so much progress has been made, much more remains to be accomplished.

That's where this book comes in. As authors, we were inspired to develop this book based on our life-long work with health and safety issues. Between us, we have 80 years of professional work, primarily in the arena of health promotion. Our work in an academic environment has provided us with opportunities to work with students preparing for work in a wide range of professions, whether health-related, business-oriented, human development focused or other specialty. We have each worked in settings outside of academics, and each of us has worked closely with local, state and national organizations. We are aware of changes in how health and safety issues are addressed and are often frustrated with the quality with which health and safety topics are discussed and addressed.

With our work with a range of groups and organizations—non-profit and profit-oriented, large and small, urban and rural—we find that knowledgeable people and organizations often seek relevant approaches for communicating their messages. We have found, all too often, that these dedicated individuals don't have the background or skills for preparing or implementing their communications work. Our aim with this book is to aid individuals and organizations to communicate more effectively with their health and safety initiatives—to be more clear, more up-to-date and, ultimately, more persuasive. We strongly believe that those communicating the health and safety messages do want to have their messages respected and followed. We also believe that, all too often, these well-intended messages fall short of their targets. Thus, we prepared this book with a very practical orientation. It is our aim to enhance the skills as well as the confidence of those doing the communication, so that the results achieved more closely match the results desired.

This is not to say the current messages are not effective, as many are. Many individuals and organizations with specialized skills are quite effective with their messaging; however, these can be costly and out of reach of the thousands of individuals and smaller groups seeking to promote healthier and safer lives with their audiences. Even in the classroom, we find gaps with students' academic preparation focusing on communication skills; while much of this comes with life experience, we seek to "jump start" these young professionals with their message development and delivery.

General considerations

In our preparation of this book, several factors were critical for our writing. Primary among our guiding principles was that we wanted an applied approach. We wanted a "hands on" resource that would be helpful for students and practitioners. The aim for our book was to be useful and practical, and to provide numerous "how to" approaches for their current and future efforts with communicating about **health and safety** issues.

Coupled with this applied approach was the fact that we wanted a resource that was grounded in current science and best practices. To accomplish this, we incorporated our varied experiences and current professional literature to help orchestrate the content and examples. Central with our thinking is that effective approaches need to be grounded with sound theoretical frameworks and good practice; we build on this and highlight effective practices based on firm foundations.

Third, our aim was to provide current examples from practitioners in the field, from all types of settings. We asked policy makers and agency heads, organizers and academics, leaders and grassroots personnel to share their experiences. The book has dozens of examples labeled "Messages from the field" that highlight a wide range of experiences and insights from these professionals. We sought to gather their insights and wisdom to help guide the book's readers with planning and implementing their efforts.

Fourth, we sought a broad focus with communications activities. We weren't limited to brochures and posters, and we didn't want to emphasize campaigns alone. We wanted to be sure that all types of communication initiatives would be included, knowing that our audience of students and practitioners would have the opportunity to share their messages in a wide variety of ways. We wanted to be sure to include workshops and speeches; we incorporated interviews on the radio or television, as well as newspapers and newsletters. We included the emerging role of social media and highlight approaches like flash lectures and blogging. While each of these could comprise an entire book (and many do!), we emphasize the breadth of approaches.

A fifth consideration is that we also addressed both health and safety together. We believe that, while safety is often omitted from a consideration of health, its topics and issues are very much based in a healthy life and environment. Consider safety belts and bike helmets; fire safety and boating safety; impaired driving and personal safety; these often do not come to mind when thinking about "health." We know how vitally important these and many other safety topics are, and we wanted to formally highlight this with both the book title and contents.

Sixth and most important, we wanted to focus on proactive, preventive approaches. Our emphasis is with individuals and organizations seeking to promote health and safety. Our emphasis is not on patients and what is typically a reactive approach, such as dealing with an illness or medical situation. Our focus with this book is for promoting positive attitudes and behaviors, so that unsafe, unhealthy and otherwise problematic situations are avoided. While dealing with patients is vitally important, and health communication is indeed an essential part of that interaction, that specific setting or focus is not the emphasis of this book. In addition, medical personnel may very well benefit from this book; this book is not about "bedside manner" or "patient communication," although some of the approaches will be helpful for these personnel. Beyond this, a medical specialist may, indeed, be called upon to offer his or her expertise in a proactive manner; imagine a dentist conducting a workshop, a nurse practitioner appearing on a television show to describe actions for reducing harm during a medical emergency, a veterinarian describing healthy habits or a doctor testifying at a public hearing. Each of these situations is quite relevant for this book, as they are envisioned as proactive in approach.

These points serve as the foundation for our approach. We emphasize praxis, where theory and background join with practical applications. We want a sound, practical approach that builds on many quality approaches, yet offers a process that is open for renewal and refinement. We are acutely aware of the changing landscape associated with the ways in which people learn. We encourage our readers to attend to sound processes such as those incorporated here and be open to embracing new strategies if they can aid with delivering a quality message and having the desired results.

Book organization

The organization of this book builds upon our approach as one of praxis—the blend of theoretical and practical approaches. As such, the book is organized into two major parts. The first part—Health and safety communications model—incorporates a strong theoretical foundation and sound planning approaches. In this part, we offer a framework that serves as a foundation for planning and executing health and safety communication efforts. This five-part model—the health and safety communications model – is introduced in the book's first chapter. Each of its five elements serves as the basis for the following five chapters.

The second part of the book—Health and safety communications approaches—addresses the primary ways in which these communications activities occur. Chapters are devoted to campaigns, print materials, workshops and working with the media. We also offer a chapter called "A public presence" where we highlight a range of individualized approaches, such as giving a speech or a TED talk, being interviewed or on a panel, or having an "elevator speech" ready. Further, we have a chapter about social media, with some fairly basic approaches such as websites and blogging, Facebook and Twitter, and other recent and emerging approaches. We end the book with some final thoughts and perspectives.

Throughout the book, even in the first part, we incorporate practical approaches and experiences shared by individuals and organizations that have worked with health and safety communications in the past. We conclude each chapter with a theme of "Forward!" as that highlights our perspectives about where we expect our readers are heading with specific efforts.

The book's audiences and context

As we prepared this book, we envisioned two major audiences. One audience encompasses the practitioner and the other is a student. With the practitioner, this is someone who may or may not be working in a health or safety setting. This practitioner may be a public health specialist, whose responsibility is one of promoting health messages as part of a defined professional responsibility. Or, it may be an individual who is working in a health profession, but whose responsibilities do not involve communications; however, based on his/her expertise, others may call upon this individual to participate in some communications effort such as a community panel, testifying, public speech or other approach. Similarly, as described earlier, a doctor or nurse may be called upon to conduct a workshop or offer a talk. Or, consider a local sheriff who is asked to do a talk about highway safety concerns, or to prepare a brochure about the use of mopeds in the community. Similarly, an engineer may be asked to lend his or her expertise to a panel discussion, and wants to be able to be more effective with the presentation. Or, within an organization with multiple or many employees, an aim is to provide better information for the employees on any of a range of health and safety topics; perhaps a newsletter or information series is wanted, and an employee is asked to provide leadership for that. For each of these individuals and so many others, this book provides practical guidance and suggestions about being more effective with planning and implementing these efforts. While the second part of the book may be of immediate relevance, the first part provides some foundational information that can be helpful for planning larger-scale and longer-term initiatives.

The other audience includes students preparing to embark on a professional career. This could be a student preparing for health promotion, community health or a related professional area. It could also be someone in the allied health professions who seeks to be able to communicate more effectively with prevention messages. It may be a student in the judicial or enforcement arena, or someone who is studying public and international affairs; it may be a student in business who wants to be prepared to promote a healthier work environment. Whatever the professional role, this book offers professional preparation with the range of theoretical and planning constructs offered in Part I, as well as the numerous practical approaches incorporated within Part II. Many traditional textbooks have identified learning objectives for each chapter, as well as quiz questions, discussion topics and related pedagogical features; this book, with its applied approach, relies on the engagement of the instructional faculty as well as the self-directed learning styles found among many students.

Our hope is that both types of audiences find this book helpful and refreshing. We hope that the blend of theoretical and practical, and exemplified by examples from a wide range of practitioners, is helpful in establishing sound foundations for more effective communications.

Summing up

Our vision with this book is to help a wide range of practitioners from all sorts of professional and volunteer settings. Our audience is not limited to those who have a professional role with health or safety communication; we know so many others will benefit from the skills and tools to be more effective with their communication efforts. With so many health and safety issues warranting sound science and more effective messages, our aim is a simple one—help individuals and organizations, with their behaviors of interest, to "move the needle"!!

We have heard the common phrase of "paying it forward," as individuals are doing good works to help make others' lives better. As individuals read this book, whether specific segments or in its entirety, we hope our readers think about how they can help make others' lives healthier and safer. We know so many people are well intended with their efforts but just don't have the time or expertise to communicate their messages in ways that resonate effectively and that make a difference. We hope some of the tools and resources here help to bring greater awareness and, ultimately, behavior change.

In preparing this book, we clearly stand on the shoulders of those who have prepared the "Messages from the field," as they share their wisdom and experiences, their heart-aches and joys, from which all of us can learn and grow. We hope the readers learn from those experiences, as well as those from us as authors, to help leave others better off as a result of our collective efforts.

David S. Anderson, Ph.D., Professor Emeritus of Education and Human Development,
Richard E. Miller, Ed.D., Associate Professor, George Mason University, Fairfax, Virginia

Part I

Health and safety communications model

1 Health and safety communications

You as the communicator

If you want to produce some type of health and safety communication, then this guide is for you. Maybe it's a newsletter, public service announcement or presentation meant to promote the health of others or reduce their risk of injury. Or maybe you'll be interviewed for a newspaper article or on a radio or television show. Perhaps you'll be leading a workshop or discussion, or even providing some testimony for a group of decision-makers, whether at the local, state or national level. Maybe you just want to write or say something, or prepare some standard or creative approach to help others be healthier or safer in their lives. For any of these situations and more, the insights, strategies and tools in this guide will help you be more effective.

This guide is for three audiences: students studying health and safety communication, employees with job responsibility in health and safety communications, and those wanting to health-and-safety-communicate as a community service. Producing and delivering materials addressing traffic safety, stress management, healthy eating and exercise, and related topics requires a sound grasp of health and safety communications. You might think putting together a flier is a simple undertaking. However, much more goes into it if you want to be successful at reaching and influencing your audience. That's where this guide comes in handy.

You are an important source of health and safety communications. You have some degree of knowledge or awareness that you think is important and helpful to share with others. Your success with getting your message across hinges on your understanding of the audience. Specifically, you need to compose your message according to what you want your audience to know, feel and do. Being successful requires sending your message using one or more appropriate channels. You have many approaches from which to choose: fliers and posters, newsletters, workshops, social media, public service announcements and so many more. Ultimately, your efforts should have an impact—that is, influence or persuade recipients to promote personal health and/or reduce their risk of harm and injury. This guide for health and safety communicators explains the "how-to's" as well as provides actual examples and tips from the field.

Communication and messages

Communication involves messages. A **message** is information sent from a source to an audience. The **source**, like you, originates the message. The message needs to be encoded. That is, the information has to be organized in a manner understandable by the intended audience. This is accomplished through composition in which the message is designed with certain structure, content and style. In order for the message to be sent successfully from the source to the audience its composition is based on **strategy**, a plan of action to create change. The message **channel** is the route of delivery (i.e., medium or approach). The **audience** is the receiver and decoder of the message. And, message **impact** is the degree of influence and persuasion experienced by the receiving audience. These are the basic components of communication and messages (see Figure 1.1).

Communication and its components have synonyms that will be used throughout this guide. The term health and safety communications also goes by: effort, initiative, production or program. The component, source, is also referred to as the communicator. Composition of the message involves knowing the intended audience and constructing the aim and goals of the communication effort. The aim is to influence and/or persuade whereas the goal is the desired change in the intended audience. Strategy will be substituted with know-feel-do at times. Think of it as a plan for changing the behavior of the audience. The channel is the route of message delivery. It requires selecting an appropriate approach (e.g., workshop, speech, billboard or public service announcement) and using it as the vehicle for implementing the strategy. The audience decoding the message can be recipients, receivers or targets. The influence or persuasiveness of the message on the audience is considered the impact; these are the results, and represent what is different with the audience as a result of your communication efforts.

Types of communication

One evident type of communication is directed at the masses. **Mass media** are used to disseminate messages widely, rapidly and continuously to a target group or audience. The **aim** or goal is to arouse intended meanings in large and diverse audiences and to influence them in a variety of ways.[1] You are likely familiar with **mass communication**. Think of it as a prepared and distributed brochure or as a displayed poster with an intended audience of more than 20 individuals. As a larger-scale example, perhaps you may have received Amber Alerts or Silver Alerts through your cell phone. Those, indeed, are safety mass communication efforts. Mass communication of health and safety messages is conveyed through public service announcements, whether on the radio, television, newspapers, billboard or through other channels. You see it in internet advertisements as well as with social media. Health and safety communications can be paid advertising or they can be incorporated within the day-to-day affairs of those involved with the media. Mass communication relies on larger-audience workshops and training. Webinars, podcasts, blogs and tweets can transmit interviews, discussions, speeches and flash mob talks to the masses. *Health and Safety Communication: A Practical Guide Forward* centers primarily on mass communication.

More venues and opportunities for applying health and safety communication skills are coming, particularly with the fast-changing nature of technology in today's society. The skill-building in this guide is foundational in nature and covers much of the state of the art for addressing health and safety topics and exploring related issues. Effective health and safety communication relies on the passion and creativity of the source—that's you!

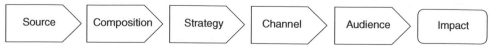

Figure 1.1 Communication and messages

The other type of communication is **interpersonal communication** during which messages are conveyed between persons to inform, instruct or persuade. Usually, a source generates the message to be conveyed to either another individual or a small group of individuals (20 people or less), all of whom represent the audience. An example of this communication is between a health professional and his/her patient or client. There is usually a two-way dynamic in interpersonal communication. The person receiving the message (audience) can process its meaning (decode) and, in turn, generate a responsive message back to the original source. During this reciprocity of messaging, professional and personal health information is shared, matters are discussed, instructions are provided and intended action is expressed. An important feature to interpersonal communication is the range of non-verbal cues. That includes impressions or feelings given to a person or small group through the use of facial expressions, body movements and other gestures.

One example of interpersonal communication is found with the interactions with a health professional, sometimes called "bedside manner." For a patient, it could appear as attentive eye-contact and cooperative body positioning. Another example is found with the delivery of workshops or speeches, and the ways in which the presenter relates to the audience. Appropriate interpersonal communication is a vital factor for effective message delivery, and for the audience feeling a sense of connection with the presenter.

While this guide has a primary emphasis on mass communication, the elements of interpersonal communication are integral for professionals as they incorporate approaches such as patient education, in-service training and public responses.

Health and safety communications

Health and safety are dynamic states of living involving degrees of personal risk, function-ality and satisfaction. Stating the obvious, health is central to your life and to the lives of those around you. Without health, life's challenges severely compromise well-being. With health, you can live a more rewarding and fulfilling life. Similarly, safety is vital to your continued survival and well-being; living unsafely is a leading cause of death, injury and debilitation.

You face health- and safety-related tasks and challenges daily:

- eating breakfast (whether you choose to and what you eat);
- washing your hands regularly;
- wearing safety belts as driver or passenger;
- working out on most days;
- drinking plenty of water daily;
- watching where you walk and properly crossing at traffic intersections;
- wearing protective gear or clothing, depending on the situation and weather;
- getting your food from sanitary locations.

Performing these tasks and facing challenges tend to become second nature with little consideration of the health and safety risks associated with not doing them. Have you ever observed a distracted pedestrian texting on a mobile device while wearing ear buds? Other issues may not be seen as vital, such as the importance of drinking plenty of water or flossing teeth. And still, other challenges may have not been contemplated by you or others, such as making responsible alcohol drinking decisions or protecting your hearing from loud noise. Whatever the situation, engaging in more healthful and safe practices can do a lot to enhance the quality and length of your life; and helping others be more healthy and safe can do the same for their lives.

Is living healthily and safely a cure-all? Absolutely not. Are there guarantees that engaging in healthy and safe behaviors will be successful? No. Even if an individual follows all the guidance and lives life with all the health principles that can be found, no guarantees exist that his/her life will be extremely long. A good example of this is the past exercise enthusiast Jim Fixx, author of best-selling books on running and fitness, who died of a heart attack at the age of 52.[2] Genetic predisposition, a congenitally enlarged heart, and being a former smoker who was obese prior to beginning his running routine, eventually caught up with him. The point is that Fixx's healthy behavior change did not prevent him from having a heart attack, but it may have contributed to his living nine years longer than his father.

Many diseases exist today without clear causal factors, and situations may emerge that result in a shortened or compromised life. In addition, as science continues with new discoveries, perspectives may shift about how to best live one's life. The advice received from the scientific and medical community continues to evolve, so it is important to stay as current as possible. For instance, it was once considered unhealthy to eat eggs due to the risk of high serum cholesterol, but more current nutritional researchers are encouraging reconsideration since they view eggs as a whole food, with positive contribution to a healthy diet.[3] Through the process of maximizing the inclusion of health considerations, one's chances of living longer, and living a life with increased quality, are enhanced. Another example is hand positioning on the automobile steering wheel; gone are the days of "10 and 2" because now traffic safety specialists recommend "8 and 4."[4]

Health and safety communication is conveying messages that raise awareness about health- and safety-related topics and encourage the audience to explore related issues. The messages are aimed at influencing or persuading recipients to develop knowledge, attitudes and skills to address these issues. This guide prepares you as an effective health and safety communicator. Designing a poster, composing a brochure, contributing to a newsletter, creating a website, conducting a workshop and other approaches are ways to communicate about health and safety topics and issues. You might be assigned communication tasks through work or you might eagerly volunteer to make these productions "happen." So to start this journey of becoming an effective health and safety communicator, whether through your work or your community service, it is necessary to understand what you are trying to do.

You might think it is easy to raise another person's awareness about a health/safety topic and engage them in related issues. Essentially, you intend to influence and persuade them to gain knowledge, reexamine their beliefs or consider changing their behavior. You may think all that is needed is to expose the audience to relevant information. In fact, many efforts to promote health and reduce safety risks fall short because the message did not reach the targeted audience. This could be explained by **selective exposure** in which the receiving audience is not the target audience but rather the audience most receptive to the message. Think of it this way: the people who listen to public service announcements, volunteer in community campaigns or actively participate in a workshop might not be the intended or preferred target audience, or the ones who need the information or inspiration you offer. That means that they were receptive to the intended message from the start and probably did not require efforts at influencing or persuading them. So many times health and safety communications end up being a confirmation or reinforcement for people who are already healthy and safe—a type of reassurance they are already doing well. Unfortunately, in these efforts, the communicator misses the people at risk who need to hear the message. One way of getting around this is to make sure your message has a novel, eye-catching or shaking feature in order to ensure the attention of the desired target audience.

An effective health and safety message does more than simply secure the audience's attention. The receiver must comprehend the information being presented, whether this is the result of a single delivery or through varied approaches or through repetition (perhaps to the point of being obsolete). Any medium, if properly utilized, can lead or assist the receiver in increasing personal knowledge just as well as face-to-face approaches. Important with this process is **media literacy** which is the ability to analyze and interpret the messages. This means helping the audience have the skills necessary to apply what is communicated, and preparing messages and approaches that incorporate the varying media literacy levels of target audiences.

A health and safety message's ability to influence knowledge gain, and to affect belief and behavioral change, rests on its meaningfulness as well as its impact over a period of time. It is one thing for a persuasive communication to trigger audience response to an immediate situation demand, and it is another matter for the message to be consequential. To obtain the desired results, the communication should be repeatedly generated from one or more sources of credibility and trustworthiness and then conveyed through a variety of media or channels. The message should engage the audience by appealing to its salient interests and needs. Accordingly, the receiver should realize the message is consistent with his/her social network and be invited to express a newly formed attitude. Just as important, health communicating prompts the receiver to plan for action and directs him/her to appropriate sources of instruction and demonstration.

A model

For health and safety communications to work, you need a recipe for success. Without a recipe or model, your effort may not reach the intended audience, whether in a physical sense or through its appeal. Can you imagine a product being designed without background work? Something complex, like an automobile, requires an immense amount of research and testing prior to release; even a simpler product, such as a pair of shoes, requires significant planning and research. How about someone writing a play or theatrical production—wouldn't the playwright need to have done a lot of preparation?

If communication is messaging, then the message represents or addresses a particular health and safety topic or issue. The composition of the message is based on persuasive communication with the aims of informing and influencing the audience's health and safety status. The channel can be one of an array of available vehicles from newsletter articles to staff in-service training workshops. The ultimate goal is for health improvement and risk reduction in the audience.

There are several health and safety communication models in practice for both interpersonal and mass communication.[5,6,7,8] A highly cited model is presented in the National Cancer Institute's *Making Health Communication Programs Work*;[9] for this guide, a simplistic yet effective model of health and safety communications is used. The model used in this *Health and Safety Communication: A Practical Guide Forward* is similarly straightforward, simple, yet effective. The content throughout this guide relies on this basic **health and safety communications model** (see Figure 1.2). The model's steps are circular and depict the start and successful end to your health and safety communications effort.

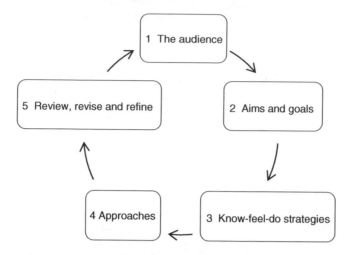

Figure 1.2 Health and safety communications model

Step 1: The audience

Health and safety communications start with knowing the audience—the intended receivers of your messages. You have to identify and recognize the audience's needs. Think of a **need** as circumstances in which something is necessary or a situation that requires a course of action. You are not going to undertake a communications endeavor simply to do so (unless it is for a class project or work assignment, for example). Your work starts with recognizing something that is not right or not as healthy as you would like it to be. Further, the issue of concern may be more relevant to one audience compared to another audience. For example, there may be health disparities among groups based on various demographic or other factors, such as level of education, socio-economic status, race/ethnicity, country of origin/immigration status or sexual orientation. You also want to know about the circumstances or context within which the audience exists, as well as different ways in which they learn best.

Step 2: Aims and goals

Next, you will decide on the purpose or intention of your effort. This is called the *aim* of the health and safety communication. The aim is not preparing posters, doing workshops or designing attractive fliers. Rather, the aim is providing influence or facilitating motivation so a change in knowledge, attitudes and/or behavioral intent (and ultimately behavior) will be achieved or reinforced. To help in this regard, think of the *goal*, that is, the desired state of the audience. You will probably envision them, overall, as having higher health and safety risk, and/or having lower functionality and life satisfaction. And then, more specifically, you will identify concrete and focused areas and issues (e.g., knowledge, attitudes, perceptions, skills) that will build on the need and then contribute to the achievement of the broader goals. Health and safety communicators commonly review relevant topics and explore significant issues related to risk reduction and life enhancement.

Step 3: Know–feel–do strategies

The next task is planning your action—just what you want your audience to know–feel–do. Health and safety communications strategies are based on behavior change theories. The messages need to penetrate the audience and encourage recipients to consider changing behaviors to improve health and safety status. For example, to promote children's dental health, your message has to be effective in getting children to brush and floss their teeth regularly. If you are campaigning for physical fitness, then you have to convince people to perform physical activity for 30 minutes on most days.

Step 4: Approaches

The **approach** is a specific health and safety communications method or medium such as a flier or a workshop. It needs to be designed by the communicator and then delivered to the audience. Designing and delivery comprise channeling. This step requires careful planning and sufficient resources. Sometimes health and safety communicators select more than one approach since one method/medium can draw upon the other, each serving to reinforce the primary messages. This is seen in campaigns that customarily are comprised of several approaches, such as print media, radio public service announcements and billboards. The health and safety message has to be consistently and effectively woven throughout these combined approaches.

Step 5: Review, revise and refine

While placed as the fifth step, this is actually not the "last" step to the model because reviewing, revising and refining the health and safety communication effort takes place throughout the preceding steps; the activities of this step are not simply conducted after the approach has been delivered to the audience. This step is based on every day evaluation, meaning the communicators determine the impact of the message while also ensuring continued improvement of the overall effort and its successful implementation.

All too often, those preparing health and safety communications rely heavily on only one or two of these steps without full consideration of the rest of the steps. With that in mind, it should not be surprising that many health and safety communications efforts are unsuccessful. But to be fair, trying to enact behavior change through health and safety messages is often challenging and difficult. At the same time, these efforts can be most rewarding. To be successful, your approach must be grounded and thoughtful. That's why each of the five steps is important, and each one serves a vital role with designing and implementing successful health and safety communications. Further details about knowing the audience, deciding on aims and goals, specific know–feel–do strategies for composing and channeling the message, and evaluation approaches for gauging success and approaches follow in subsequent chapters.

As you think about using this model, a final reflection is that it is, indeed, a lot of work. You may also wonder about whether it is worthwhile to do, since your health and safety communications effort will generally not be perfect. Those are valid concerns, yet they should be recognized. Just imagine what your effort would be like if you did *not* engage in thoughtful planning, but just threw together a brochure or flier. As you critique current campaigns, fliers, workshops or other communication approaches currently available, you can often find ways that those efforts could have been improved. Further, even though you go through a thoughtful and grounded process, this does not guarantee that your results will be 100 percent successful; the reality is that you are working with human beings, each of whom has different perspectives and ways of being motivated to know, feel or do what you want them to. If you and your effort can increase the likelihood of success, and that's exactly what this process is designed to do, then you should feel satisfied that it was worth the effort.

Messages

The success of health and safety communications rests on the message reaching its intended audience and influencing the recipients to know, feel and do, and to do so in the desired directions that you seek. While communicating, it is important to remember that there are no guarantees of success. Just because you are clear does not mean that your audience will understand your message, or that you will, in fact, achieve the results that you desire. What is important to remember is that you will be more likely to achieve your desired results if you are clearer with your aims.

There's another perspective that is vitally important—it is unwise, unhealthy and unnecessary to set yourself up for failure, whether in your eyes or in the viewpoints of others. If you set out to affect behavior change on a specific topic or issue, with a particular audience, but you do not achieve your intended outcome, then you (or others) may view this effort a failure. That is just not fair. However, if you aim to increase the knowledge of a specific audience then you should assess whether or not that audience did, in fact, increase its knowledge. It is not appropriate to evaluate the communications effort solely on behavior change (which may be your ultimate goal) when your aim was actually to increase knowledge; however it is fair to assess changes in knowledge when that was your aim. Later in this guide, you will find a chapter on evaluation; this emphasizes the needed congruence between your aims, your know–feel–do strategies and your measures of success. Throughout this guide, examples of actual health and safety messages are inserted.

Forward!

In summary, communication specialists rely on messages sent from a source to an audience. Originating the message is the source. The message comprises structure, content and style designed for the intended audience. Accordingly, the message is channeled through a delivery medium (e.g., pamphlet, presentation, public service announcement). The audience is the receiver of the message. If effective, the message will impact, influence or persuade the audience. This guide centers primarily on mass communication methods and emphasizes the importance of well-planned and clearly communicated messages. To be an effective health and safety communicator, you need to be competent, confident and committed.

In this chapter you were introduced to the health and safety communications model. A brief description of each step was provided. More will be covered about this model in subsequent chapters. Overall, the challenge for you as a health and safety communicator is to apply this model in order to influence and persuade your audience. The health and safety communications effort must, to maximize its impact, be planned and carefully orchestrated. This process might seem daunting. After all, as will be emphasized throughout this guide, there is no one set strategy, and no single magic answer, even for a specific health topic. The idea is to become better prepared and skillful in implementing an approach that is more likely to have the impact that you want. Your involvement with health and safety efforts is not a pointless one; you have some level of commitment to seeing your efforts be successful, or as successful as possible.

Notes

1 DeFleur, M.K. and Dennis, E.E. (2002). *Understanding Mass Communication*. Boston, MA: Houghton Mifflin Harcourt.
2 Altman, L. (1984, July 24). The doctor's world; James Fixx: the enigma of heart disease. *New York Times*.
3 Herron, K.L. and Fernandez, M.L. (2004). Are the current dietary guidelines regarding egg consumption appropriate? *The Journal of Nutrition*, 134, 187–190.
4 VADOE (2011). *45-Hour Parent/Teen Driving Guide*. Richmond, VA: Virginia Department of Education.
5 Patient Safety Assertion Model (2015). *Assertion—Communication & Patient Safety Speaking Up for Patient Safety—Communication Skills for Healthcare Professionals*. Safer HealthCare. Retrieved February, 2015 from http://health and safety communications.saferhealthcare.com/high-reliability-topics/communication-and-patient-safety/.
6 OSHA (2003). *Model Plans and Programs for the OSHA Bloodborne Pathogens and Hazard Communications Standards*. Washington, DC: Occupational Safety and Health Administration, U.S. Department of Labor.
7 NYU (2015). *Overview of the Structure and Sequence of Effective Doctor Patient Communication*, NYU Macy Initiative on Health Communication. New York, NY: NYU School of Medicine. Retrieved February, 2015 from http://nyumacy.med.nyu.edu/curriculum/model/m00a.html.
8 MHCPW (2015). *Making Health Communication Programs Work: A Planner's Guide*. Retrieved February, 2015 from www.cancer.gov/publications/health-communication/pink-book.pdf.
9 McKenzie, J.F., Neiger, B.L. and Thackeray, R. (2013) *Planning, Implementing, & Evaluating Health Promotion Programs: A Primer* (6th ed.). San Francisco, CA: Benjamin Cummings.

2 The audience

Step 1

Applying the health and safety communications model starts with a sound working knowledge of your audience (Figure 2.1). In fact, having knowledge and insights about your audience (or audiences) is an essential aspect of preparing your messages and having the results that you seek.

Imagine if you are trying to learn a new language, but to do so you are thrust onto an advanced conversational course. The language is difficult to process at that level of proficiency. Another example is reading Shakespeare's plays. The scripts are in early modern English, very timely for when he wrote them, but now they sound funny and can be difficult to understand. Despite these challenges, you can learn a new language by knowing sentence structure, vocabulary or tenses practiced by the conversationalists.

Similarly with health and safety communications, you want to make sure that your message reaches and resonates with your audience. If you are trying to connect with

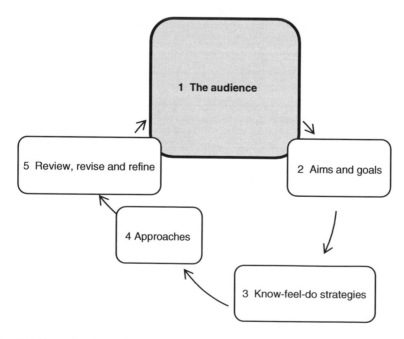

Figure 2.1 Knowing the audience

those in a large urban setting with illustrations about farmland and open spaces, this may not be relevant or appropriate (unless, of course, your aim is to illustrate differences with these distinct settings). If your audience is primarily visual in style, or the cultural values and perspectives are strong in a certain direction, you will want to make sure your approaches honor these orientations.

To know your audience means realizing its interests and needs. What are your audience's needs? Think of a need as circumstances in which something is necessary or a situation that requires a course of action. You are likely not going to undertake a communications endeavor simply to do so; you have something that you want to accomplish and some difference that you want to make. Your efforts with communication center first on recognizing something that is not healthy or safe among your intended audience. Whether it is from data, experience, or your general feeling, you know that some changes or improvements are needed. You may also know that the gap or area of concern is greater in one audience when compared with another; for example, within a certain age group, males may have a greater incidence of the identified health or safety issue than females. Further, health disparities may exist among different groups of individuals, based on a range of demographic factors (e.g., age, gender, education level, socio-economic status, race/ethnicity, country of origin/immigration status, or sexual orientation/gender identity). Accordingly, attending to specific audience(s) of need as well as distinct needs among audiences is important because of numerous factors. You may believe that these gaps are due to inattention or lack of prioritization of that audience; you may further believe that this difference is unethical, or at least unwarranted.

Another factor for consideration is that different audiences may have different needs; you may find that a health issue is higher in a particular audience but it is not found in another audience; thus, the need commands greater attention. For example, first-year college students, when compared with other students, have higher needs regarding appropriate study habits, or healthy decision-making about alcohol use. Or those in certain geographic regions of the country may have been exposed to certain experiences based on the weather, topography, climate, natural resources, culture and numerous other factors; this awareness makes a difference for you as you plan for your communication efforts to resonate positively with your target audience.

Related to awareness about the audience is knowledge about the issue. It is vital to be as current as possible, as knowledge continues to evolve. It is helpful to know what the science surrounding the issue reports. In other words, what is the latest research? It is also important to know the latest approaches to be used. For example, learning about cardiopulmonary resuscitation (CPR) using the latest techniques is so important that certification needs to be renewed every one to two years; in fact, in 2009, the American Heart Association started a campaign promoting Hands-Only CPR, designed to minimize brain damage while awaiting professional assistance. This change also addressed many individuals' concerns with artificial respiration, as some people did not want to do "mouth-to-mouth" on a stranger because they did not know if they could get infected or because of their own lack of comfort using this approach. Having quality facts and current information is important for a quality communications approach.

There are some issues for which the need may be fairly universal among the range of audiences; however, the message composition and channeling to reach specific audiences or subgroups will need to vary. For example, if the objective is to increase the use of automobile safety belts, the strategy would likely vary based on a whole range of factors. With soon-to-be juvenile drivers, the approach may be based on a game or challenge opportunity. With youth just learning to drive, the emphasis may be based on legal responsibilities and linkages to a new driver's license. With young adults, attention to perceived invulnerability or **optimism bias**—this is, "a crash will never happen to me"—may be warranted. It was once thought that safety belts would cause pregnant women to miscarry in the event of a car crash, so a campaign to combat misinformation may be best for this audience; this would include evidence that the primary cause of fetal death during traffic crashes is death of the mother because she was not wearing a safety belt. The approach used to engage middle age adults may focus on professional or family responsibilities and elderly adults may be encouraged to use safety belts because of increased fragility of their bodies.

Some communication approaches require the involvement of multiple individuals with varying roles. Consider the issue of dental health habits of children. To achieve appropriate dental hygiene at home, the parent may receive a set of messages that includes tips for using know-feel-do strategies appropriate for the child's age group; at the same time, the child may receive different yet consistent messages, using know-feel-do strategies appropriate for the particular age group. These messages are all designed to accomplish the same goal, but are composed and potentially channeled in different, yet complementary, ways.

Central to effective health and safety communications is targeted segmentation. This might seem obvious based on the examples provided above; however, in actual practice, it is forgotten all too often. What often happens with health and safety communications is contamination by two broad misconceptions. The first misconception is "one approach fits everyone" and the second is "I know my audience." This chapter tackles these two misconceptions while providing greater detail on understanding the audience.

Audiences

Your audience is understood within a universal, selected, or indicated context (see Figure 2.2).[1] The universal approach is used when all audiences are included and a single message is used for everyone. Commonly, federal agencies such as the National Highway Traffic Safety Administration issue standards that are adopted as state laws. For example, the legal alcohol concentration is set at a blood alcohol concentration of 0.08 percent. It is a uniformly accepted standard communicated to the universal audience—the public. The selected context is when specific sub-populations or groups of interest are targeted, whether based on specific need or issue. In this sense, your efforts are to reach those of automobile driver licensing age. Good examples are safe teen driving campaigns or efforts to reach older drivers. A universal message would not be appropriate in this situation, as it would not maximize the opportunity to reach the desired audience most effectively. The same message—safe driving—would be offered in different ways for different audiences, whether new drivers, those with some experience (two–three years), those just turning age 21, those with many years of driving history and older drivers. The indicated strategy is more individualized and based on unique needs while working with an individual in that group. For example, recidivist drunk drivers may receive messages that are targeted to them; similarly, those seeking counseling for a specific mental health issue may benefit from communications efforts that would resonate most effectively for them.

If you think about it, the universal approach would be the easiest to implement. Conversely, it is more challenging to have targeted, focused messages based on an

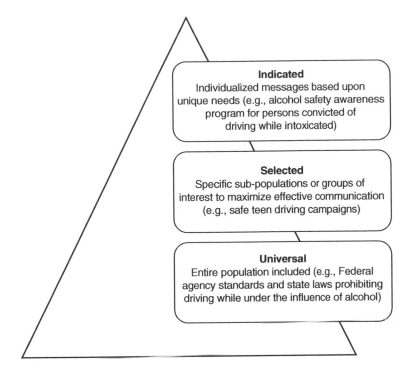

Figure 2.2 Audiences

individual's or subgroup's needs. Thus, many health and safety communications efforts are universal in nature, rather than being targeted. You will see in this chapter how it is more appropriate and helpful to segment your audience to obtain the maximum impact of your communication. Segmenting the audience produces a deeper and richer understanding of its needs, aspirations, hopes, issues, culture and more.

As the audience gets defined for the health and safety communications initiative, the main consideration now is to know more about them. You will want to know what characteristics might be important to understand, so that your health initiative will have the greatest likelihood of success. Why is this important? The answer is fairly obvious, as you want to be able to communicate—to resonate—with the audience you are trying to reach. You want to communicate in the best ways, using the most appropriate approaches that work for meeting your goals with the communications effort. You want your message to be "heard" by them. You want to be understood. You want your audience to "decode" your communication in the way you intend. You may have a very well-designed initiative, but if it is not heard well by them, or is not perceived as being credible, your efforts are, to a large extent, wasted. Similarly, consider the way different generations speak to others. A group of retired seniors will not understand current slang and today's youth won't understand examples that resonate so well with these retirees.

So how can you best learn more about your audience? You will want to conduct some assessment activities, incorporating as many as are reasonable and appropriate based on your timeline and available resources. These may be formalized or very informal. This will also depend on your existing familiarity with the audience. More detail about learning about your audience is found in Chapter 6 which focuses on evaluation activities; the range of approaches useful for evaluation are also applicable for needs assessment activities and can be most helpful as you formulate your strategies and approaches.

It is also vital that you stay up-to-date. For example, if you work with college students on a regular basis, you are likely fairly up-to-date with their thinking, patterns, lifestyles and more. They demonstrate changes from year to year, but many of these are slow and evolving. If you leave the campus, and return in ten years, you will probably notice major changes. Similarly, if you provide examples of or linkages to various things, you will want to be sure they are relevant to your audience. Beloit College has a list of experiences and frames of reference for each entering college class, a listing that has been published annually since 1998. Table 2.1 shows selected items from the listing of 50 items for the class of 2019.[2]

As noted earlier, your work with a specific subgroup may evolve from data collection that has already occurred. That is, you may have decided to target a specific audience because of the differential needs that emerged from some data that shows a higher need or area of concern; that provides an excellent starting point for your planning activities.

Table 2.1 Mindset list of the class of 2019

For this generation of entering college students, born in 1997 …

Hybrid automobiles have always been mass produced.

Google has always been there, in its founding words, "to organize the world's information and make it universally accessible."

They have never licked a postage stamp.

Email has become the new "formal" communication, while texts and tweets remain enclaves for the casual.

Hong Kong has always been under Chinese rule.

They have grown up treating Wi-Fi as an entitlement.

The announcement of someone being the "first woman" to hold a position has only impressed their parents.

Color photos have always adorned the front page of *The New York Times*.

Cell phones have become so ubiquitous in class that teachers don't know which students are using them to take notes and which ones are planning a party.

If you say "around the turn of the century," they may well ask you, "which one?"

The therapeutic use of marijuana has always been legal in a growing number of American states.

Fifteen nations have always been constructing the International Space Station.

The Lion King has always been on Broadway.

First responders have always been heroes.

Poland, Hungary and the Czech Republic have always been members of NATO.

Humans have always had implanted radio frequency ID chips—slightly larger than a grain of rice.

TV has always been in such high definition that they could see the pores of actors and the grimaces of quarterbacks.

However, you may decide that you need to understand more about why this group has a heightened need in this topic area; this may warrant discussions or focus groups to probe deeper into the issue.

- With the data gathered, you see that males are more likely to drink heavily than are females. Why do you think that is the case?
- It has been reported that student-athletes feel more stress than other students; do you agree with this? If so, why do you think this occurs? If not, why?
- How would you describe the different perspectives of various groups so they best understand the topic of aggressive driving and ways of avoiding doing it?
- In what ways would you motivate people a few years younger than you to take better care of their health?
- What messages are most appropriate for reaching groups of people like you about this health issue?
- What approaches would be best for reaching older adults on these specific health concerns? What approaches or know-feel-do strategies would be best?
- What sorts of incentives or disincentives exist regarding getting your peers to pay attention to this health or safety topic, and how do these vary based on the specific topic?

As you think about the issue that you will be addressing with your health and safety communications effort, there are numerous elements that you might want to know about. In fact, as you start to think about it, you may easily get overwhelmed. The important thing is to prioritize what you learn and what you want to know from and about your target audience. One way of thinking about this is to "fast forward" to some of your general outcomes in a more deliberative manner, as you build your communications effort. That is, think now about what it is that you believe you will want the audience to "know, feel or do"; with that in mind, you can start to query their levels of knowledge about various aspects of the topic, their feelings about it, and their current skills as well as perceptions about their own confidence in addressing the issue.

Numerous frameworks and guides can be helpful. As you start to think about the issue, consider the following as trigger points for you to further refine the nature and scope of your questions:

- knowledge about the topic area and sub-topics within this overall topical issue;
- attitudes about the issue or aspects of it;
- reasons that they or others do or don't do the specific behavior;
- awareness about current practices, policies, programs;
- perception of various consequences and associated harm or benefits;
- helpfulness of resources and know-feel-do strategies, messages and referral services;
- understanding of this issue and its importance;
- information desired;
- ease of access for helpful or problematic factors;
- challenges in understanding the new behaviors;
- the role of the cultural context, including family, friends, peers, groups and society;
- health considerations about the issue;
- existing leadership on this issue;
- messages heard about the topic or related topics;
- what is important to them in their lives;

- what types of messages resonate best;
- perspectives of others' engagement in the behavior;
- what communication vehicles are most helpful, and what should be avoided.

One typical outcome that emerges from a data collection process about a specific audience is that it often generates more questions than you started with. As you gather information, you may find that you want to probe further and more deeply, so that you gain a more complete understanding. What you can always remember is that full knowledge about a group of people is never feasible with this type of work (nor will anyone approach work for all individuals within that grouping). The context within which you are gathering information is to maximize further the effectiveness of your efforts. When you gather information about a subgroup, you are gaining further insight and elucidation about what is important to them and, ultimately, what might be triggers or factors that would be associated with behavior change. Thus, you will, in fact, be more knowledgeable; you will also be more aware of all that you do not know.

Once you gather this information, you are poised to start organizing it in some meaningful and helpful ways for the communications effort. You may need to go through several rounds with this, as you gather information and begin to formulate your communications; you may then realize that you need some more information, which you can obtain and feed that back into your planning and development process.

This entire process is just that—a process. You are formulating approaches that have the greatest likelihood of making a difference. You are working to prepare materials that will resonate with your audience. So you are continually tinkering with it, until you release it, or your time is up and you just need to finalize it.

Intermediary audiences

Another important factor while thinking about your audience has to do with **intermediaries**, those persons linking others in order to reach agreement or reconciliation. These persons are important because they can help your message to be heard; similarly they can block the access to as well as the impact of the message you communicate.

For example, if you are working with student-athletes on campus, your effort will benefit from an understanding of the important role that various intermediaries can play on your behalf. These individuals can reinforce your message; alternatively, they can block it. They serve as a gatekeeper role, where they may not permit the distribution of your messages. Consider each of the following within this context:

- Director of Athletics
- Senior Woman Associate
- Compliance Coordinator
- Sports Psychologists
- Sports Dietitians
- Life Skills Coordinators; Academic Advisors
- Faculty Athletics Representatives
- Coaches
- Student Athlete Advisory Committee/Student Athlete Mentor Peer Educators
- Athletic Trainers
- Others.

This can be the same in other settings, where you are working to get your message across. Your efforts benefit from knowing about these intermediary audiences, so that they serve as a helpful and positive "gatekeeper," that they further reinforce your message with the ultimate audience and that their messages are consistent with your message. Each of these is important.

Intermediary audiences are important for several reasons. Essentially, getting your message communicated to your target audience is not as simple as you just providing the message and having the audience receive it. Typically, intermediaries are part of this process of communicating the message. One aspect is that the intermediary may be an approval agent. You may need his/her sign-off or buy-in so that the message can be communicated. Think of a parent, who reviews the message before it is viewed by his/her child. Also, think about the principal of a school; she/he will likely need to approve the message and strategy before it is distributed.

For example, consider a health campaign that you plan to implement within the high school setting. You may have done numerous planning activities, working with the target audience with knowing their needs, pilot testing the messages and much more. However, if your approach has not involved the school principal, or the appropriate approval bodies such as the parent–teacher association, school board, counselors or others, then you may not get the necessary go-ahead to implement the initiative. Involving the gatekeeper or intermediaries in the process of planning can help assure you that you are on the right track. Further, they become more invested in the process and can provide the necessary support and guidance at various points along the way.

Second, the intermediary may be a communications vehicle. You may be relying on this individual to get the message distributed. For the example with the principal again, you may rely on this individual to distribute the message to the audience, whether that be teachers, counselors, parents or students.

Third, it would be helpful to have the intermediary buy into your message and approach. In that way, they could offer supporting information to the audience, as well as additional encouragement for the audience's participation and engagement in the desired outcome. This could be as simple as them saying "Did you see the message about this health topic? I think this is a good thing." At a minimum, you would hope that the intermediary would not say or do something that would conflict with your message, which might point the audience in a different direction, that could confuse the audience, or that might otherwise undermine your efforts.

Finally, consider the fact that the intermediary may be your specified audience, as they are the access point for ultimately reaching the final audience. That is, your communications effort may have some individuals as the audience to be reached, while your attention for your effort is more focused on a different level. An example would be with medical doctors; these professionals may be the group you reach directly and your communications efforts may be directed specifically at them. However, the ultimate audience you seek to reach is actually the patient and his/her decisions about a specific health issue. Within this, consider that your communications effort is designed to get the medical doctor to engage in a deeper conversation with patients about their use of tobacco or alcohol or other drugs; so the focus of your strategy is with the doctor. Your aim is to get the doctor to have more conversations with their patients, to provide the doctor with some speaking points and trigger statements, to enhance the doctor's confidence about the appropriateness of having these conversations and to provide the doctor with some resources that can then be used by them or shared by the patients. Ultimately, your audience for the initiative is the patient—but your direct and focused audience for your efforts is the doctor specifically.

Within this context, it is not only the composition of the message that may need the support of the intermediary, but also the channel or approach used to get the message out. The message may be very straightforward, but the approach may be what generates the appeal. As you strive to reach your ultimate target audience, you may be using know-feel-do strategies that are most appropriate for them, but with which the intermediary may not be familiar. A classic example of this is with emerging technology and approaches currently found with social media. To include your message on Facebook, or Twitter or Instagram is something that would not have been possible a few years ago; in fact, many intermediaries may not be familiar with these communications and social networking know-feel-do strategies. Further, some intermediaries may not trust these approaches as valid and may not view them as helpful. What will be important is to garner the support of the intermediaries, particularly with know-feel-do strategies about which they may not be familiar or conversant. This may require some education as well as convincing information, so that the intermediary becomes a supporter, and at least not a roadblock, for your overall communication strategy.

Messages from the field

Creating empathy through intergenerational dialogue

Chris Delatorre, Senior Digital Content Manager, SAGE
Christina DaCosta, Assistant Director of Communications, SAGE

Lesbian, Gay, Bisexual and Transgender (LGBT) older adults are often invisible in our communities and their needs are often missing from important conversations about health. To help change attitudes and increase advocacy for this issue, SAGE (www.sageusa.org) participated in two Twitter chats during LGBT Health Awareness Week. These bridged older and younger generations with content that focused on common issues. We sought to promote empathy with the younger generations, since they are more likely to share and act. For #MillennialMon we linked participants to an LGBT-friendly provider directory, reiterated Affordable Care Act protections and showed how access to healthcare has improved for all LGBT people. Two examples are "The #ACA protects trans folks by prohibiting sex discrimination in hospitals and other health programs. #MillennialMon #TransHealth" and "The rate for uninsured #LGBTQ folks has been cut in half since 2013: http://bit.ly/1RKipP5 #MillennialMon #ACA." With #WellnessWed we focused on the LGBT older adult experience before tweeting about cultural competence trainings and trending preventative measures that improve health for all ages; one example was "Cultural competence trainings, cultural competence trainings, did we say cultural competence trainings? #WellnessWed #LGBT #TransHealth." Over 5 days SAGE gained 62,644 impressions on Twitter and 1.3 million impressions on Facebook by 1.2 million users. In addition to elevating the needs of LGBT older adults in discussions about health, bridging generations may also help to compensate for a lack of traditional family structure in many LGBT homes, providing both a way out of social isolation and a conduit through which elders can impart wisdom to younger people.

Audience segmentation

Your health and safety message will be tailored to the specific audience(s) you are seeking to reach.

- If you are reaching a certain age group, you will use examples that make sense to that group. For older adults, examples involving youth will probably not be appropriate.
- If you are trying to engage a specific audience, incorporate language appropriate for them. This includes words or phrases that resonate for them. If you are trying to reach employees in the railroad industry, ground your efforts in ways that make sense to this group.
- Use illustrations that link to your audience. If you are working with traffic safety personnel with an enforcement orientation, use visual and verbal illustrations and support materials that work for that group.
- Make sure your language is appropriate for the audience. Some groups vastly prefer visual illustrations; some groups have a lower reading comprehension level. Attend to the audience's reading level; most audiences will not understand a college reading level.[3]
- Your examples may not be precisely of the age of your target audience. Since some groups, such as youth, aspire to those a little older than themselves, your examples may be "several years above" those whom you are seeking to reach.
- If your efforts are designed to address an issue that is primarily gender-specific or focused on a particular race or ethnicity, you will want to have know–feel–do strategies appropriate for that audience. If the topic is about a women's health issue, you may benefit from testimonials from women; you may include men as valid sources if that complements your strategy. Similarly, with race or ethnic considerations, make sure your spokespersons and know–feel–do strategies are appropriate for your planning and content implementation.

This does not mean that your efforts need to be entirely "pure" and only linked to the group or audience you are trying to reach. What it does mean is that whatever you do needs to be grounded and should make sense to your audience. As an example, if you are directing a message of substance abuse prevention to college students, you have to determine which portion of the general college population is more likely to abuse which substances (see Figure 2.3). This requires segmenting the audience. Research evidence indicates that females graduate from high school and college more than males. Further, males are diagnosed with learning disabilities more than females and people with learning disabilities succumb to substance abuse at higher rates than those without these challenges. Also, people with learning disabilities drop out of college at much higher rates than those without such disabilities. In response to the needs of the audience segmentation you could provide useful resources for keeping people with learning disabilities from dropping out from college.[4]

The issue of audience segmentation is grounded with the basic concept that people do not all respond in the same way. Their behavioral intention is a function of not only their view of the relevance or importance of the message but also how they perceive others' attitudes toward the same message. This notion is in keeping with the theory of reasoned action and planned behavior that will be described in Chapter 4 on know–feel–do strategies. Marketers of commercial and social products are cognizant of the needs and interests of market or audience segmentation. At the same time, the marketers also assess the needs and interests of others who might influence the target segment's preferences.

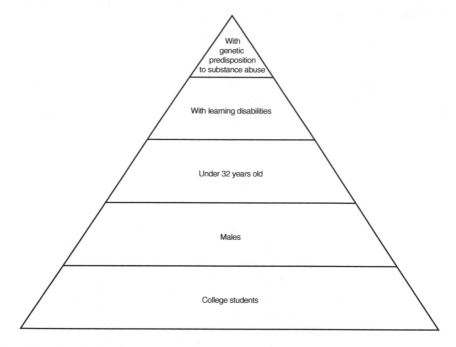

Figure 2.3 Example of audience segmentation

Another aspect of audience segmentation is that your effort may be trying to reach multiple audiences, all at the same time. This may be the case when you have a topic that has multiple strands, such as with youth. If you are initiating a bicycle safety campaign, you may have some approaches that focus directly on your target audience, another approach that complements this and highlights how parents can be involved and a third strategy that engages others active and influential in the lives of youth, such as community leaders, educators and other adults who surround the youth.

As you do the segmentation of the audience, and attempt to include multiple audiences, you will want to be sure that your messages and know-feel-do strategies actually do complement one another. This sounds like an obvious factor, but it is important that it is incorporated in your planning efforts. As you have a specific message or strategy for youth, for example, you may be saying other things for the parent or adult. These additional messages would complement the youth messages and would be consistent with them also. You may just be saying things in a different way and making suggestions or offering tips for adults that would help the youth—the specified target audience—best implement the desired outcomes.

The segmentation of your audience can be based on many different factors. Consider the following:

- Age
- Affiliation groups (clubs, organizations)
- Culture
- Gender
- Race/ethnicity

- Religion
- Occupation
- Region of the country
- Language
- Country of origin
- Education level
- Areas of interest (sports, culture)
- Other.

As you start to think further about audience segmentation, it can appear somewhat overwhelming. That is, what are the primary factors or determinants affecting how individuals will respond to the messages? Is it based on age? Race? Language? Occupation? Further, would this be based on a blend of factors? Think about an effort where you are trying to reach a group of student-athletes—the topic of concern is with a specific team, focusing on women and further highlighting younger students. With adults overall, the body of literature on adult learning theory is helpful and provides useful guidance about ways of best reaching the adult audience as a whole. The end result may be so narrow that it becomes cost-inefficient or inappropriate to implement some initiative. It may make more sense to step back and be a bit broader with your focus.

Audience segmentation is a great concept and one that should be considered as you prepare your efforts. It is something that you could do with various complementary approaches. It is also something where you may include one or more messages for different audiences within a single overall strategy. It is also an approach where you can back off the narrow, specific approach of segmentation and do whatever you can to maximize the appropriate approaches with your audience.

Messages from the field

Adult learning from a presenter's perspective

Kathryn Bedard, MA LCADC, Sojourner Consulting LLC

Children are new to the world. They react; they explore and learn through sensory experiences. If you are providing information to children, and they perceive you to be an authority, children will believe you. Providing information to adults is very different because the adult learning process is complex, uniquely personal and is a subtle dance of power and control, so adult learners offer many variables to consider when developing presentations. The field of adult learning was introduced to the United States in 1968 by Malcolm Knowles.[5]

Adult learning is where theory, experience and practice all crash together: presenters offer their new information with hope (theory). The audience studies the presenters' theory and style of presenting and decides the credibility of the information and its relevance for future use. If the presenter seems credible, information may be put into practice. Part of delivering information effectively, and getting the audience to want to use the information, involves understanding various factors about adults.

Cultural appropriateness and competence

An important part of knowing the audience is attending to culture. Cultural appropriateness in health and safety communications is tailoring the message based on the audience's language, manners of speech, norms and mores, religious beliefs and practices and other ethnic distinctions. Cultural competence in health and safety communications is the ability to design and deliver messages that are culturally appropriate for the audience and, hopefully, ultimately successful. What is important for you as the health communicator is to have a basic understanding of cultural distinctions in your audience.

What is meant by "culture"? It is learned, socially patterned habits of thought and behavior that are characteristic of a group. Other definitions include the following:

- the beliefs, customs, arts of a particular society, group, place or time;
- a particular society that has its own beliefs, ways of life, art, customs;
- a way of thinking, behaving or working that exists in a place or organization (such as a business);
- the integrated pattern of human knowledge, belief and behavior that depends upon the capacity for learning and transmitting knowledge to succeeding generations;
- the customary beliefs, social forms and material traits of a racial, religious or social group;
- the set of shared attitudes, values, goals and practices that characterizes an institution or organization; and
- the set of values, conventions or social practices associated with a particular field, activity or societal characteristic.

The term "culture" is used within various other contexts, with terms such as "pop culture" and the "culture of a region." There are references to "organizational culture" or "corporate profit-seeking cultures" as well as a person having a "lack of culture." For the purposes of health and safety communications and this chapter, the focus is actually about the issue of more global and intrinsic cultural factors for individuals and groups, as cited in the bullets above. Culture thus focuses on the habits of thought and behavior affiliated with a group.

Within this broad construct of culture, an initial consideration focuses on examples of culture. The first issue that comes to mind is factors associated with race and ethnicity. This may include Hispanic, African-American, American-Indian and Asian/Pacific Islander. Even within each of these, additional groupings or considerations will be important and relevant. For example, within the Asian/Pacific Islander designation, different cultural perspectives will be found among Thai and Vietnamese; and differences among those in mainland China and Hong Kong. On Guam, you will find those who have located there as well as the native Chamorro; further, these Pacific Islanders are different from those on the Marshall Islands or Yap or Palau. Related to these are considerations with respect to language, as well as to country of origin.

Another issue with culture has to do with gender; there may be cultural considerations appropriate for men, others for women and still others for transgender individuals. Culture is a consideration with sexual orientation and/or gender identity, whether it be straight, gay, lesbian, transgender, transsexual, queer, questioning or other consideration. Age may play a role with culture, with youth cultures being different from young adult, mature adult and elderly groups. Another factor may have to do with culture associated with individuals in recovery from substance abuse or psychiatric disorder. And many more cultures exist.

Beyond this basic "listing" of cultures, there is blending of cultures. Of course, this can be found within each individual—a person of color, female, whose primary language is not English and who is in recovery from an eating disorder. Another type of blending that occurs is with relationships; consider a married couple with different cultural backgrounds (whether by race or ethnicity, country of origin, language or other factor).

Another consideration is that some cultures may be less obvious and/or more hidden than others. For example, there may be an individual who is a person of color, but "passes" and may be known as a "marginal person." It may not be obvious if a person is in recovery from addiction, but this may be a strong cultural factor for his or her life; this can be the same as a person who drinks or uses drugs excessively as that could be a strong cultural influence. For a gay or lesbian or bisexual individual, this cultural influence is not necessarily expressed or obvious; some individuals may not be "out" with their lifestyle, or may be selective with whom they disclose or share their cultural perspectives. The list can go on and on, so it is important to acknowledge that culture is important, but is not always clearly observable.

It is important to acknowledge that the cultural group or subgroup you are attempting to influence may not be reachable or accessible through normal channels or channels used with others; there may be different channels, or no specific channels may exist. Also, perhaps these individuals are not going to react to the same behavior change theory—for example the subjective norms from the theory of planned behavior are going to be different for someone who is leading a guarded lifestyle or for whom cultural norms are different from the overall societal norms.

The important focus for any of these situations and for reaching individuals who comprise the target audience address the defining cultural considerations appropriate for maximizing your impact. Earlier in this chapter, attention was provided to factors that may resonate well for your audience—so if you are attempting to reach student-athletes, you would be well served to provide examples and illustrations from student-athletes or from those respected by the student-athlete. With issues of diabetes, involve those with experience and expertise with this disease. Similarly, for topics associated with recovery from substances such as drugs or alcohol, engage people in recovery as well as professionals with a deep and compassionate understanding of the processes and struggles associated with recovery issues. Within this cultural context overlay, consider what it is within the cultural context of your audience that may be relevant and appropriate. When trying to reach women, who are the best, most trusted communicators and experts, what are the best examples and illustrations appropriate for reaching this group? When trying to reach gay men or women in recovery or the 1.5 generation of Chinese (those who immigrate to a new country by their early teens, sharing characteristics of both first and second generations), what would be the most appropriate resources and references for achieving your goals?

So the question now arises, why is culture important and how does it matter? As established with a resource on substance abuse issues prepared decades ago,

> Each of our multicultural communities offers a rich and diverse ethnic heritage that, if fully explored and understood, will play an important role in the development of [alcohol and other drug] prevention programs that focus on strengthening cultural resiliency and protective factors.[6]

While this focuses on drugs and alcohol, the context of this is that attention to cultural issues is helpful in understanding the audience. This understanding can lead to the inclusion of know–feel–do strategies and approaches that are more helpful in reaching the audience. Imagine what it would be like to try to reach an audience without an appropriate understanding.

Culture matters because individuals identify strongly with a specific cultural group or several groups. With your efforts in health and safety communications, it is vital that you attend to cultural factors to the extent that they make a difference in the lives of the audience you seek to affect. Your efforts in doing so are important in communicating the respect you have and feel toward your audience. Even though your quest to be culturally competent is never complete, your effort in attempting to maximize your understanding will be helpful in achieving your desired goals with communications efforts.

Today's world is pluralistic and much celebration of diversity is found. Figuratively, American culture has gone from a "melting pot" to a "salad bowl." Individuals within a culture or grouping often view their own culture in ways that are different from those "on the outside." In this sense, culture and diversity go hand in hand. With the presence of various cultures is found diversity. While many similarities exist, differences are also present, thus creating diversity within the overall setting, whether it is a work setting, community, affiliation group, organization or other.

Attention to culture and diversity can be manifested in a variety of ways. **Cultural competence** refers to an ability to interact effectively with people of different cultures and socio–economic backgrounds.

Moving forward within the issue of culture and diversity, two key questions remain. First, what can you do as a health and safety communicator to maximize your cultural competence? Second, how might you apply this to your work? From a professional development perspective, here are some specific things you can do to enhance your cultural competence.

1   Acknowledge that increasing your cultural competence represents a commitment to growth and improvement. Realize that this is not an "endpoint," but rather a process.
2   Make specific efforts to heighten your own personal awareness. Look for opportunities to learn about different cultures and lifestyles. Realize that this may be a personal challenge, as you may learn of practices or perspectives that are quite novel for you.
3   Be aware of all that you do not know. Know that you have limits and that it is not realistic for you to be an expert on all cultures. Also realize that culture may change over time, so various traditions or practices or values may evolve for a group.
4   Attend to your own values. Try to understand your own culture and what is important to you. This is a challenge, as it is hard to fully understand your own culture. As the old maxim says, "a fish doesn't see the water around it."
5   Try to be aware of the culture that affects you. As you understand this, you can gain a better perspective about what might affect others, also.
6   Listen, ask questions, query, probe and strive to better understand others' cultures. Try to understand what aspects of a person's culture are important and why.
7   Strive to have a balanced approach when thinking about cultures. In this, understand cultural differences as well as cultural similarities. Try to acknowledge individual differences within the broader construct of a culture (that is, all individuals within a cultural context or group are not the same on all aspects of their lives). Strive to not

stereotype; while broad cultural considerations are important, that does not mean that all individuals within a cultural grouping are the same.

As you work as a professional in health and safety communications, specific know-feel-do strategies will be important for your work to demonstrate your cultural sensitivity and awareness. Here are some tips that may be helpful in this regard.

- Incorporate, to the greatest extent possible, your understanding of the cultural context of the audience you seek to affect.
- Use language that is respectful and inclusive.
- Choose materials, images and illustrations that best resonate with the cultural perspectives and values of your audience.[7]
- Engage individuals with personal backgrounds or cultural representation of the cultural groups you wish to influence. This may be in the planning and/or pilot testing phases of the process.
- Incorporate a variety of approaches and learning styles with your communications effort.
- Realize that your efforts may face challenges, resistance and lack of understanding. It is thus helpful to acknowledge that discussions of culture may be awkward or uncomfortable for individuals.

As you prepare your efforts, it is critically important to understand the role of culture in the lives and minds of the audiences you seek to reach. You want to acknowledge the important role that culture plays in the minds and lives of individuals and to find ways of dovetailing your communications efforts within the context of their lives and their cultures.

Try for a moment to imagine the opposite perspective. That would be one of highlighting "one message for all" or "one approach for everyone," consistent with the "universal" approach highlighted in the chapter on theoretical groundings. How effective would your efforts be if you ignored cultural factors, or if you attempted a singular strategy designed to reach everyone? In fact, your efforts would likely not work at all; at best, they would not be as effective as if they were more inclusive or acknowledging of cultural considerations.

The practical side, however, is that you will not be able to have a uniquely appropriate approach that addresses all the cultural factors for each individual. That would be virtually impossible, as it requires a full understanding of these various cultural factors and then tailoring the know-feel-do strategies and materials in a way that would be different for each person. That is just not practical or reasonable. However, the important consideration is that you attempt to include cultural considerations, at least at the broadest level, within your efforts to communicate in a reasonable and appropriate way with your audience.

Culture is important for health and safety communications, because culture is important to the people whom you seek to influence. Culture and diversity can be exciting, as this can create healthy interaction among individuals. Culture can be vibrant, as culture affects individuals, groups and the surrounding world. To acknowledge and embrace culture can make a big difference with the impact of our work; to do otherwise is to ignore the obvious.

Messages from the field

Getting to know your audience

David Closson, M.S., Illinois Higher Education Center/Eastern Illinois University

Essential for preparing a health and safety message is knowing your audience and understanding who they are. Where are they spending their time? What do they care about? What are they talking about? Where do they get their information? To what extent do they rely upon newspapers, TV, radio, posters or online via social media for information?

My experience working at a campus police department, with the college student target audience ranging from age 18 to 25, incorporated increased messaging on social media since we found that 9 out of 10 people in the age range 18–29 use social media.[8] However, current work at the Illinois Higher Education Center, with a target audience of professional staff members who are older than college students, necessarily uses other methods to share our message to be more effective. This is because research shows that between 25 percent and 65 percent were not using social media.

Here are some strategies to get to know your audience:

- Your website analytics
  - Where visitors are spending their time on your website tells you what they are most interested in.
- Facebook insights
  - For Facebook pages, their insights will tell your audience demographics, languages, location, when they are online, how they interact with your posts and how many saw your posts.
- Twitter analytics
  - This will show your audience demographics, location, interests and how they interact with your tweets.
- Listen
  - This can be done in person by talking to your audience and/or online. Paying attention to what they are talking about, sharing and watching on social media is valuable information as you create your messaging.
- PEW Research and other data sources
  - Provides valuable data on social media usage by age, gender, education, household income, race/ethnicity and whether they live in a rural, suburban or urban environment.

Knowing your audience will guide you about what platform to use and how to hone your message for maximum effectiveness.

Getting started

By learning more about your audience, you are ready to start a health and safety communication initiative. However, there must be some reason for the initiative. Maybe it is based on an expressed felt interest or concern by yourself and your group. For example, your group volunteers for the American Diabetes Association to prevent type 2 diabetes in all women and to support women in managing their diabetes. As you address this matter of importance, you will not be able to do everything with all audiences, as you will have limited resources and time. You can decide which segment would benefit most from your attention. Is it preventing the disease, for instance, or is it providing support to those with diabetes?

Messages from the field

Considering the audience's needs

Diana Karczmarczyk, PhD, MPH, MCHES, American Diabetes Association
Evelina Sterling, PhD, MPH, MCHES, American Diabetes Association

One of the initiatives of the American Diabetes Association (ADA) is to work to prevent type 2 diabetes in all women and to support women in managing their diabetes. Since the emotional impact of living with a chronic disease, like type 2 diabetes, can have a significant impact on women, the ADA developed the educational booklet *Coping with Diabetes: A Handbook for Women and their Families*. Each section of the booklet was carefully designed to provide information to women in an easy to read format on a wide variety of topics. It was important to explain the connection between stress and diabetes management. The booklet includes a short quiz to assess stressors and provides practical know-feel-do strategies for coping with stress effectively. The booklet also addresses seeking out medical care and communicating effectively with health care professionals. Although the content was important, the images that the booklet included were also critical. The target audience for the booklet was women, but it was important that the images included were women of diverse racial and ethnic backgrounds, varying ages and body types. Each image included in the publication was therefore hand selected with great care.

So it's important to consider all the serious side effects and complications and not just focus on the obvious or stereotypical. If health educators and experts don't know about the disease, how can others be expected to do so? The lesson learned is that it is so important to consider the audience.

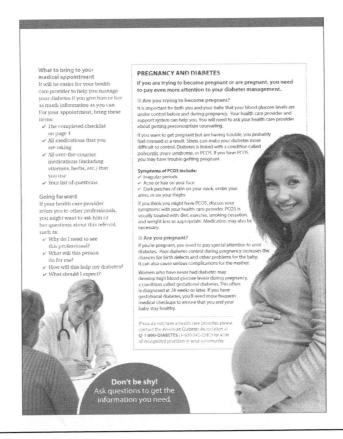

Another way of "getting started" is when you are working with an audience on one particular matter only to notice another pressing concern. For example, you may be collaborating with a faith community, recreation center or athletic team to address high school students on the proper use of social media (i.e., Facebook postings, Twitter tweets) when you overhear members of the audience reveal violent experiences in their lives. Essentially, you have come across a specific group within your original audience that would benefit from a violence prevention initiative.

In either case, you need to prioritize your efforts. You have to determine what areas within the larger concern and what segments within the audience deserve the greater attention. Your decision may be based on funding or priorities as established by the group's leadership. Your decision may also rest on "what the data says." Audience segments can differ in their experiences—whether with diabetes or with violence. Similarly, each segment has a respective way of receiving messages based on age, or gender, or race/ethnicity, or level of education, or some other factor or some blend of factors. In the next chapter, you will learn about aiming messages in order to effectively influence and persuade your audience.

Forward!

This chapter addressed the importance of knowing about your audience. It is vital, as a health communicator, that you strive to learn about your audience and to reach them in the most appropriate and effective ways possible. You should not presume that others will respond in ways that work for you or your own circle of influence. You want to work to identify factors and approaches that will work best for your audience, as best you can. While this can be complicated, subsequent steps in the health and safety communications model will clarify how this is done.

The health and safety communications approach may provide guidance and direction about specific action steps an individual would be well advised to follow in various situations. These can illustrate best practices for health and can also be developed within the context of age and culturally appropriate approaches.

In short, knowing the audience is helpful in connecting with them. This understanding can help you be more effective in understanding what motivates them, whether it is images or symbols or language or some other factor. Further, having this understanding, and using this understanding, can help your effort by demonstrating your commitment to them as a group and as individuals, and perhaps as a culture. Your effort can have dramatic effects through itself by being relevant, but also by demonstrating your respect for them. That can serve you and your efforts to a very high level.

Notes

1 Springer, J.R. and Phillips, J. (2007). *The Institute of Medicine Framework and Its Implication for the Advancement of Prevention Policy, Programs and Practice*. Washington, DC: Institute of Medicine, US Department of Health and Human Services.
2 Nief, R. and McBride, T. (2016). *The Mindset List*. Beloit College, Beloit, WI. Retrieved May 15, 2016 from www.beloit.edu/mindset/
3 Centers for Disease Control and Prevention (2013). *CDC Clear Communication Index: A Tool for Developing and Assessing CDC Public Communication Products*. Retrieved May, 2016 from www.cdc.gov/healthliteracy/developmaterials/guidancestandards.html
4 Troiano, P.F., Liefeld, J.A. and Trachtenberg, J.V. (2010). Academic support and college success for postsecondary students with learning disabilities. *Journal of College Reading & Learning*, 40(2), 35–44.

5 Knowles, M., Holton, E. and Swanson, R.A. (2005). *The Adult Learner* (6th ed.). New York: Butterworth-Heinemann.
6 Center for Substance Abuse Prevention (1992). *Cultural Competence for Evaluators*, p iii. DHHS Publication No. (SMA) 95–3066.
7 Plimpton, S. and Root, J. (1994). Materials and strategies that work in low literacy health communication. *Public Health Reports*, 109(1), 86–92. Retrieved April 20, 2016 from www.ncbi.nlm.nih.gov/pmc/articles/PMC1402246/?page=1
8 Perrin, A. (2015). *Social Media Usage: 2005–2015*. Pew Research Center. Retrieved April 2, 2016 from www.pewintcrnet.oɪg/2015/10/08/social-networking-usage-2005-2015.

3 Aims and goals

Step 2

What are you trying to accomplish through your health and safety communication? The answer would be the aim of the communication. Aim means purpose or intention. So the likely aim of your health and safety communication is having a persuasive influence on the target audience. It is important to be clear on this. The aim is not to prepare the posters or conduct workshops. Likewise, the aim is not designing packets or publishing newsletters. Your aim is having an impact on recipients of your health and safety message. You are providing information and enhancing motivation so a change in knowledge, attitudes and/or behavior takes place in the audience receiving your message (see Figure 3.1).

A related but different term is **goal**. The goal of your health and safety communication is the desired state of the receivers of your messages. Essentially, it is what you want them to know, feel and do after being exposed to the communication. Know–feel–do strategies are explained in the next chapter. So if the goal of your health and safety communications is good dental health in children, then your aim is to influence and persuade children to brush and floss their teeth regularly. If the goal is adult physical fitness, then your aim is to convince people to perform physical activity for 30 minutes on most days.

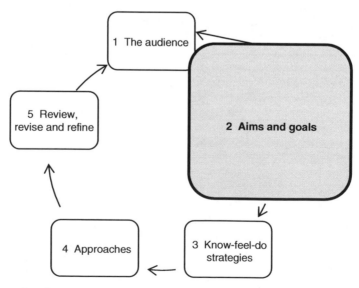

Figure 3.1 Aims and goals

Topics and issues

A sure way of aiming your message would be to set your sights on relevant topics and issues. **Topics** are matters or subjects for discussion. Health and safety messages are based on topics. When you think of a topic, keep in mind its several sub-topics. For example, with the topic of substance abuse, you may have sub-topics of underage alcohol use, mixing drugs and alcohol, gender issues, age or gender differences, high risk use, substance use and driving, responsible decisions, dependence, recovery and many more. There will also be overlap among topics and sub-topics; consider traffic safety with topics such as drinking and driving, young drivers, distracted driving, aggressive driving, pedestrian safety, speeding, bicycle safety and more.

Some topics are more appropriate for the college-age student, some are appropriate for infants or children, some are appropriate for teens, some are appropriate for elderly people and some are appropriate for all audiences. From a larger societal perspective, a helpful starting point is Healthy People, the nation's health policy.[1] Healthy People is organized around 42 topics (see Table 3.1). Noteworthy in this listing are three points: one is the broad reach of topics associated with health and safety, each providing opportunities for effective and appropriate communication within the context of strategic initiatives. A second is the inclusion of

Table 3.1 Healthy People 2020 topics

Access to Health Services	HIV
Adolescent Health (new)★	Immunization and Infectious Diseases
Arthritis, Osteoporosis and Chronic Back Conditions	Injury and Violence Prevention
Blood Disorders and Blood Safety (new)	Lesbian, Gay, Bisexual and Transgender Health (new)
Cancer	Maternal, Infant and Child Health
Chronic Kidney Disease	Medical Product Safety
Dementias, including Alzheimer's Disease (new)	Mental Health and Mental Disorders
Diabetes	Nutrition and Weight Status
Disability and Health	Occupational Safety and Health
Early and Middle Childhood (new)	Older Adults (new)
Educational and Community-Based Programs	Oral Health
Environmental Health	Physical Activity
Family Planning	Preparedness (new)
Food Safety	Public Health Infrastructure
Genomics (new)	Respiratory Diseases
Global Health (new)	Sexually Transmitted Diseases
Health Communication and Health Information Technology	Sleep Health (new)
Healthcare-Associated Infections	Social Determinants of Health (new)
Health-Related Quality of Life & Well-Being (new)	Substance Abuse
Hearing and Other Sensory or Communication Disorders (new)	Tobacco Use
Heart Disease and Stroke	Vision

★ Those items marked "new" were not included in the listing of topics in Healthy People 2010.

13 new topics in the Healthy People 2020 listing that were not included in the Healthy People 2010 listing; this illustrates the continuously involving science regarding issues of importance and also highlights the importance of remaining up-to-date with the most current knowledge, highlighted in Chapter 2. Third, there will be topics of a health or safety nature that are not included in this listing; for example, boating safety, fire safety and traffic safety, among others, are not included on this listing. This does not diminish their importance; it simply means these topics were not part of the criteria used in developing the Healthy People listings.

Important topics for discussion and debate are considered **issues**. There are numerous issues related to the Healthy People 2020 topics (see Table 3.2). Whereas

Table 3.2 A sampling of issues related to Healthy People topics

Practicing dental health	Complying with required vaccinations
Preventing childhood obesity	Not smoking
Promoting responsible college drinking	Not drinking and driving
Adhering to medical prescriptions	Lowering risk of sexually transmitted infections
Exercising on most days	Getting enough sleep
Eating healthily	Practicing dental hygiene
Protecting oneself from the sun	Reducing cardiovascular disease risk
Practicing mental health	Managing diabetes
Managing high blood pressure	Clicking safety belts
Wearing motor/bicycle helmets	Appreciating clean water
Swimming safety	Volunteering at homeless shelters
Taking part in regular cancer screening	Contributing to community sanitation
Following food safety guidelines	Practicing stress management
Accommodating mobility impairments	Avoiding overmedication
Being cautious of antibiotic resistance	Adjusting to arthritis
Self-medicating appropriately	Appreciating holistic medicine
Considering alternative/complementary health care	Managing asthma
Avoiding allergy triggers	Selecting appropriate video games
Moderating caffeine consumption	Being aware of pregnancy issues
Practicing internet safety	Advocating responsible gun control
Preventing teen pregnancy	Recognizing medical quackery
Coping with addiction	Developing healthy relationships
Understanding alcoholism	Eliminating children's tobacco exposure
Being aware of radiation sources	Protecting hearing
Realizing veteran homelessness	Reporting family violence
Knowing poison control	Evaluating organic vs. non-organic
Reporting child abuse	Protecting against bioterrorism
Discouraging bullying	Performing hand-washing
Heeding public health alerts (i.e., epidemics)	Rehabilitating lower back pain
Reducing exposure to contagious diseases	Discouraging texting while driving

the public is aware of many health and safety topics, you as a health communicator need to be in tune with issues. Staying up-to-date on the health and safety issues with which you are working is itself a big challenge. Further, it is important that you remain aware of controversies associated with various issues, and what the latest scientific evidence shows. Staying current is further complicated by how viewpoints and perspectives vary between yourself, your colleagues and your audiences. For example, effective health communication strategies have been developed to help the audience stay up-to-date on the issue of bullying in school populations. The strategies primarily rely on social media.[2]

Key elements for being knowledgeable

Preparing communications about health and safety requires you to be as knowledgeable as possible about the issue you are addressing. That does not mean knowing everything, but it means being aware of what you know as well as what you should know. It means being current, factual and truthful. It means understanding some of the controversies surrounding the issues, and some of the nuances of language. It means being deliberate and careful. It is reasonable to expect that you have a significant amount of knowledge on specific health topics. It is also reasonable to expect that you remain up-to-date and that you acknowledge what you do not know.

Knowing the issue is a theme that permeates all of your work on health and safety communications. By knowing the issue, you can create appropriate, succinct, visual and impactful messages that make an impression on the audience. This is called **tailoring** the communication in that the message is appropriately designed for the readiness of the target audience to make a change.[3] As you implement a workshop session on a specified topic, you will want to be sure that you are correct and current with your data, that you understand what it says and does not say, and that you are clear with your explanations. It is important that you know your information. Further, as you implement communications efforts, whether preparing a print document, public service announcement (PSA) or a talk, or being interviewed by the media or making a funding proposal, you should be prepared to address questions that go beyond the specific and sometimes narrow content of your topic. You should also be prepared to acknowledge what you do not know, or what scientific research has not yet addressed or resolved, so you can share those insights as questions arise.

Seven areas of importance are highlighted to help guide your thinking as you plan your health and safety communications initiative. These areas are helpful, whether you are on the "front end" of building knowledge, or generating some "renewal" or "refresher" content for yourself:

1   Truthful information
2   Staying current
3   Dominant paradigms and perspectives
4   Controversies and unresolved issues
5   Emerging issues
6   Staying realistic and reasonable, and
7   Being believable.

Truthful information

As a person communicating about health and safety issues, a vital quality of your professionalism is being truthful. To the best of your ability, you must share what you know to be the facts. This is embedded in your profession's code of ethics—the importance of you being factual, truthful, honest and trustworthy. Another way to put it is to have integrity.

Step back for a moment and think about the audience listening to you, whether during a workshop, a speech, a television interview or with something you have written such as a brochure or poster. Would you, if you were in the audience, believe what is being said? What does it take for you to believe the speaker or the source? Do you want to know the credentials of the speaker or organization? Do you ask about where they got their information and whether that source is unbiased?

Further, as you think about working with the media on some initiative, covered in this book's chapter on the media (Chapter 9), you will learn that the media likes elements such as a controversy, a hook or angle, something current or local, or something new. The challenge for you is to maintain the standard of being truthful and striving to be newsworthy at the same time. To be newsworthy requires something different, which may seem a bit foreign or inconsistent with current knowledge, and thus may be viewed as being of questionable trustworthiness.

So, for you as the communicator of health and safety issues, you want to be as truthful as possible. Based on the audience's needs, and the complexity of the issue, you will later decide how best to communicate awareness of information related to the issue. For now, however, the focus is on how you get your knowledge in the best possible way. An example of this is when you are given a work assignment for developing communication on a particular topic about which you do not know much. Where do you start? Where do you get your information? What are your criteria for determining what are reputable and appropriate sources of information?

Probably the best place to start is with the government agencies, primarily those at the federal level. They conduct a lot of research and deliberate substantively over the findings before they publish them. Thus, these reports are vetted to be sure that science stands behind them.

Consider the following agencies, for your purposes with health and safety issues:

1   U.S. Department of Health and Human Services
2   U.S. Department of Education
3   U.S. Department of Agriculture
4   U.S. Department of Transportation
5   National Highway Traffic Safety Administration
6   Centers for Disease Control and Prevention
7   Government Accountability Office.

These are the lead public sector agencies at the national level; others exist at state and local levels. Likewise, there are several useful sources of health information within the private sector starting with non-profit community health organizations. Another good source of information includes research organizations. Some of these are found within universities and others may be independent, free-standing research entities.

Consider becoming a member of a professional association that specializes in health and safety communications. At the broadest level, examples would be the American Public Health Association, the Coalition for Healthcare Communication and the

Health & Science Communications Association; for specific thematic areas, topics and issues, professional associations and affiliation groups abound.

You can also examine professional journals that publish articles in the area in which you are interested; there, you will find the names of organizations or centers, as well as those of authors. The professionals or specialists with whom you may be most interested are those who are often authoring or co-authoring articles. These articles can be helpful in providing solid information for you and also for specifying resources of a reputable background. Some professional journals have public outlets and free viewing, but most require subscription-based access. You can always go to a library and search through their shelved periodicals. If you join a professional association, you should have access to its publications. While reviewing the professional literature, you may consider writing or calling some of the publishers or authors to ask for advice about where to find specific publications and resources that you can use to gather reputable and reliable background information for your initiative.

All of this sounds like a lot of work. The point is that you want to find reputable sources. You do not need to look at all sources identified here. But what is important is to look at more than one source. You may find a quality government publication and generally that would be the most trustworthy source. But it is always good to look a little more broadly to see what else you can learn on your topic.

As you plan your efforts, one of your major constraints or guiding factors is how much time you have to gather the factual information. For your purposes, you very probably will not have the luxury of time nor the resources to do a thorough literature review to garner all the various points of view and key content for your topic. You will probably have time constraints; this is not only the time during which the preparation of the communications effort will be made, but how much of that preparation time is for information gathering alone. You may have only a few days, a few weeks or a few months, during which you can gather the important information that can guide your efforts with your communication know-feel-do strategies.

Also, as you do this information gathering, you would be well served to do this in phases: gather the main information you need and then start to pull together the communications approach. Then, as you and others review the planned communications, gaps will be revealed and questions raised; this will point to some additional information gathering. As you work more on the communications effort, and as you do the final preparation, you'll want to be sure that your data is correct, so some additional information gathering may be in store for you.

What is important as you gather this is that you are not guided by simplistic summary findings that you may find on commercial websites. While the internet does provide the opportunity for quick and easily obtained information, you must exercise great caution with what you need to be sure it is appropriate and valid.

Overall, as you start to review, look at the source. It is much more trustworthy if it is published by a federal agency or office. Similarly, it is likely to be a valid source if it is based in a state agency or office, although most state agencies do not have the resources to fund research at the level of the federal government. Other resources typically reliable are those based at research institutions such as colleges or universities; these can be very helpful, particularly with grounded, independent research studies that have their own good reference materials. Once you see a study or a source, it is important that you determine the funding source of the study or report. If the report comes from a group with a vested interest in a particular outcome on an issue, you will want to pay particular attention to the methodology and independence of the data and its interpretations, to be sure they are scientifically grounded and valid. For instance, you should question published research findings funded by a group with a vested interest in the results (especially if the results are in favor of the funder's desires).

As you do more information gathering on a specific topic, you will find sources that may be independent in nature (i.e., not government or industry funded) but without a bias with the methodology or findings. Some sources pride themselves on this reputation and you will learn which sources you find most reputable, based on your own experience. As you get accustomed to a topic area, you will become more and more conversant with what the valid sources are, what information overlaps with other information and what different perspectives are found with different sources. You'll want to continue your monitoring of these sources, to garner new ones and to stay up-to-date on their neutrality, as you continue in this work. Further, as you talk with experts and specialists, continue to ask them what sources they find most helpful and appropriate.

This type of neutral data collection is important. You know this from your own experience with various news organizations, commentators and columnists, whether these are television, radio or print media. You have undoubtedly found some that are more liberal in their orientation and reporting and others that are more conservative in their focus. These sources are all reporting on the same news event or series of events, so which is most valid and truthful? You find that they have different slants or perspectives offered; they also incorporate different experts and commentators to make their key points.

For you as a health communicator, you want to do the best you can to gather information from valid sources. Then, you will incorporate other factors based on your knowledge of the audience as well as the nature of the overall communications effort.

Staying current

Parallel to gathering information from valid sources is the matter of staying current. As you'll see in the next section, paradigms and frameworks change over time. So you'll want to be sure that the information you communicate stays current. As you look at the journal articles or government publications, you'll want to assess when these were published. It may very well be that information published ten or twenty years ago, or longer, is still current and valid; it may also be that some of the knowledge, even that from just a few years ago, is no longer current or valid based on new scientific findings or changes in paradigms or methodology.

The process for staying current is to continue to do a scan of the research around your topic area. Use the same approaches, and the same valid sources, as identified in the previous section. If you have prepared some communications effort, whether it is a workshop, a talk, a poster series, brochures or other approach, you'll want to be sure the information provided is the most current. Some studies are conducted annually, so their data gets updated very regularly; it will be important for you to do the same with updating your materials with the most current data!

Periodically, you may wish to share your materials with those whose opinions you value; these would be content experts in your field, whether as a formally constituted advisory board or some colleagues from the region or around the country who are aware of the latest research and trends. Ask them where they get updates and new information and how they make sure their information and resources are current.

With this updated information, you can prepare trend charts, easily updated from one year to the next. Sometimes it is helpful to organize those into illustrations that demonstrate the changes (or lack of changes), not just the point in time data. For example, you might show the extent of growth or reduction over a given period of time, provided that this illustrates key points that you wish to highlight.

Another way of making sure you are up-to-date is to query colleagues on a regular basis. One way of doing this, if you want to help ensure that you are current, is to ask key individuals, whose opinion you trust, questions such as the following on the issue or topic of interest:

- What is new this year with this issue?
- What new information or research, if any, emerged this year?
- What new approaches have been used?
- Is there a new source of information that you value and trust?

On a periodic basis, it may also be helpful to ask the following questions:

- What did you know earlier that you now no longer believe? Why is that the case?
- What message or information is most important to communicate to a specific audience, such as youth, parents, decision-makers or others?

Messages from the field

Staying current

Beth DeRicco, Ph.D., Drexel University and Caron Treatment Centers

Periodically, I would take a random sample (not a formal one!) of colleagues and reach out by phone and/or email to a representation of folks (stakeholder groups, higher education professionals, etc.) to hear what their concerns were about substance abuse issues, student life and other issues. I would ask what they thought trends were in terms of issues and what were "one hit wonders," and what responses they were using at the individual and environmental level. I would also look at various survey results to see if responses pointed in a certain direction. I would read current research papers on approaches and interventions to see how what they were doing measured up to the research.

As you hear new information or a new phrase with your work, it is important that you don't simply adopt it. You should take these clues about the topic and investigate further. You may hear something on the news that piques your interest; see if you can get the transcript of the news item and track it down with the original source of the information (such as a research study). You may find, with your critical eye, that what was reported is not simply what the research found; the news report may be incomplete or misleading. That fact is something that you can then communicate, to correct misperceptions among the audiences you serve.

All of this can get very confusing. With health and safety issues, in particular, scientific discoveries continue to occur and breakthroughs are happening quite often. Studies with small and large sample sizes, and studies in different countries or settings, can be very helpful with new information. For example, saccharin was banned temporarily, but it has been found not harmful to humans in multiple studies. Currently, there are ongoing questions about other sweeteners, such as aspartame or sucralose. Those will be addressed, undoubtedly, for years to come. And, currently, recent research shows that salt may not be as harmful as previously thought; how will that unfold with further research and what will be the consequences for different individuals, based on other individual factors to be discovered or identified?

Frankly, the changing scientific discoveries with these health and safety issues can get very confusing, as new information comes through all the time. It is, clearly, a challenge to sort through all of this and to decide what is valid and what is meaningful and appropriate for your audiences.

The important thing with staying current is to be vigilant. Listen, monitor, probe and be as up-to-date as possible. Facts and perceptions continually change. Further, as you work with various groups, whether they are colleagues in your organization, those in the field or your actual target audience, you'll want to inform them, in an appropriate way, that what you are sharing is the latest information or facts.

Dominant paradigms and perspectives

A **paradigm** is a pattern or template of thought. Somewhat similar to this discussion is one of dominant paradigms and points of view that guide a particular field. Many fields have specific frames of reference and ways of thinking of the issue; further, some of these change over time and others are difficult to change.

For example, there's a classic paradigm with traffic safety, with its three Es— Enforcement, Engineering and Education. With marketing, there are the four Ps—Product, Place, Price and Promotion; these have been used with social marketing, with some refined definitions of what these four Ps are. In public health, there's the public health model, with the Agent, Host and Environment elements. There is the medical model with Primary, Secondary and Tertiary Prevention. An evident paradigm shift is with health promotion efforts mediated by digital technologies, incorporating such features as mass customization, interactivity and convenience.[4]

For various fields, changes occur over time. Just as in the previous section with the discovery of new scientific foundations, changes occur with paradigms or dominant approaches for addressing situations. For example, the disease concept is prominent with dependence; however, a moralistic or educational approach, which, many decades ago was popular, is still sometimes found.

Similarly with your work in health and safety communications, more current approaches evolve based on new findings and documentation of results. With addressing problematic substance abuse behavior, individualized motivational interviewing has evolved into a dominant approach. With various problematic behaviors, attention to bystander behavior (and empowering people to not be bystanders and to speak up and speak out) has become more dominant. With attention to sexual orientation, views about this have evolved over recent decades from a moral issue to one of a human rights focus; much more is happening with this issue in recent years.

Remember the AIDS crisis of the early 1980s and how it was viewed then? Sadly, many young people have no memory of this and only know of it from what they read. The scientific approach then discussed the four Hs of HIV/AIDS and how it was spread; these were that HIV was found with homosexuals, Haitians, those with hemophilia and heroin IV drug users. That knowledge changed substantially with new scientific discoveries and how it was and is talked about and treated (and thus education about prevention and treatment) has evolved with new paradigms.

With various psychological issues, the *Diagnostic and Statistical Manual of Mental Disorders* (*DSM*) prepared by the American Psychiatric Association serves as the primary guide for understanding, diagnosis and treatment of a range of disorders. For example, with the *DSM V*, the most recent edition published in 2013, "substance abuse" has been replaced with "substance dependence." Currently, the focus is not on autism, but the autism spectrum; Asperger's is no longer present, but it is placed under "autism spectrum disorder." The *DSM V* also includes a new disorder—caffeine use disorder—that was added with this edition. Revisions also include many more changes, including how eating disorders and post-traumatic stress disorder are addressed.

Many of these views are scientifically grounded. These are what guide the medical community, as well as specialists in various fields of study. Even the language you use can have meaning; thus it is vital that your language and how you approach your topic and issues are current and reflect the appropriate paradigms for your area. For example, with drunk driving, all-too-often the term "drunk driving accident" was used; but professionals in traffic safety talk about a "drunken driving crash." Further, the language is expanded to cite "impaired driving" rather than "drunk driving," as the term "impaired" includes illicit or prescription drugs, as well as lower amounts of alcohol that can impair a person's driving ability (without being classified as legally drunk). The term "binge drinking" is confusing—does it mean the definition associated with alcoholism or dependence? Or is it the more recently adopted government definition of five or more drinks at a setting, for men (four or more for women)? And "distracted driving"—that includes talking on a phone, texting, use of social media, talking with others (thus laws about teen drivers and passengers) and so much more.

With paradigms and frameworks comes the issue of myths; cited above were the four Hs associated with HIV/AIDS in the earlier days of this disease. Those "facts" of the 1980s are myths of today. How many other areas have myths based on old, outdated or faulty paradigms? What information is accepted as current today, yet will be discarded or replaced tomorrow? The message here is to remain vigilant and up-to-date with the latest science surrounding your health and safety topics and issues.

Moving beyond the scientific realm, another perspective has to do with whose point of view is being considered. Is the issue being assessed from the perspective of parents or youth? Health professionals or law enforcement? Teachers or parents? And, if it is a set of professionals, whose code of ethics will be used? This is particularly the case if these are competing (e.g., a health orientation of "do no harm" or a safety orientation emphasizing "peace and tranquility" or a secure and safe setting).

The importance of understanding the overall framework or paradigm is important for you, as a person who is planning and orchestrating helpful health and safety communications. It is vital that you know where you are heading—know the overall context. If all you know are the facts and figures, this good knowledge about your topic really won't be sufficient if you are doing a workshop or engaging in a discussion, if a question or issue outside that framework is raised. It is important that you see the larger picture yourself and know how your information fits into that overall context. Other, related questions and issues will undoubtedly arise and it is important, for the understanding of your audience, that you be able to help them "connect the dots" to show how their question or myth or misunderstanding fits into the larger framework. While they may or may not agree with your perspective, you can be helpful in assisting them to understand the larger picture of this issue.

Imagine a history teacher who can state clearly the facts, but does not know ways of showing the relevance of a historical understanding, or how history tends to repeat itself.

Or with substance abuse issues, the teacher may be able to report what is important for a specific topic, but may not see the interconnectedness of various topics, such as prevention versus intervention versus treatment versus recovery. What is helpful is to see and understand, and then communicate, the larger "roadmap" of how things link together. Then, you can, with your work and with your audiences, show the linkages and show the connections between today and tomorrow.

Another way of thinking about paradigms relates to the data you gather and how you stay current. What sorts of data do you trust and use? Do you use what you are used to using? How do you feel about using data, for your own understanding, that is from sources different from those with which you are familiar? How about the use of quantitative data if you are used to qualitative data (or qualitative data if you are used to quantitative data)? What may be most helpful is to incorporate a blend of these, as well as triangulating the results for best understanding the issue. Once you have a more holistic perspective, you may be better able to communicate this to others.

It is also important within this context that you are aware, to the extent that you can be, of your own paradigms and frameworks; that is, be cognizant of your own biases. Then, you should attempt to be as aware as you can of the frameworks that guide those around you, whether that is co-workers or peers, or other colleagues in your line of work. Finally, be aware of the existing frameworks and issues of importance to those whom you are seeking to influence; by understanding their paradigms, you can better address their insights and find ways of moving them forward with the desired outcomes. Only by understanding their perspective and foundations can you help to move them from their current perspectives and ultimately to the desired outcomes.

Controversies and unresolved issues

Many health and safety issues have related controversies. For you to communicate a message, assuming that everything is resolved and clear, is fine, as long as that is actually the case. However, if controversies exist, or if issues remain unresolved, it is important that you acknowledge these and put these in perspective. If your aim is to engage an audience, and you seek to maximize their opportunity to affect their behavior or knowledge, you first want to promote their trust in you and what you have to offer. For you to acknowledge that controversies exist, or that some issues remain unresolved, can be very helpful in promoting that honesty. The fact that you put this fact out there, and then address it in some way, is likely to result in positive regard for you and your overall messages.

Many controversies exist throughout health and safety topics. Consider the following:

- How helpful are diets? Which diets are most helpful?
- What are the health benefits of vitamins? Are there safety concerns?
- Should men have PSA tests conducted?
- Is addiction a disease? Is it different for alcohol, drugs or tobacco?
- What are the benefits and drawbacks regarding the use of statins?
- When should vaccines be used? Should they be mandatory for public school attendance?
- What are the benefits and drawbacks with e-cigarettes, considering quitting smoking and enticing individuals to smoke?
- What role does religion play with health?
- Should "junk food" be regulated?

- Should bike safety helmets always be used? Should this be for everyone, or just children?
- What are the benefits and drawbacks of breastfeeding?
- How should eating disorders be viewed and treated?
- Should safety belts be mandated?
- How much salt is too much? How much sugar is too much?
- Under what circumstances should an older driver be required to give up their driver's license?
- Should the government be involved with managing portion sizes, such as with carbonated, sugary drinks?
- Should telephone apps that prevent texting while driving be mandatory on all cell phones? Or, should this be only for those under a certain age?
- Should traffic cameras be used? Should this be limited to monitoring traffic? Or, should they be used to document violations such as not stopping at a red light, or speeding?
- Where should restrictions on smoking exist? Enclosed spaces? Hotels? Restaurants? Bars? All public areas? Parks and beaches?
- Should motorcycle helmet use be required by a law?
- Should ignition interlock devices (car start breathalyzers) be mandatory in all cars?
- How helpful are "alternative" therapies, such as acupuncture, aromatherapy or massage therapy?
- Should genetically modified organisms (GMOs) be labeled as such?

These are just some of the controversies; countless others can be identified. Some controversies have existed for many years; others may be a controversy because of some new scientific discovery that challenges the way the issue is viewed. Controversies can exist because of the way that different groups or individuals view an issue; sometimes this is because of their perspective due to their professional role (e.g., law enforcement versus health professional) and sometimes it is due to a personal orientation. Sometimes, the media inadvertently perpetuates unfounded health claims such as with the controversy over early childhood immunizations and the risk of autism.[5]

The important thing with the controversies is to acknowledge that controversies exist. You may decide that you want to highlight the various sides of the controversy; alternatively, you may also determine that you simply want to acknowledge that the controversy exists and then move ahead with your health and safety communications initiative.

Emerging issues

Through the process of health and safety communications, it is helpful to be straightforward and truthful with what you do and do not know. As noted earlier, you may be expected to "know everything" since you are a "health specialist" or "safety specialist" or have expertise in a specific topic area; some people may expect you to know about all of health, or all of safety. That is, in fact, unreasonable; but it does not stop others from expecting that. Similarly, if you are a specialist in one specific topical area, it is unreasonable for you to know everything about other areas. Thus, acknowledge your limits and do not seek to promote your expertise beyond what is appropriate and valid. This may be something where you state "that is another area of study" or "I am not a specialist in that area."

If you go back in time, into fairly recent history, there was a time when ...

* Cars did not have safety belts.
* Roads did not have rumble strips to alert the driver that s/he is going over the edge of the roadway (or in some settings, crossing the middle line of a two-lane road).
* Cars did not have airbags.
* Medications did not have child-proof caps.
* Food did not have nutrition labels.
* Cigarettes did not have warning labels.
* Smoking was allowed fairly widely, including in restaurants, airplanes and more.
* Beer was sold in vending machines at government office buildings.

Whatever the health issue, expect that change will be occurring. You will hear of new scientific discoveries, some of which become more widespread and mainstream. Others will be something that is exciting and promising, but may not be ready to bring to scale or may be too expensive to implement widely. Some new research will occur that suggests helpful ways for addressing medical conditions or health concerns and will be reviewed by other scientists and professional groups before it is widely adopted. Some new research may not be reviewed favorably, because it is done with unconventional or typically non-traditional approaches; it may not be within the current accepted paradigm for addressing the issue. An example of this relates to a ban on chocolate milk in some schools; a study found that children drink a lot less milk when they do not have the option of drinking it with chocolate flavoring.

The question for you is how to handle emerging issues. This is viewed as different from staying up-to-date with new information; this is the type of information that is "out there" and may, indeed, become new accepted information. But, for now, it is new, it is emerging and it may or may not be validated.

This is quite important, as needs emerge during contemporary topic discussion and issue exploration. For example, a couple of decades ago, the public was unaware of organic foods and their distinction from conventional foods; at that time, communicating claims about the health benefits of organic foods might reach a targeted audience. This is coming into further public awareness with scientific results surrounding genetically modified organisms (GMOs). Another example is that, not long ago, the public was unaware of safety concerns associated with "distracted driving." Some drivers shaved, put on makeup or disciplined unruly children while driving. Now, "distracted driving" is very often associated with the dangers of texting while operating a vehicle.

Current now is the relatively recent introduction of e-cigarettes. Some argue that their use can be helpful for a cigarette smoker who is trying to reduce the level of smoking; rather than having all the various ingredients and additives and carcinogens, the e-cigarette becomes a different kind of nicotine delivery system. On the other hand, does their availability promote tobacco use among non-users including, but not limited to, youth? Further, does the existence of e-cigarettes make more vulnerable the danger of ingestion of their contents? The answer, today, is that it is not known. The research just hasn't been conducted; however, this may be resolved in the years to come.

Another example is with the potential health benefits of some of the active ingredients of marijuana. The implementation of medical marijuana laws and the legalization of marijuana have changed the landscape surrounding this substance. Scientific research will elucidate more clearly the extent to which medical benefits actually exist; and further insights will emerge regarding which part of the marijuana plant and which active ingredients in the plant have what effects, and for which people and for which conditions. All-too-often in public discourse, the dialog is emotion-laden and not grounded in sound research. The research will undoubtedly differentiate the effects of several active ingredients in marijuana known as cannabinoids. In addition, what will be learned about the effects of many of the other cannabinoids found in marijuana?

Consider also the efficacy of nicotine use for addressing Alzheimer's disease. Since nicotine has been linked to memory with humans as well as animals, the question is whether its ingestion may be helpful to protect against or reduce the effects of Alzheimer's disease. This may affect certain types of memory (e.g., attention, information processing), but not others. Further, there may be negative consequences associated with nicotine use with Alzheimer's patients that offset potential benefits achieved with memory. Just as with other issues, this can cause controversy and concern. The point here is to be aware of this as an area of research and potentially changing know-feel-do strategies for addressing this disease (and possibly other diseases).

How does this translate for you? To be valued and valuable as a health communicator, it is important that you remain ever vigilant to what is emerging, and what is on the cutting edge. This does not mean that you accept everything you hear, but you are open to the new information and insights. Some new information may not necessarily, or not yet, represent new "knowledge"; however it is helpful to remain aware of what is on the horizon and monitor it as the science becomes clearer. It may be that it takes years to get resolution on the issue, which is fine. As you work with your audiences, whether it is with colleagues or with the ultimate audience you seek to influence, you will decide the extent to which you include these issues.

For each of these statistics, some readers will say "I didn't know that" and others may say "Well, here's a setting where the results are worse." Further, some readers may say "That's not as important as this other issue." The point is that health and safety concerns surround us. And controversies and new information, as well as idiosyncratic results, will remain. And further, individual differences and unique circumstances will remain. What is important is to acknowledge that many of these issues can be addressed better and that improvements throughout the realm of health and safety topics are continually occurring, some through scientific discoveries and others through changes in approaches.

Staying realistic and reasonable

As a health communicator, you are undoubtedly striving to be knowledgeable, staying up-to-date and being open to new information. However, as is obvious from some of the examples cited in this chapter, you cannot be expected to know it all. Further, you will probably be a specialist in one or more (but not all) areas of health. As cited earlier, some of those people reached by you may expect that you know it all, "since you are in the safety field" or "because you are a health educator."

The question now focuses on how you can be reasonable with your own expectations and how you can manage the expectations of others, as you move ahead with communicating about the health and safety issues.

One perspective noted is that it is important that you strive, to the greatest extent possible, to stay current and up-to-date. You should read the public media, including news clippings, newsletters, newspaper articles and professional journals. Listen to the news, and when you read or hear something that is related to your area of specialty, seek out additional information about the topic. See if you can find the actual research upon which it is based and see if the news article addressed it properly and fully. If the article is something about which you are not sure, you may be well served to contact other specialists or researchers to determine their take on the research. And, if you think the findings were misrepresented, this is something you might address with your communications work; you may use this as an opportunity to reach out to your media relations personnel or the media directly (see Chapter 9 on media relations for more on this).

Another approach, linked to the earlier discussion about staying current, is to solicit, periodically, comments and suggestions from colleagues or others whom you trust. Ask for their perspectives, ask what is current, suggest that they identify emerging issues and areas of controversy, solicit promising know-feel-do strategies and request anything that will help keep you current. For example, a team of researchers surveyed a community regarding preferred ways to be informed about available health resources; internet web sites was most preferred followed by newspaper and then U.S. mail.[6]

A third perspective with this is that your biggest challenge may, in fact, be that of meeting your own expectations. Said differently, you may be your own worst critic. After all, you know what it is that you do not know; you know where you are unclear and where you may not be up-to-date. You know the controversies and the issues, and you may just know too much. So keep the perspective that you do know a lot and that you are striving to stay up-to-date with the issue (assuming that you are!).

Fourth, acknowledge that things do continually change. You can only do so much. As long as you are diligent with your efforts to be knowledgeable and current, you are being most appropriate and ethically sound.

Fifth, there may be some things that, while true, may just not be appropriate to share because of how they can be misinterpreted. Of course, this will depend on your audience. For example, with fetal alcohol syndrome, it is known that this is caused by a pregnant woman drinking during pregnancy, and that greater risk of more serious damage to the child occurs the earlier in pregnancy that alcohol use occurs. But how much alcohol is too much? Some will advise that no drinking should occur if a woman is pregnant or thinks she might be pregnant; others will say that a periodic drink may not be harmful. How appropriate, and how ethical, is it to share this distinction; rather, is it better to say clearly "no drinking during pregnancy"? This becomes a dilemma, as fetal alcohol syndrome is obviously linked to alcohol consumption, but that does not mean that any or all alcohol consumption during pregnancy will definitely result in fetal alcohol syndrome. This isn't resolved here, but simply illustrates the types of dilemmas and challenges that you may face as a health communicator about how much to state to your audience.

Finally, it is helpful to remember your role as a health communicator and the difference between your knowledge and what it is that you want from your audience. Recall, continuously, that your audience is at a certain place with their knowledge, their beliefs, their attitudes, their intentions and their behavior (see more with the stages of change theory in the next chapter on know-feel-do strategies). Your aim is to help them move from one place (or stage) to another. Your aim is to provide information, to ultimately have some effect or impact—what you want them to "know, feel or do." Your aim is not one of imparting all of your wisdom and the complexities and related issues associated with your area of focus; your aim is to move them systematically and deliberately from one place to another. If you keep in mind this perspective, then it shouldn't be as daunting as you work with your communications effort. You do know the issue, you are up-to-date and now you are determining how to affect your audience in the most desirable and appropriate way.

Messages from the field

Hone your message for maximum effectiveness

Annie Elble Todt, PhD, MPH, Give Hope, Fight Poverty

The mission of Give Hope, Fight Poverty (GHFP) is to foster philanthropy domestically by designing service-learning programs that engage US students & professionals with rural communities in Swaziland, Africa. Three features of Facebook Pages aid with providing relevant and time-appropriate messages, thus enhancing the effectiveness of our posts.

First, through using the data we are able to see when our audience members are active on Facebook. This valuable information about when to post is welcomed by our organization since we work in multiple time zones.

Second, by using the drop down menu next to the "publish" feature on Facebook, we can schedule the post to become active during our popular 12pm and 9pm CST periods, even if we are in Swaziland.

Third, we study the audience's likes, shares and comments so we can drive up the reach of our posts. Through studying the analytics, we have found three simple things drive up our pages' reach.

1 Posts incorporating photos of our orphans reach a greater audience than posts without photos. Photos (and particularly those of our children rather than scenery) tend to drive up the post's activity.
2 Posts with a plea or task often results in more shares and higher reach. This does not mean simply asking the viewer to like or share—but a specific plea for help. For instance, we asked in one post if the viewer knew an author or illustrator.

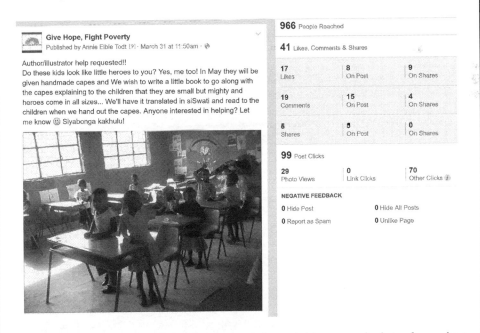

**As you can see, this post was published during our peak time period, incorporated a photo of our orphans and asked for help in networking. Any one of these pieces alone would not have reached the success rate of incorporating all of them together.

3   Who doesn't love free? An easy way to drive your numbers is to advertise something free. One example is our charity challenge: Win a Trip to Swaziland. We had the highest activity reaching 1,400 people as well as the most post clicks compared to any other post within that month. Additionally, this resulted in a sharp increase in both "suggested page likes" and "organic page likes" increasing our overall audience.

Date		Post			Reach		Engagement	
03/29/2016 3:37 pm		Hoping to WIN A TRIP TO SWAZILAND? Some easy fundraiser	🔗	🌐	858		56 5	🚩
03/29/2016 12:02 pm		Purdue! Join us next Wednesday April 6th Give Hope Fight Pove	💬	🌐	26		0 1	
03/29/2016 8:39 am		Mark your calendars for May 29th.... join us for our favorite semi-	🔗	🌐	61		0 2	
03/23/2016 7:52 am		Crazy busy next two days recruiting service learning volunteers a	🖼	🌐	309		0 2	
03/22/2016 5:18 pm		Here are the first batch of capes for our preschoolers in at our Ne	🖼	🌐	875		51 53	
03/20/2016 8:56 pm		Win a trip to Swaziland - Charity Challenge	🔗	🌐	1.4K		147 36	
02/27/2016 1:17 pm		For a $33 donation, this pair of bracelets can be yours (shipping i	🖼	🌐	517		12 18	
02/21/2016 3:46 pm		Elementary School Teacher Friends - anyone have a school with	🖼	🌐	985		55 37	
02/15/2016 11:17 am		Being totally transparent! Here are is our final accounting from 20	🖼	🌐	959		107 24	

Overall, engaging posts are crucial. For us, it's introducing our audience to an intimate detail or major success of one of our orphans—or asking them for direct or indirect help in some manner. We have found that very few people engage with our day to day activity such as recruiting at a specific university or starting a new program. If we have too many unresponsive posts we also run the risk of having someone unlike the page and therefore reduce our audience. Post during your peak time period, incorporate a powerful photo or video, and try to be as interactive as possible urging your audience to share or comment without directly using those words.

Being believable

The final consideration within this chapter of aims and goals focuses on being believable by the audience. With the assumption that you do know the current information on your topic, and that you are conversant with the controversies and emerging issues associated with this, how do you "translate" this in ways that are understandable and believable to your audience? In fact, as you think about your audience, you are thinking about the ultimate audience as well as the intermediaries and gatekeepers affiliated with reaching your target audience.

Start with the following questions: When you are listening to someone, or reading something, who or what do you believe? Why? What are the specific factors there that suggest that you ought to, or do, believe what is being communicated? Is it the clarity with which the information is conveyed? Is it the fact that the information is current? Is it due to the illustrations provided, whether graphic or data or testimonial? Is it the nature of the presenter(s)? Does it have to do with the linkage to national, state or local needs, data or issues? Is it because it is tied into an external campaign (such as an awareness day, week or month)?

As you start to discern what makes the communication believable for you, those insights can be helpful for determining how to prepare your information. This becomes a type of starting point for you. Further, you will think about the audience you seek to affect, and what might be influential or important for them (see Chapter 2 on knowing your audience). Again, there are no magic answers, but the consideration about what YOU believe, and what leads you to believe it, can be helpful as you seek to have your perspectives and information believable by your audience. So, as you are communicating with others, whether through personal interaction (such as a workshop, lecture or interview) or product (like a brochure, poster or public service announcement), make sure that you and your messages are relatable.

A big part of being believable is communicating what you do know and not communicating what you do not know. If there is the opportunity (whether time or space), you might acknowledge unresolved issues or controversies. But with the general communication overall, realize where your audience is and then focus the message on their current state of awareness. To be believable, you want to be sure that you resonate with them, through know-feel-do strategies, language, illustrations and examples that make sense to them. You want to be sure to not overstate or exaggerate the topic, even if it represents a slight overstatement; this can affect the respondents' views of your truthfulness and that of your organization. The American College Health Association surveyed thousands of college students nationwide on "most believable sources of health information." Respondents indicated the following sources as being more believable: health center medical staff, health educators, faculty or coursework and parents. Interestingly, of these four sources, medical staff, health educators and faculty were underutilized compared to how often college students rely on parents for health information. The researchers concluded that awareness of use and believability of health information sources can help professionals design more effective health campaigns.[7]

To further your believability, it is helpful to blend both quantitative and qualitative approaches. Building up the theories undergirding your effort, consider appealing to both the reason (logos) and feelings (both pathos and ethos) of your audience. To do so, you may include the rational foundation for them engaging in your desired outcome; this is the logic and will typically include a quantitative approach. This may involve facts and figures; it may be the sound reasoning behind your recommendation. Further, it is helpful to incorporate some qualitative approaches also to connect to their emotions, as well as with their sense of right and wrong and even social justice. This may include testimonials from those who are similar to your audience about their perspectives, as well as endorsements from those in knowledgeable positions (such as health professional experts).

Messages from the field

Storytelling

Amr Abdalla, Ph.D., Institute for Peace and Security Studies, Addis Ababa University; Vice Rector for Academic Affairs, University for Peace (2005–2014)

Over the last two decades, I have taught and conducted courses and workshops worldwide on topics related to peace, conflict resolution, social science research and multiculturalism. I also conducted several research and evaluation missions of various development and peacebuilding projects. Through it all, I encountered numerous situations and heard stories which have enriched me as a person and as a professional. Many of these stories and situations served very well as real-life practical examples and stories to illustrate some complex or abstract concepts during my teaching and training. Over the years, I found that my student evaluations have constantly emphasized how they particularly enjoyed the stories I brought to my classes and workshops, and that such stories enhanced their learning experience and made it most enriching and relevant.

That constant positive feedback about using stories in my classroom and workshops led me to expand my pool of stories to include not only ones I have come across during my work, but also ones that I have encountered in any situation, as long as I found a clear relevance of the story to a topic about which I am teaching or training. I continued to receive praises for the stories and I have witnessed over and over again how students and workshop attendees—from all walks of life and from all parts of the world—listened attentively to those stories with eyes wide-open and anticipation.

Beyond blending both quantitative and qualitative approaches, ways of maximizing your believability include demonstrating your understanding of and empathy with the audience and their needs. For you to acknowledge your awareness of where they are, and how you want to be helpful for improving some aspect of their lives, can be helpful.

It is also helpful for you to acknowledge clearly the limits of your knowledge. You have probably been to workshops or talks where it is clear that the session is "all about them"; this may be a speaker who is focused on impressing you with his/her level of knowledge. For you to be believable, yes, you do need to be knowledgeable and communicate your awareness of the issues within the topic of concern. It is also helpful, in terms of believability, to communicate where you see limits. It is helpful to acknowledge when you do not know something. It is helpful to provide the larger context of specific issues, whether that involves paradigms or conceptual frameworks, emerging issues or controversies. This is not designed to overwhelm an audience, but to communicate that many health and safety issues are not as cut and dried as they may seem; the idiosyncrasies and individual differences are important to communicate. For example, you may communicate the following:

- "The answer to your question really depends on some personal characteristics, such as ..."
- "In responding to that, it is helpful to provide a brief historical context."
- "In fact, there are two very different lines of thinking on that issue."
- "It used to be common that people would do a specific activity to address that; however, more recently, the approach involves the following effort."
- "While the general public believes that a certain approach is the way to go, the [medical or safety] professionals are in strong agreement that this is the way to approach that issue."

So, to be believable, it is vital that you do know your information and that you communicate this knowledge and the limits of this knowledge as you work with your audience. Try to envision listening to the information and its approaches, as if you were sitting in their place or standing in their shoes. Provide information that you believe to be helpful and appropriate and offer suggestions about where they may go for additional information. Depending on the nature of your approach, you may include the references and background you acquired to make yourself knowledgeable.

Forward!

In summary, health and safety communication is conveying messages to raise awareness of health and safety topics and issues. The message is based on what you want the audience to know, feel and do. Important health topics are provided by Healthy People, although additional health and safety topics exist that are not incorporated in this helpful framework.

How can you summarize the state of knowledge, when knowledge is constantly changing? How do you communicate clearly information that is, actually, quite complex? In what ways should you communicate limited information in a focused period of time or space, so that it is timely, accurate, as complete as possible and appropriate?

You want to be sure that your message is understandable and that it points them clearly toward a next step. You do not want to be misleading or provide misinformation; however, you need to be succinct and provide as much information as is reasonably appropriate considering your approach. Sometimes too much information, while accurate, is just not appropriate or needed. That's where you, as a professional, are pulling together the information and resources and offering your audience the information in a way that is relatable and usable by them. Hopefully, through this process, you become a valuable and valued resource and the audience wants to come back to you for more information and insights in the months and years to come.

Notes

1 Healthy People 2020. *Topics & Objectives Objectives A–Z*. Retrieved February 15, 2016 from www.healthypeople.gov/2020/topics-objectives
2 Edgerton, E., Reiney, E., Mueller, S., Reicherter, B., Curtis, K., Waties, S. and Limber, S.P. (2016). Identifying new strategies to assess and promote online health communication and social media outreach: an application in bullying prevention. *Health Promotion Practice*, 17(3), 448–456.
3 Noar, S.M., Harrington, N.G., Van Stee, S.K. and Aldrich, R.S. (2010). Tailored health communication to change lifestyle behaviors. *American Journal of Lifestyle Medicine*, 5(2), 112–122.
4 Neuhauser, L. and Kreps, G.L. (2003). Rethinking communication in the e-health era. *Journal of Health Psychology*, 8(1), 7–23.
5 Dixon, G.N. and Clarke, C.E. (2013). Heightening uncertainty around certain science: media coverage, false balance, and the autism–vaccine controversy. *Science Communication*, 35(3), 358–382.
6 Colby, S.E., Johnson, A.L., Eickhoff, A. and Johnson, L. (2011). Promoting community health resources: preferred communication strategies. *Health Promotion Practice*, 12(2), 271–279.
7 Vader, A.M., Walters, S.T., Roudsari, B. and Nguyen, N. (2011). Where do college students get health information? Believability and use of health information sources. *Health Promotion Practice*, 12(5), 713–722.

4 Know-feel-do strategies

Step 3

If the aim of your health and safety communication is to influence and persuade the audience, then the ultimate goal is for the audience to change its behavior. This calls for a strategy—a plan of action—to create change. You will see, however, that actual behavior change is a complex process. So, maybe the more prudent strategy for change is to focus on more proximate results, which can be seen as connected together along the way toward behavioral change. Your strategy may thus emphasize raising awareness, increasing knowledge and urging the audience to examine its beliefs. Behavior change on any scale is best tackled through know-feel-do strategies (see Figure 4.1).

Typically, no automatic, magic switch gets thrown so that the change in behavior occurs. Think about some behavior that you changed. For example, did you stop biting your nails? Did you start turning the light off when you left a room? Did you stop texting

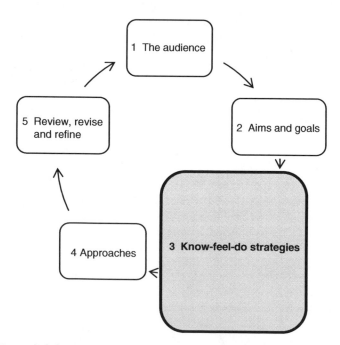

Figure 4.1 Know-feel-do strategies

while driving? Have you begun eating healthier? With each of these efforts, what did it take on your part? Was it as simple as having more knowledge and then, voilà, the behavior changed? Probably not. Was it having your attitude modified and then the behavior was automatically altered? Probably not.

To make matters more complicated, some behaviors seem to be changed by one strategy, while other behaviors are affected through another strategy. For example: not biting your nails might require knowledge about germs, applying bitter-tasting nail polish and finally getting a manicure and not wanting to mess it up. Another example is stopping texting while driving. It could have been as simple as keeping your cell phone out of reach while you are driving. And, there are still other health or safety concerns for which your behavior has not yet changed. Eating healthily can be a lifelong challenge. This is the same with your efforts working with others—you know your ultimate goal is their behavior change, but your more immediate focus includes having them accomplish results in one or more of the areas along the way.

With your work in health and safety communications, the mantra stressed throughout this guide is being clear with what you want your audience to know, feel or do. Specifically, you may want them to know some facts through a particular health and safety communications initiative. Or, you may want them to feel a particular way, or to have a different type of attitude about an issue. In the bigger picture, you want your target audience to do something different in order to engage in healthy and safe behavior.

Strategies

Know-feel-do strategies are used while composing the health and safety message. What happens with the process of understanding the needs of the audience and planning is that you become much clearer with what it is that you want for the audience, as a result of whatever it is you are doing with your health and safety communications initiative. These desired endpoints may be in the area of knowledge, they may be in the arena of feelings or they may emphasize action steps or behavioral results—thus, the "know, feel and do" distinctions.

For what you want someone to *know*, any of the following may be helpful:

- The *fact* that services to address a certain condition or issue are available. For example the Substance Abuse and Mental Health Services Administration (SAMHSA) runs the National Suicide Prevention Lifeline. The number is 1–800–273–8255 and the website includes a crisis chat center.[1]
- The *cost* (or lack of cost), the available hours, or the location of resources. For example the National Directory of Designated Driver Services website has a list of 1215 designated driver companies in 42 states, where searches can be done by state and county, with phone numbers and websites of companies for a safe ride home in a local area.[2]
- The *types of symptoms* that might suggest the beginning of a particular health condition. If someone is having a stroke, for example, they will experience numbness or weakness on one side of the body and it can be in the face, arm or leg. They will also be confused and have trouble speaking, they may be blind or have difficulty seeing from one or both eyes, they will have trouble balancing or walking and may have a sudden headache (NIH). A person having a stroke has the best chance of survival if a witness to these symptoms calls for emergency care quickly.

- *Ways of starting* a difficult conversation. This may be with a person about whom you are concerned such as a significant other, a friend or roommate who seems to have severe depression or a substance abuse problem.
- *What to look for* when selecting a product (or when reviewing information on the internet). For example, with understanding nutrition labels to select healthy foods, "partially hydrogenated" means the food contains trans fats.
- *Quick tips* for addressing an emergency situation. This may include learning to count the number of doors between your hotel room and the nearest emergency exit in case of a fire, because you would not be able to see the "Exit" sign when smoke rises and if you know the number of doors you can count them as you crawl to the fire escape.

For each of these examples, increased knowledge can help with the person's progress to the next step in behavioral change. Knowledge about the availability of services, or its hours or costs, may be all that is needed for the person to avail him/herself of the resource. Likewise, things to look for, conversation starters, tips and related items can be all that is necessary to be better informed.

When you want to focus on what someone *feels*, here are some examples:

- A greater *sensitivity* to the needs and issues faced by the vulnerable homeless population.
- Whether it is *fair to pay* a very high price for medication to treat a serious medical condition.
- Increased *confidence* in speaking up or not being a bystander when witnessing emergency situations where multiple individuals are present.

Helping your audience with enhanced feelings can be a significant step along the way to behavior change. By emphasizing an individual's understanding of others' perspectives, the result may be that he/she will be more likely to actually do something about it (the behavior change). By having a different attitude about him/herself (such as increased confidence), an individual may be more likely to speak up or speak out with specific situations. Feelings are not a magic bullet for affecting behavior change, but they can be an important factor in this process.

Being clear with what you want someone to *do* is another area of focus within the framework of health and safety communications. For example:

- *Starting the process* of exercise with short, non-strenuous activities.
- Highlighting *how to prepare* food, whether a dish or a meal, from scratch.
- *Demonstrating* specific skills for conducting a breast self-examination.
- *Illustrating* clearly the steps for safely installing a child safety seat—correctly.
- *Practicing* self-control and sound decision-making when faced with an irrational request.
- *Learning* specific steps to take in an emergency situation involving an earthquake or other weather-related situation.
- *Practicing to remember* "stop, drop and roll" as a measurement to take when someone is on fire.

The distinction between the various aspects of what you want the audience to know, feel and do can be somewhat artificial. Often, the focus is on just one of these three elements.

Just as often, overlaps among these three broad areas do exist. For example, emphasizing increased knowledge-based skills may help increase the confidence in using those skills (consider tips for confronting an abusive person, you need to know ways to confront him/her before you do it). Similarly, when promoting greater empathy with a situation, you may also highlight some of the factual aspects of it (it is difficult to feel empathy toward others if you do not know about their struggle). This blend of areas of emphasis is fine, as each can play off of the other. Further, it may take both of them to have the ultimate desired outcome for your communication effort.

The important thing for you as the health communicator is to be clear with what it is that you seek with your audience at this point in time. As you design a brochure or prepare for a talk, it is most helpful to be crystal clear with what you want them to know, feel or do as a result of them engaging with your communication approach. It doesn't matter whether you are actually interacting with them—it is an extension of what you want to communicate. The clearer you are with what you want, the more likely you are to get your message across.

Relating back to the issue of segmented audiences highlighted in Chapter 2, note that different groups can be best addressed using different examples or know-feel-do strategies. If you are targeting high school aged youth, you will undoubtedly use different approaches than when targeting elementary aged youth. And, targeting society's first generation citizens will incorporate different know-feel-do strategies to those used with those whose ancestors have been in the country for centuries.

Turning to some considerations within this step, the development of communication know-feel-do strategies that involve both the composing and channeling of the effort will be based on whatever you define as the need. For example, think of a high traffic road near a school zone. If drivers do not know there is a school in the area, they will not be on the lookout for students, so signs may be placed near the school and flashing lights may also be installed; the speed limit may be reduced during certain times of the day and school crossing guards and/or a police car presence may be in sight at the start and end of the school day. This precaution is to raise awareness among the vehicle operator audience. There may not have been any collisions involving students or the drivers may not have children who go to that school and this would result in a low level of awareness and concern. For perception of invulnerability, neighbors may think "I grew up in this neighborhood, nothing bad happens here." Or parents may believe their child would never cross the busy street without looking both ways even if he/she is distracted. Other factors could include the road being used as a shortcut, so speed bumps may be needed. A child at the school could be blind and would need crosswalks with tactile paving and pedestrian alert sounds so they will know when to cross—or perhaps a crossing guard is needed to help direct traffic and keep kids safe. So in addition to the traffic control device of flashing yellow lights, there may be a need to launch periodic safety messages with the involvement of the crossing guards or directly to parents and children about the necessity of cautious driving through school zones.

The issue of behavior change can be quite complex; these distinctions about know-feel-do are ultimately interrelated and such that your efforts can be more focused, deliberate and achievable. The aim is for your efforts to be more intentional and planned. Another aim is for your efforts to be more grounded in the experience of others, including what they have found to work or not work; these results may or may not be based on formal evaluation activities. What's more, you can strengthen your strategy for change by basing it on behavioral change theory. The next section of this chapter summarizes some of the dominant theories helpful for planning health and safety communications efforts.

Theories

Strategies are used to change recipients' awareness, knowledge, beliefs, attitudes, intentions and practices. Strategies work best if they are based on theory. Think of a **theory** as a set of related ideas explaining a situation or justifying a course of action. Applying theory strengthens the communication effort or product. You want the target audience to experience some change, based on what you define for them to know, feel and/or do. After all, that is the intent of this professional guide to health and safety communications. Numerous theories are helpful for your communications, with some more popularly used than others. The National Cancer Institute has compiled a succinct overview of theories relevant to health.[3]

Could it be that one theory is more appropriate than another? Absolutely. You may also find that you want to proceed in a certain direction, yet with the pilot testing activities, find that that didn't work out too well or test well with that audience. What is most important with these theoretical foundations is that your communication planning, and ultimately the effort, is grounded in some theory, and that you are thinking of these theoretical approaches as part of your work. It is important that you have SOME foundation for your efforts. This is certainly better than the alternative—doing a communication effort that is based on what "seems to be good" or what "feels good" or "feels right."

Here is an example of how theory is considered while following the steps of the health and safety communications model. Consider the situation where you are developing an initiative to encourage testing for HIV. What do you want to communicate? Your aim is probably that you want to have more people tested and your message will be about whatever are relevant factors, such as access, availability, cost, confidentiality, consultation as needed, importance or others that emerge from your understanding of your audience. As you develop your communication, think about how to reach the audience and what is important to them. What do they already know, where do they have information gaps or misinformation and what perceptions do they have about getting tested? This is, in part, a needs assessment. Next, consider some basic assumptions such as what knowledge they have about testing. What questions do they have and what concerns do they have? As you think about these, you can incorporate this knowledge in your efforts to draw more people into the process of getting tested. Your efforts should be based on one or more of the theories described in this chapter. For instance, you might prepare your product or approach according to the stages of change theory. This requires fashioning your intervention based on the audience's readiness to change. Similarly, you could incorporate the tenets of the health belief model. In doing so, your efforts would be designed around salient beliefs of the audience in order to obtain the results you want. As you will see, there are other theories from which to adopt.

This section provides brief summaries and illustrations of the more popular behavior change theories applicable to effective health and safety communications.

Health belief model

The **health belief model**[4,5] is an apt theory for health and safety communicators who want to appeal to an audience's beliefs (see Figure 4.2). It especially relates to the "feeling" component of know–feel–do strategies that address areas of potential concern, as well as to bolster the audience's likelihood of engaging in or reinforcing the desired behavior (see Table 4.1). The focus is **salient health beliefs**. Salience means immediate, important or conspicuous. The health belief model includes four factors as predictors

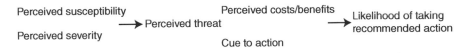

Figure 4.2 Health belief model

Table 4.1 Health belief model applied to know–feel–do strategies

Belief or factor	Definition	Know–feel–do strategies
Perceived susceptibility	Beliefs about the chances of getting a condition	Define what populations(s) are at risk and their levels of risk Tailor risk information based on an individual's characteristics or behaviors Help the individual develop an accurate perception of his or her own risk
Perceived severity	Beliefs about the seriousness of a condition and its consequences	Specify the consequences of a condition and recommended action
Perceived benefits	Beliefs about the effectiveness of taking action to reduce risk of seriousness	Explain how, where and when to take action and what the potential positive results will be
Perceived barriers	Beliefs about the material and psychological costs of taking action	Offer reassurance, incentives and assistance; correct misinformation
Cues to action	Factors that activate "readiness to change"	Provide "how to" information, promote awareness and employ reminder systems
Self-efficacy	Confidence in one's ability to take action	Provide training and guidance in performing action Use progressive goal setting Give verbal reinforcement Demonstrate desired behaviors

of adopting a health behavior: perceived susceptibility to disease or disability, perceived severity of the disease or disability, perceived benefits of health-enhancing behaviors and perceived barriers to health-enhancing behaviors. So if people perceive they are susceptible to a severe unhealthy or unsafe condition, can benefit from adopting a selected health behavior and can overcome barriers during the adoption, they are more likely to undertake this positive action to improving their health. Two additional factors can also play important roles: cues to action and self-efficacy in terms of one's ability to take action.

Stages of change

The **stages of change** (or **transtheoretical**) **model**[6] determines where a person "is," or where a group of individuals are, when it comes to changing behavior (see Figure 4.3). This theory explains a continuum from not even knowing about or considering a behavior change, to a place where his/her behavior change is maintained. With tobacco smoking, for example, someone may not know about the harmful effects of tobacco (you might wonder how that could be the case now, considering all the knowledge about tobacco and its harmful effects). If the individual was totally unaware, and then becomes somewhat aware of the harm, this could be an example of moving from the precontemplation stage to the contemplation stage. In fact, with the relatively recent introduction of e-cigarettes, the extent of harmful consequences is, currently, not known. With greater scientific attention to these products, and more time for them to be available, knowledge of their health effects (harm and/or benefits) will evolve. That information could be sufficient to move an individual from one stage to another. With the cigarette smoker who has quit, the aim is to help him/her stay away from the use of cigarettes; this would be to reinforce the maintenance stage with this situation. Ultimately, following maintenance the issue may be totally finalized, representing a state of termination. Thus, the know-feel-do strategies used in health and safety communications to help move someone (or a group) from precontemplation to contemplation are different from those used to help those in the maintenance stage. Similarly, if an individual is aware of the risks associated with a behavior, but is considering a change, then they are in the contemplation stage, pending any other changes they need to make to be able to move onto the preparation stage (see Table 4.2).

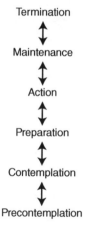

Figure 4.3 Stages of change model

Table 4.2 Stages of change model applied to know-feel-do strategies

Stage	Definition	Know-feel-do strategies
Precontemplation	Has no intention of taking action within the next six months	Increase awareness of need for change; personalize information about risks and benefits
Contemplation	Intends to take action in the next six months	Motivate; encourage making specific plans
Preparation	Intends to take action within the next 30 days and has taken some behavioral steps in this direction	Assist with developing and implementing concrete action plans; help set gradual goals
Action	Has changed behavior for less than six months	Assist with feedback, problem solving, social support and reinforcement
Maintenance	Has changed behavior for more than six months	Assist with coping, reminders, finding alternatives, avoiding slips/relapses (as applicable)

Messages from the field

A community's readiness to change

Beth DeRicco, Ph.D., Drexel University and Caron Treatment Centers

I think that some of my most successful work has been around community readiness to change—based on the work of Prochaska and DiClemente. I have worked with campuses and communities to use readiness models to understand and act in a way that reflects these models—there is always something to help move toward public health goals, as long as the preventionist or public health practitioner can figure out what a community is willing and able to commit to within the logical frame of action steps toward reaching a long term outcome.

Aristotle's proofs

A third theoretical underpinning for health and safety communications efforts is based on Aristotle (see Figure 4.4). In short, the model has been described and applied by several scholars[7] and highlights know-feel-do strategies that can be helpful in making a difference to individuals' perspectives about a health or safety behavior (see Table 4.3). Are they motivated primarily by logic? Or does their emotion drive their activity? Alternatively, is it a sense of right and wrong that makes a difference for them?

So, with Aristotle, three forms of proof are attributed to his teachings. For the reader who did not have to take a philosophy or Latin class, Logos is framed around logic and involves an individual's ability to reason rationally. The individual is presumed to be able to accomplish this and will most likely be persuaded by a logical, rational argument that incorporates facts and figures. To accomplish this, the health and safety communications effort emphasizes data, charts, tables and samples that demonstrate the importance of engaging with a particular behavior. This may include the prevalence and incidence of a problem; it may also highlight the success rate for engaging in specific proactive, positive, healthy or safe behaviors.

The second area emphasizes Ethos, or ethic. This highlights the character or values associated with an individual. The health and safety message would convey a sense of "right or wrong" or "good or bad," which can be done through highlighting contrasts among various choices. This can also emphasize the consequence of behaving in a certain way, so that the audience is drawn toward positive results and away from negative results.

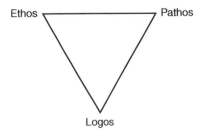

Figure 4.4 Aristotle's forms of proof

Table 4.3 Aristotle's forms of proof applied to know-feel-do strategies

Proof	Explanation	Know-feel-do strategies
Logos	Emphasizing a rational and logical approach, building upon scientific foundations. Often used to highlight assumptions upon which decisions are made, including challenging faulty assumptions.	Behavior based on faulty assumption: A person doesn't wear a bicycle helmet, because they believe they can see and hear around themselves better without wearing this.
Pathos	Addressing the emotions, aims, feelings, and social desires of individuals. Can tie into insecurities. Often linked to tragic events without attention to rational arguments.	Action stimulated by tragedy: A community wants strict crackdown on cyclists moving in and out of traffic and ignoring traffic signals after the tragic death of a young bicyclist.
Ethos	Promoting a quality character among the audience, through engaging in trustworthy sources. It is helpful to evoke good sense, good moral character, knowledge, and authority to gain the confidence of the audience.	Confidence promoted by authority: Promoting a bicycle safety campaign with testimonials by law enforcement, medical and research personnel.

The health communicator and safety communicator can also stress what is appropriate within the frame of reference with the audience, such as with an affiliation group, a community or neighborhood, a culture or other contextual audience. Attention to increasing the knowledge base of the audience can be helpful, by pointing out consequences, or a sense of judgment, about which the audience may not have previously known.

Third, attention is provided to Pathos, or passion. With this area, attention is provided to images, examples or testimonials. The health communicator may emphasize priorities and demonstrate the positive consequence of health decisions, as well as the negative results associated with behavior that is not health oriented. The aim of the communicator is to draw upon a sense of excitement or positive regard for a specific outcome and to gain the support or endorsement of the audience to engage in that behavior.

Theory of reasoned action and planned behavior

The theory of **reasoned action and planned behavior** is based on the combined work of Fishbein[8] and Azen[9] (see Figure 4.5). The theory offers a different construct helpful for designing communications efforts. The theory assumes a person makes reasonable and systematic use of information when deciding how to behave. His/her intention to act is the immediate determinant of the health or safety behavior. However, intention is shaped by personal attitude toward the behavior as well as perception of the social pressure to perform the behavior (subjective norm). Perceived behavioral control over the behavior is also an important part. Therefore, this theory is applied primarily in feeling and doing strategies (see Table 4.4).

The first aspect of this theory is an individual's behavioral intention. How strong is this? How committed is the person to carrying out the behavior? For example, if the issue is one of wearing a safety belt when driving a car, is this something that an individual is really committed to doing? Or, if the behavior is one of quitting smoking cigarettes, how committed is the person to doing this? You know of people who say they want to quit smoking, but do they really intend to give up? So this starts with the issue of commitment or intent.

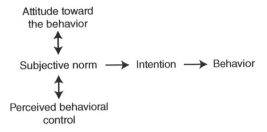

Figure 4.5 Reasoned action and planned behavior

Table 4.4 Theory of reasoned action and planned behavior applied to know-feel-do strategies

Concept	Definition	Know-feel-do strategies
Behavioral intention	Perceived likelihood of performing behavior	Are you likely or unlikely to perform the behavior?
Attitude	Personal evaluation of the behavior	Do you see the behavior as good, neutral or bad?
Subjective norm	Beliefs about whether key people approve or disapprove of the behavior; motivation to behave in a way that gains their approval	Do you agree or disagree that most people approve of/disapprove of the behavior?
Perceived behavioral control	Belief that one has, and can exercise, control over performing the behavior	Do you believe performing the behavior is up to you, or not up to you?

Undergirding this behavioral intent are two factors. One of these is the person's attitude, as to whether he/she sees the behavior as good or bad, desirable or undesirable, or neutral. Of course, these attitudes are not discrete points ("good" or "bad"), but rather placement along a continuum from extremely positive to extremely negative. This represents a type of self-assessment, regarding why the individual wants to engage in a specific behavior; this is a type of value orientation for the individual. The other factor relates to a subjective assessment regarding others' views about the behavior. This aspect examines how the individual sees others' views of the proposed behavior. The emphasis here is that individuals assess how others view their potential involvement in this behavior; these other people include individuals (such as friends, family members, colleagues) or organizations (such as neighborhood groups, professional associations or work settings). The individual targeted with your communication efforts would incorporate how others would view the potential behavior and also make a judgment about how important those perspectives are. Thus, if others who are held in high regard by an individual have a belief that the proposed behavior is desirable, then the individual is more likely to engage in it. All of these factors contribute to the individuals' behavioral intent and thus influence the likelihood of a specific behavior.

The final factor associated with this theory is perceived behavioral control. This represents a self-perception about one's own ability to control the specified behavior. In a sense, this is related to self-efficacy. The issue of behavioral control addresses how a situation and factors beyond a person's control affect their behavior and behavioral intent.

Thus, if a person felt that they didn't have control over a behavior, they may not want to try very hard to accomplish it; more realistically, if they felt that they actually had control over the behavior, then they would be more likely to work hard to accomplish it, as they would believe that would thus have a greater likelihood of success, at least with getting a sense of accomplishment.

Social (cognitive) learning theory

Originated by Bandura,[10] **social (cognitive) learning theory** shifts the frame of reference from the individual and incorporates greater context of the social environment within which the behavior occurs (see Figure 4.6). Through the interaction a person has with his/ her external context, continual feedback and perceptions occur that affect an individual's decisions about his/her own behavior.

Within this theory are six basic concepts. The first is known as reciprocal determinism, which emphasizes the interaction between the individual and his/her environment. The individual may receive messages or have perceptions that encourage a particular behavior or attitudes; similarly, the influences may be more of a direction that discourages or detracts from the viability of engaging in a behavior. Second, behavioral capability addresses an individual's actual capacity; this focuses on his/her skills, knowledge and capabilities to do the desired behavior. This means that the knowledge must be accurate and current, and that the skills, whether simple or complex, are appropriate for accomplishing the desired behavior. This provides a rich foundation for health and safety communications, including correcting myths and misperceptions, demonstrating appropriate skills and documenting specific foundations and know-feel-do strategies for the behavior (see Table 4.5). This is linked to the factor of self-efficacy, to be discussed shortly.

The third aspect is expectations, emphasizing what the individual believes will happen as a result of engaging in the behavior. Expectations for a prescription drug are that the medication will work better if the consumer abstains from consuming alcohol. For a pregnancy, expectations would be that the baby would be born as healthy as possible, without any risk of fetal alcohol syndrome. If a person believes that wearing a safety belt when in a car will enhance safety, that will contribute to engaging in the behavior; however, if a person has expectations that wearing a safety belt may have a negative effect, whether for his/her clothing, comfort or ability to exit an automobile if a crash occurs, then these expectations could detract from the behavior. Another perceived negative effect as mentioned previously is the misinformation about a seatbelt causing harm to a fetus if a woman is pregnant. Ultimately, the aim is to focus on the positive outcomes associated with the proposed behavior, to couch the results to be achieved within the

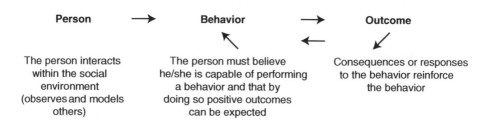

Figure 4.6 Social (cognitive) learning theory

Table 4.5 Social cognitive theory applied to know-feel-do strategies

Concept	Definition	Know-feel-do strategies
Reciprocal determinism	The dynamic interaction of the person, behavior and the environment in which the behavior is performed	Consider multiple ways to promote behavior change, including making adjustments to the environment or influencing personal attitudes
Behavioral capability	Knowledge and skill to perform a given behavior	Promote mastery learning through skills training
Expectations	Anticipated outcomes of a behavior	Model positive outcomes of healthful behavior
Self-efficacy	Confidence in one's ability to take action and overcome barriers	Approach behavior change in small steps to ensure success; be specific about the desired change
Observational learning (modeling)	Behavioral acquisition that occurs by watching the actions and outcomes of others' behavior	Offer credible role models who perform the targeted behavior
Reinforcements	Responses to a person's behavior that increase or decrease the likelihood of reoccurrence	Promote self-initiated rewards and incentives

framework of these anticipated results. The opportunity for health and safety communications know-feel-do strategies here can focus on expectations, such as modifying the expectations that may be faulty, or actively comparing competing expectations to facilitate good decision-making.

Fourth, self-efficacy is an important component of this model, similar to what is found in other models. This emphasizes a person's belief in his/her own capability of achieving the desired behavior. This includes self-confidence, resiliency, persistence and ability to modify behavior to overcome challenges or obstacles that appear. The fifth area is observational learning, emphasizing how individuals learn from others. This can be through the experiences that others have had in addressing or accomplishing the desired behavior and can be accomplished through testimonials or expert opinion. This can be envisioned with personal statements from individuals similar to the target audience, illustrating their achievement as well as challenges and how they overcame them; this type of approach can demonstrate how reasonable it is to address a behavioral outcome such as that which is proposed and how a "person like them" can achieve this. Another aspect of this can be through the guidance or advice of someone who would be considered an expert or highly knowledgeable and respected for this issue.

Finally, the model includes reinforcements, which is important to sustain and maintain the change. This is done particularly after the person has made the behavioral change, so that this change will "stick" or be maintained. As with many behaviors, the experience of using new approaches can feel awkward, at least initially. It's somewhat like a new pair of shoes; the old, worn out pair of shoes are very comfortable, as they have been broken in quite well, and the new shoes are stiff and hard, may cause pain or blisters and are such that the user just wants to discard them. For the model, positive reinforcements are helpful in maintaining the behavior change; these can be both internal and external.

Ultimately, the aim is to have internal reinforcements, as the external reinforcements will undoubtedly not be sustained over time. The external reinforcements can be helpful at least initially, but with an aim for ultimate internally generated reward systems.

Strategy and impact

A health and safety message's impact on the audience hinges on the properly devised know-feel-do strategy. The strategy, itself, does not have to be based on the ideal theory; after all, what is the best theory? What it does mean is that you are thoughtful and incorporate theoretical foundations as part of your efforts. What will happen is that your efforts will be more grounded and thoughtful—they will be more intentional. This does not necessarily translate into having your communication know-feel-do strategies work perfectly. What it does do is create a greater likelihood of your know-feel-do strategies having the desired impact; involving a theoretical foundation brings your efforts closer to achieving the results you actually want to achieve.

Is it possible to influence behavior change in an audience through communications? Can a message be so effective as to sway recipients to take it upon themselves to change? The answer to each of these questions is "yes"; after all, this book is based on the premise that change is possible. While a lot of effort can be required to achieve the desired results, the foundation of having this practical guide is to facilitate health and safety communication efforts to be more grounded, planful and engaging, thereby achieving progress and moving forward.

When you think about healthy and safe behavior, one of the obvious points is that a wide variety of reasons exist regarding why individuals do not engage in these behaviors. That is, if knowledge was all that was needed for behavior change, then the behavior you would see would be much different. As you know, behavior change is much more complex than this. Think about what people say about why they do not engage in healthy or safe behavior regularly: how often have you heard these reasons? In fact, what additional reasons can you think of?

If you want to increase knowledge, your content will emphasize the facts about an issue or situation. You may provide examples, illustrations, samples and other factors that will aid in achieving this outcome. You may engage shocking approaches, or stories with a heartfelt message or delivery process. Similarly, if the aim is to increase participants' confidence, attention will be provided to both the skill as well as the attitude. An individual may have a skill, but not feel confident; the focus will thus be on practicing the skill so that results are sound and the individual receives feedback so that their feelings about the skill are enhanced. The focus on confidence is all about having a good feeling about what is being done; ideally, you would want to have confidence and skill together, rather than confidence without the skill. On the other hand, if your aim is to increase the skills of a participant, you will want to illustrate specific ways of implementing the strategy, show common errors or mistakes and give individuals a chance to practice and receive feedback. To be able to end up with a skill means that the individual will have to know correct and incorrect approaches, and be able to demonstrate its implementation, and to do so accurately. The point is for you to be clear with what you are seeking to achieve with the communication strategy and then to design the content and approaches with know-feel-do strategies that support the desired goals.

Messages from the field

Applying theory

Richard E. Miller, Ed.D., GMU's Center for the Advancement of Public Health

Evidence in the professional literature confirms that well-designed communication interventions do impact the audience. For example, I was instrumental in designing a smoking discouragement poster series for employees of a multinational corporation. The strategy for the posters was based on reasoned action and planned behavior.[11] That is, each poster conveyed a message asking the viewer to compare his/her attitude with the attitudes of co-workers. The posters were distributed to two hundred employee representatives who displayed the posters in strategic locations within their worksites. The representative employees were then asked to report the degree to which the posters seem to have an impact on the workforce at that site. Feedback from the representative was convincing and specific examples of employee reactions to the poster series were captured in qualitative statements.

Within any health issue, the need may be a lack of awareness, a low level of concern, the perception of invulnerability, or some other factor that you would like to see addressed. Important within this area of need is to be as specific as possible; the reason for this is that a full understanding of what makes this "a need" is most helpful in defining the nature and scope of your communications effort. This specificity provides a good foundation for your later efforts of defining what you want the audience to know, feel or do. Thus, if you want to increase awareness, your approach will be more informational based; if you want to improve upon the feelings of your audience, your know-feel-do strategies will have more of an affective flavor. Think back to public service announcements about heeding the stop signs on buses—children were filing off of the bus, talking to each other and not paying attention, then something happens—a screech of tires maybe—and a lone backpack is left in the middle of the street. It is possible that drivers who have recently immigrated to the United States might not understand the importance of stopping for school buses even though it is a traffic law. Plus, the laws about pedestrians in crosswalks, and who has the right of way legally, may vary from jurisdiction to jurisdiction and country to country.

With greater resources and an interest in research, you might expand your efforts to test your theoretical grounding. For example, if you have the time and resources, as well as a large enough audience, you might consider engaging in parallel processes with different audiences. Specifically, you might design, with a single goal and similar audiences, a communications initiative based on one set of theoretical foundations and a different communications initiative based on a different theoretical background. These could result in different know-feel-do strategies, based on different foundations. The question is whether, and how, the results obtained on the desired outcomes (what you want the audience to know, feel and/or do) are different. The audiences would not be overlapping, but would be similar in characteristics and needs. The audiences would receive different communications messages and may ultimately have a different impact. This may sound like a dream, as most of us do not have the luxury of resources and time, nor access to parallel audiences that help establish a type of experimental design. What it does suggest is that your work in health and safety communications is not performed in a laboratory where you can test out different theories. Your work does, however, benefit from being enhanced with a strong foundation that is based on what you deem to be the most appropriate theory or theories possible.

As you move through other chapters in this guide, you'll find a wide range of elements that are part of the overall "toolkit" appropriate for designing helpful and appropriate health and safety communications. You won't be using all of these tools; you'll be selecting what you believe to be the most appropriate to meet the audience and its needs. Some of your work will be experimental, some of your work will be creative and all of it should, ideally, be grounded in order to maximize its impact. In this way, your planned initiative will be prepared with a sound process, enhancing the likelihood of achieving the desired results.

Forward!

In summary, this chapter on know-feel-do strategies stresses the importance of a theoretical grounding for your health and safety communications efforts. At this point, you should have a greater respect for incorporating theory as part of the planning process. And while this chapter introduced the dominant theories, other theories do exist beyond what are presented in this guide, such as the precaution adoption model and self-efficacy approach. Further, undoubtedly additional behavioral health theories will be forthcoming in the years to come and theories from other fields of study may be appropriate for adaptation for your health and safety initiatives.

Notes

1 Substance Abuse and Mental Health Services Administration. National Suicide Prevention Lifeline. Retrieved May 15, 2016 from www.suicidepreventionlifeline.org
2 DrinkingAndDriving.Org. National Directory of Designated Driver Services. Retrieved August 22, 2016 from www.drinkinganddriving.org/designated-driver-services/
3 National Cancer Institute (2005). *Theory at a Glance; A Guide to Health Promotion Practice. Second edition.* Washington, DC: National Institutes of Health, US Department of Health and Human Services.
4 Hochbaum, G. (1958). *Public Participation in Medical Screening Programs.* (DHEW Publication No. 572). Public Health Service. Washington, DC: US Governmental Printing Office.
5 Becker, M. and Rosenstock, I.M. (1984). Compliance with medical advice. In A. Steptoe and A. Mathews (Eds.) *Health Care and Human Behavior* (pp.135–152). London: Academic Press.
6 Prochaska, J. and DiClemente, C. (1983). Stages and processes of self-change in smoking: toward an integrative model of change. *Journal of Consulting and Clinical Psychology*, 5, 390–395.
7 Jaqua, L. (2010). *Discovering the Arguments: Artistic and Inartistic Proofs.* Classical Writing, WordPress. Retrieved February 10, 2016 from www.classicalwriting.com/blog/2010/01/12/discovering-the-arguments-artistic-and-inartistic-proofs/
8 Fishbein, M. (1979). A theory of reasoned action: some applications and implications. *Nebraska Symposium on Motivation*, 27, 65–116.
9 Azen, I. (1991). The theory of planned behavior. *Organizational Behavior and Human Decision Processes*, 50, 179–211.
10 Bandura, A. (2001). Social cognitive theory: an agentic perspective. *Annual Review in Psychology* 52, 1–26.
11 Miller, R.E. (1992). Health communication through workplace smoking discouragement posters. *Journal of Health Education*, 23, 250–252.

5 Approaches

Step 4

As the communication source, you have learned about your audience and its needs. The aim of your communication effort is to influence and persuade the recipients of the health and safety message in order to change their behavior. To do that, you have to strategize what you want the audience to know, feel and do. Now it's time for you to prepare the approach—in other words, channel your message (see Figure 5.1). An approach is a delivery medium or vehicle for conveying a message, it may be a poster, brochure, newsletter, website, workshop or other initiative. Preparing the approach is called the **production** whereas implementing the approach is known as **channeling**.

This chapter introduces common approaches in successful health and safety communications. Whether it is a brochure, a poster series, public service announcements, a workshop, a radio interview or other approach, you will learn about the basics of preparing and implementing these approaches. The second part of *Health and Safety Communication: A Practical Guide Forward* devotes chapters to producing and channeling specific approaches.

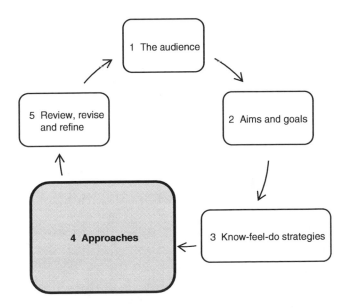

Figure 5.1 Approaches

This chapter describes preparatory components to a communication approach that is aimed at influencing and persuading an audience regarding its health and safety. Commonly employed approaches are listed in Table 5.1. Probably the best example of an approach is the **campaign**. A campaign is an organized course of action to achieve a particular goal. It is actually a composite of approaches or channels for health and safety messages. If you are preparing a campaign, how extensive will it be? Campaigns typically use more than one approach, incorporating efforts such as a press announcement, a kick-off event and a variety of printed materials (i.e., brochure, fact sheets, public service announcements, posters). The campaign is described in Chapter 7.

It is one thing to prepare or produce the approach. And it is another thing to implement or channel it. Doing so starts with covering some assumptions. After that, you are introduced to utilizing people, resources and tools necessary for producing as well as implementing the approach. Subsequent chapters in this guide detail these common communication approaches. Another matter of channeling centers on the route of message delivery. This is an exciting part of the health and safety communications process.

Production and channeling

Prepare yourself for using various tools and resources as you work toward delivery of your product. Since you have the overall intended outcomes specified (what you want the user to know, feel and do), you now have to start framing the approach. With a brochure, you will start a general mock-up. With a television public service announcement, you will start with a type of storyboard. And with a talk, you will be thinking in terms of the overall themes and approaches that you will be using to make your points. Similarly, with your brochure, your public service announcement, your workshop, your talk or other strategy, simply go ahead and get started. You have already done the foundational thinking, so now it is time to do something concrete. At least that, then, gives you something that you (and others) can critique.

With the brochure example again, think about the cover. You might have several ideas about what might be appropriate and strategic for your audience and your plans for distribution. You may also think that there is a cute slogan or catch phrase that you would like; this is the time to put these down on paper. However, if your mind is blank

Table 5.1 Common communication approaches

billboard	pamphlet
booklet	panel member
brochure	poster
campaign	press release
editorial and op-ed articles	public service announcement
emergency guidelines	social media
flyer	speech
lecture	testimony
media interview	workshop
newsletter	

and you are not able to do this, then simply skip over it and come back to that part later. Developing your content for your brochure (and similarly for other approaches or delivery media) is a process, so you will put in some parts now, and other parts later, until you end up with a coherent whole.

If you think about this with a talk that you will be giving, you will start with your general constructs (from the first three steps) and then you will pull together more specifics. In this step, you will be preparing the outline and also the content that will be the details that fill in that outline. You will be preparing the supporting materials needed to make your point. You will also be thinking about what visual illustrations you may need, whether visual images or props that you can use during the talk. The specifics will evolve as you fill in the details on the talk. Then, and this links into the next step, you should share what you are doing with others—this could be the outline, the supporting evidence, the materials and illustrations. It may also be that you have the opportunity to do a practice talk and let colleagues provide their feedback to you. All of this, regardless of the health and safety communications approach used, is part of the process of building and refining, through reflection and continual development of the final product.

Assumptions

A good way to start to implement your approach is to clarify assumptions. If you do not take the time upfront to clarify these assumptions, you may be required to revisit them later in the implementation, thus resulting in additional work for redesigning or developing your communications. More specifically, the assumptions, once clarified, become part of the roadmap to further composition and channeling your important message.

Let us say you want to launch a campaign to reduce the risk of fetal alcohol syndrome (FAS). Perhaps you first assume that some groups within the country's population were more likely to experience this syndrome and thus be the target audience for your communication effort. Did you know that, in the United States, the greatest prevalence of FAS is among infants born to white, employed, highly educated women 35 years or older? This realization might make you change your original intended audience.

A helpful starting point with the assumptions is thinking about who will be involved with the development and implementation of the communications approach. Will this be you alone, or will you have a team working on this? Will others be involved as key developers, as advisors or as specialists for various aspects of the process? Do others need to be involved for approval efforts? Is approval needed at various phases throughout the process, or just at the end?

Another factor related to this builds upon the specifics associated with the health and safety topic or issue. Are there idiosyncrasies associated with the topic about which you need to be aware? In a similar way, do trigger words or phrases exist about which you need to be sensitive? Some examples include:

- With drunk driving, safety specialists talk about a "crash" rather than an "accident."
- With this situation, they also talk about "drunk and impaired driving" rather than just "drunk driving" because lower levels of impairment can also contribute to a crash.
- When thinking about young people consuming alcohol, the attention is often upon "underage" when referring to "under the legal age of 21 for purchase of alcohol"; for many people, they think of "underage" as "under the age of majority" which is 18 in the United States.

As you think about your assumptions, try to clarify any limitations that may be appropriate as a result of your communications effort—you may seek to raise awareness, or increase knowledge or challenge the audience's belief but not necessarily try to change their behavior. Think also about the limitations of the audience. You may ultimately wish to affect a group of young people, yet the audience for the communications effort is comprised of those individuals or groups who serve as intermediaries (such as teachers, parents, counselors, mentors or other adults).

It is also important to address what it is that you might have included, or not included, in the communication approach. For example, you may decide to include scare tactics; alternatively, you may say that it would be inappropriate, or undesirable, to incorporate scare tactics for this communications effort. Your rationale may be based on any of a number of factors, including your previous experience, your understanding of what might be effective with this audience, your own priorities about that with which you want the sponsor to be associated, or other consideration. It can be as simple as wanting to steer clear of scare tactics and to be known for knowledge-based approaches. Similarly, you may decide that humor is a good way of reaching your audience; however, you may determine that you do not want your sponsoring group associated with a humor-based approach. These all serve as assumptions that help clarify your effort.

Practical considerations

In preparing the approach, keep in mind what the target audience is to know, feel and do—what might motivate them to attain the desired state. Remember, strategies are based on theory. For example, your approach might want to appeal to the audience's salient (immediate) health or safety beliefs; or you may want to focus on your delivery medium so that it matches the recipients' readiness to change.

Practical questions need to be answered during this step of the model. If you are preparing a brochure, then will it be in color, in black and white on colored paper, or some other format? What images and illustrations will be included? How do you plan to distribute it? If you are preparing a public service announcement, will it be for the radio or television? If so, how long will it be? What will it entail, in terms of preparation and complexity for development?

As you prepare to implement your communication effort, consider practical matters such as budget and timing; think also of legal matters, health considerations, safety precautions and ethical decision-making. This requires anticipating other important practical matters as you move ahead: timelines, sponsors or co-sponsors and more. You may want certain individuals or groups involved and you may need the approval of different individuals or offices.

With the budget, a helpful starting point is centered on the funding associated with the design and implementation of the communication approach. If you have a very limited, "shoestring" budget, your initiative will be rather different than if your budget is more robust. The limited budget will require local resources and the approach may be restricted to publicly available materials and software programs. With a larger budget, you may be able to hire design or artistic professionals. What budget is allocated or available? The budget available for print materials, in particular, can help guide the artistic and graphic design and preparation of your materials. If you or your agency has limited resources, your graphic design may rely on standardized templates, publicly available artwork or clipart and limited color production (perhaps black and white printing on color paper). You may also find stock photo images available for a modest fee. With a larger budget, more can obviously be done and a basic design can be enhanced significantly with professional artistic assistance. However, even with a limited budget, you may be able to obtain the services of a volunteer or a talented individual without having many expenses; some individuals or organizations will offer their services on a pro bono basis, or as a way of building their repertoire or reputation as a resource in the community. An example of this may be a celebrity who feels strongly about the topic due to a close personal relation being affected.

Regarding timing, if your timeline requires materials to be prepared quickly, perhaps due to the need to have a prompt response to a crisis or emergency situation, your efforts will need to be truncated and expedited. However, if your timeline allows for more review and reflection, more people can be involved and a variety of options can be considered. In this latter situation, which is really the norm as well as the ideal, the full process with the health and safety communications model can be incorporated.

Remember, you are likely to have a variety of people involved in the implementation of your approach. They can serve as **approval agents**, or **gatekeepers** in the process. Think of an approval agent as someone playing an active role and from whom permission is needed to proceed with the process. A gatekeeper is someone you must work with before you can reach an intended audience. As you consider their role, clarify what is important to them. For example, you may have law enforcement personnel, health professionals and educators all working together; each of these individuals may have different perspectives about how the health and safety issue should be addressed. It is important to have "buy-in" from all individuals, which requires some consensus and perhaps some compromising about what you will prepare and what your key message will be.

Consider the role of intermediaries. You may be seeking to reach an audience on a specific behavior, yet you have to work through someone else. One example highlighted earlier in this guide was the role of a parent with a child in addressing dental health. More broadly, you have to realize that the relationship between the ultimate target audience and the intermediary is not as close or clear as it should be. For instance, you may want to reach student-athletes on a college campus, yet you have to work through the coach, the trainer, the academic advisor or the team physician. Similarly, you may seek to affect teens' bicycle safety (i.e., wearing bike helmets). To do so, the intermediaries could be parents, teachers, physicians, older youth, adult neighbors or police officers. Certainly, you may want all of them saying the same thing, providing one consistent message. However, for your communications effort, you need to consider which intermediary (or intermediaries) would be most likely to have the desired effect and with which ones you will have access as well as which ones have the attention and respect of the teens. This is important because it is not always you and your effort that have the higher likelihood of making a difference. While your communication initiative may reach the audience, its message may not be "heard" by them; one reason is that you may be an unfamiliar source from their perspective, and that you are not necessarily a trusted source.

What political or other considerations or constraints are relevant? You may know that certain issues must be included, or other issues may not be included. Some of these are based on political considerations of the sponsoring organization or agency and some may be based on sensitivities of the group being reached. These are considerations that may change over time, with increasing or lessening need to include or exclude the specific topic.

Sometimes a communication effort is specified to you. For example, your supervisor may ask for a brochure and that is what is needed. Similarly, you may be invited to do a keynote address and you are informed that you have 30 minutes with the audience; that defines the general constraints and overall plan in terms of the approach. However, some elements may be variable, even within this context. With a keynote address, you may wish to incorporate some videotaped clips, or some music. You may have some interaction with the audience, such as querying them with a show of hands, or using decision software to poll them regarding their opinions on a topic.

One other consideration—a big one—is the overall context of the communication approach. Is this a one-shot deal, such as a brochure or poster? Is this a campaign? Is it envisioned as part of a series? Is it a single item, with the possibility of expansion later, depending on the results achieved?

On a related issue, allowing the necessary and appropriate time for preparing your materials is vital. As you know at this point, preparing materials with appeal and impact is something that you cannot throw together. While you may work well with brainstorming and creative development, it is important that you allow enough time for further conceptualization, review and development of your materials. You may have learned this when writing a paper: allow enough time for you to outline it, write it and then put it away for a few days or weeks. Many people do not do that with their efforts and the preparations may be done at the last minute. However, the ideal scenario is that you work through your planning processes and allow enough time for developing a quality product. When you have creative ideas, use them. But also allow time for you to put these away and then review them days or weeks later with a different and perhaps fresher perspective. To not feel rushed is most helpful with designing meaningful communications activities.

What contingencies should be anticipated? With any preparation, consider the use of equipment and software that may have problems. This could be power failure, corruption of files, equipment malfunction or other problem. It is important to have contingencies, such as saving your drafts regularly, storing your files in multiple locations (including emailing your files to yourself or others), having a timeline that is ahead of schedule and preparing materials in multiple formats (e.g., having hard copies if equipment for presentation doesn't work).

People resources

A **resource** involves a supply of assets from which to draw while designing and implementing health and safety communications messages (e.g., referenced material, data sources). Central to these resources is the reminder that you do not have to embark upon an approach alone—you can always engage other persons and their resources. For example, an **advisory group** is a good resource since it makes recommendations on the course of action. You can benefit from having others' perspectives and insights. This may be a formally constituted group, such as a defined advisory group or communications team. Or, it may be as simple as getting some colleagues involved for this specific project. You may ask them for their input or feedback as you move along on the planning activities. You may engage them in a process where you have them think through a series of questions and issues, particularly those identified in the next step. You may have the advisory group members respond privately, or in a group discussion. Your advisory group should be comprised of individuals representing a diversity of perspectives. You will want experienced viewpoints and you also want perspectives that will consider your communications effort from the perspective of the audience being reached. The main point of having an advisory group is that you should not expect to do the communications effort alone. While the effort may be your sole responsibility, and no one else at work or in the community or in your family is "officially" working on this, it is very important that you get input from others along the way. It is great if you can have a formally constituted group, particularly with work or community-based efforts. Without that, however, you should gather the input and reactions of colleagues, co-workers, friends, family and others. Ideally, these individuals should be as neutral as possible; however, sometimes you just have to involve others who are most convenient.

Another resource for getting insight or advice is to have a brief electronic query. This can be done by emailing trusted colleagues, where you ask them for their guidance or reactions. You may involve a select group (perhaps a group that is organized for a related purpose, such as state officials or regional representatives for an affiliated cause). Another way of doing this is with a listserv, where your query is more open to whomever is a participant.

There are times when you can get others involved with your effort, at no cost to you; these are volunteers (see Table 5.2). One example is having a volunteer help on various tasks, whether it is making telephone calls, organizing files or preparing a mailing. You might find a retired person who can provide technical assistance, such as keeping your accounting records straight or preparing legal documents.

Recruiting **spokespersons** can be helpful for gaining the attention of your target audience. You will need to determine what type of spokesperson would be appropriate—a researcher, a community activist, an elected official, a celebrity or someone else. You may also want the person to speak on their experience with the topic or issue being addressed. Your spokesperson has to be credible and respected in the eyes of the audience.

Similarly, it might be helpful to your efforts to secure **expert opinions**. That would include statements by, or reference to, an expert or specialized organization; this individual or organization would provide specific and specialized knowledge about the topic.

Table 5.2 Getting others involved

Ask a budding artist or graphic designer to prepare materials.

Ask someone to prepare materials if they seek to build a portfolio.

You may ask those around you, such as children, to prepare a picture that you could use.

If you are in a setting where you can give assignments (e.g., homework), you might ask others for examples that they see around them. This may include advertising that uses a particular approach or addresses a particular topic.

Ask for examples or situations that will help make your case with your audience.

Reach out to colleagues and ask them to give you a scenario, an example, or a situation.

With a dedicated person (such as a volunteer), identify ways in which s/he can be involved.

Prepare the overall design of what is needed, and have the volunteer accomplish the tasks. For example, students who need community service hours may be asked to use the internet to update public mailing addresses or research information.

With the person with whom you will collaborate, ask for their opinion, reaction, endorsement or other involvement.

There may be some specific tasks that can be relegated to another group.

Another organization or agency's employees, who are otherwise not occupied with job responsibilities, could perform specific tasks such as stuffing envelopes or preparing materials. Of course, this would add to the timeline of when you need to have materials finalized.

Further, it is important that this individual or organization is perceived as having that knowledge. For example, when talking about medical situations, it is helpful to have a statement prepared by a professional with medical training, such as an M.D. This could be a person who has national reputation, such as the U.S. Surgeon General; it may also be someone who is a local authority on the issue (such as a local doctor). The important factor is to make your choices based on the credential or reputation that would be most appropriate and convincing for the audience whose opinions you seek to affect. Likewise, the situation may be such that a reference to a national, state or local organization (such as the World Health Organization, American Medical Association, or the state or local affiliation of doctors) would be appropriate for your purposes. In a related way, when dealing with an issue that is focused on traffic safety, you would want to have a specialist with highway safety issues, such as a police officer or sheriff, involved to offer some comments. The involvement of this reputable individual or organization brings a tremendous amount of credibility to the issue.

The use of experts, particularly those individuals with credibility due to their position in an organization, is also found with the preparation of press release or press announcements about an initiative. For example, a press announcement may include a quote from the chairperson, director, lead researcher, expert or someone who will be viewed as having expertise on the issue. Including this type of quote can generate a significant amount of power and influence for the health and safety initiative.

Testimonials address the needs of those in the audience who are particularly moved by specific examples of storytelling, or ways in which the issue has affected the lives of individuals or groups. The examples can be positive in nature—how an approach has been helpful in making a difference in their lives; similarly, the examples can be negative, by documenting the need through illustrations of negative consequences that could have been avoided if something, such as the proposed action or activity, had been in place. A variety of examples of this type of qualitative approach can be found with various health and safety issues. The "personal face" associated with various movements can make a difference. Whether this is an actual story or a situation used to illustrate a need can vary from issue to issue.

Messages from the field

"Hunger bites"

Amr Abdalla, Ph.D., Institute for Peace and Security Studies, Addis Ababa University; Vice Rector for Academic Affairs, University for Peace (2005–2014)

During an evaluation mission in Rwanda in 2002, we were assessing the effectiveness of a rural development program conducted by OXFAM. The program provided financial support to rural citizens. Some members of the destitute, impoverished and ostracized ethnic group, Batwa, received funds to purchase vegetables and fruits to sell in the market. After buying, and on their way to the market, they ate all the vegetables and fruits before reaching the market! I decided to interview them to better understand their story. I met with 5–6 of them—men and women. All were evidently so impoverished beyond any standard I have seen before. I asked them about their relationship with OXFAM and how the project of selling produce in the market was developed. They confirmed everything I knew. When I asked them whether they ate the produce on their way to the market, they confirmed that as well. I asked "why?" This is when their leader, a very old man, as impoverished as any of them, with the pain of the years of suffering reflected on his face and body, looked me straight in my eyes and said to me, "hunger bites!"

Hearing those two words from that old man continues to give me shivers today. I felt that he was able in one second to teach me a deep lesson in how to try to understand even the most absurd behavior by understanding where people are in their lives. Their poverty, hunger and suffering were all far from any experience I had ever been through. How could I set myself as a judge of their action? Perhaps a better understanding of their conditions would have resulted in offering them a different type of support which takes into consideration the degree of suffering and starvation that they have lived with for so long.

I used that story on so many occasions. Its impact on any audience is powerful. Once they hear me repeat what the old man said, "hunger bites," the audience usually falls into deep silence and tears come down from some of them. This sets a perfect stage for the teacher or presenter to relate the story to the message of empathy and to be confident at that point that the audience is more than ready to embrace such a message, having had a clear example of how it looks in real life. This can also trigger similar stories from the audience, which would enrich the learning experience by including, in a participatory way, more real-life examples which in turn help the audience relate to the concept of empathy.

In overview, the concept of getting others involved, and getting other resources engaged, is focused on the concept that you don't have to do it all alone and that you don't have to "reinvent the wheel" as you proceed with your efforts. Further, particularly if you have a limited budget, you can find ways of getting various aspects of the communication effort addressed with "in-kind" resources from other organizations or agencies. Finally, and most important, the involvement of others, whether individually or organizationally, can be helpful with enhancing the quality of your work and thus potentially enhancing its impact.

Other resources

You may also be able to get **in-kind donations**, such as free paper for printing a brochure (see Table 5.3). For example, you could approach a printer and ask for a donation of print services in exchange for printing the company's logo and ad on the back of your

Table 5.3 Other resources

Prepare artwork or illustrations that can complement your strategy.
Utilize software templates available for production work (e.g., Word, PowerPoint).
Invite an organization to sponsor the artwork or design with their resources or from within their membership.
Ask merchants to provide gift cards or coupons (e.g., 50% off; 2 for 1) that can be offered or included in mailings.
Request free advertising in print publications, on websites, on the radio or on public or cable broadcast.
If you are doing a mailing, determine whether this is something for which another organization or agency could finance the postage.
Ask for funding for specific aspects of the project, by breaking up the initiative into discrete parts (e.g., printing, folding, mailing, prizes).

intended brochure. The printer might counter that the donated paper stock would be whatever was left over from other jobs and would vary in color based on availability. This is a "win–win" because the donated paper may otherwise have not been used or discarded, and it provided free advertising for the printer with an audience they may not have otherwise reached. Plus, the printing fee for the brochure would cost you $0. Similar to in-kind donations are pro bono (free for the public) services.

Another resource helpful for preparing your approaches is linking it to already-established days, weeks or months of observation. That is, release the approach during widely-recognized times scheduled at the national, state or local level. Every calendar month has numerous recognized days of observation. If you affiliate your effort with an already-existing event, you may also find resources that can complement your efforts or upon which you can expand. Highlighted in Figure 5.2 is a sample month, with topics linked to specific dates or weeks (or an entire month) for the United States (see the Appendix for all 12 months). A listing of those activities for the United States is available at https://healthfinder.gov; for Canada, see www.hc-sc.gc.ca/ahc-asc/calend/index-eng. php and for the World Health Organization, go to www.who.int/mediacentre/events/en. A calendar with the UK is found at http://learning.wm.hee.nhs.uk/events and, for South Africa, at www.gov.za/events/health-awareness-events. Depending on what is relevant for your organization and target audience, review the wide range of existing celebrations and events to find an appropriate fit. Noteworthy is that some months have many more activities and events scheduled than others, a factor you may wish to consider when planning your campaign.

Sponsorship is a valuable asset. There may be another organization that would be interested in co-sponsoring or otherwise helping with the implementation of a communications effort; you may provide the expertise and they provide funding, a mailing list or other assistance that facilitates the process.

You will benefit from thinking about others' involvement, such as those inside or outside your organization. You may ask, "Who has experience with this issue and could share some expertise or insight with the planning activities?" This would require you reaching out and asking for advice or comment(s), which may be intimidating or overwhelming. However, asking key people for their involvement can then be helpful in gathering further support for your effort.

Data

Having data or other types of documentation will be most helpful in implementing your approach. The use of data is a fairly straightforward approach. With this, you highlight the nature of the problem that you are addressing. This can involve a number of methods:

- The prevalence of the issue. This refers to how widespread a problem or issue is, at a particular point in time. This would highlight how many people have a disease or illness, or are affected by a specific health issue.
  - If a population of 100,000 people shows 5,000 living with cancer and 1,500 newly diagnosed with cancer, the prevalence would be 0.065 (or 6,500 per 100,000 people).

- The incidence of the issue. This highlights the rate of the problem occurring, during a period of time. The incidence would be the probability of a person being involved

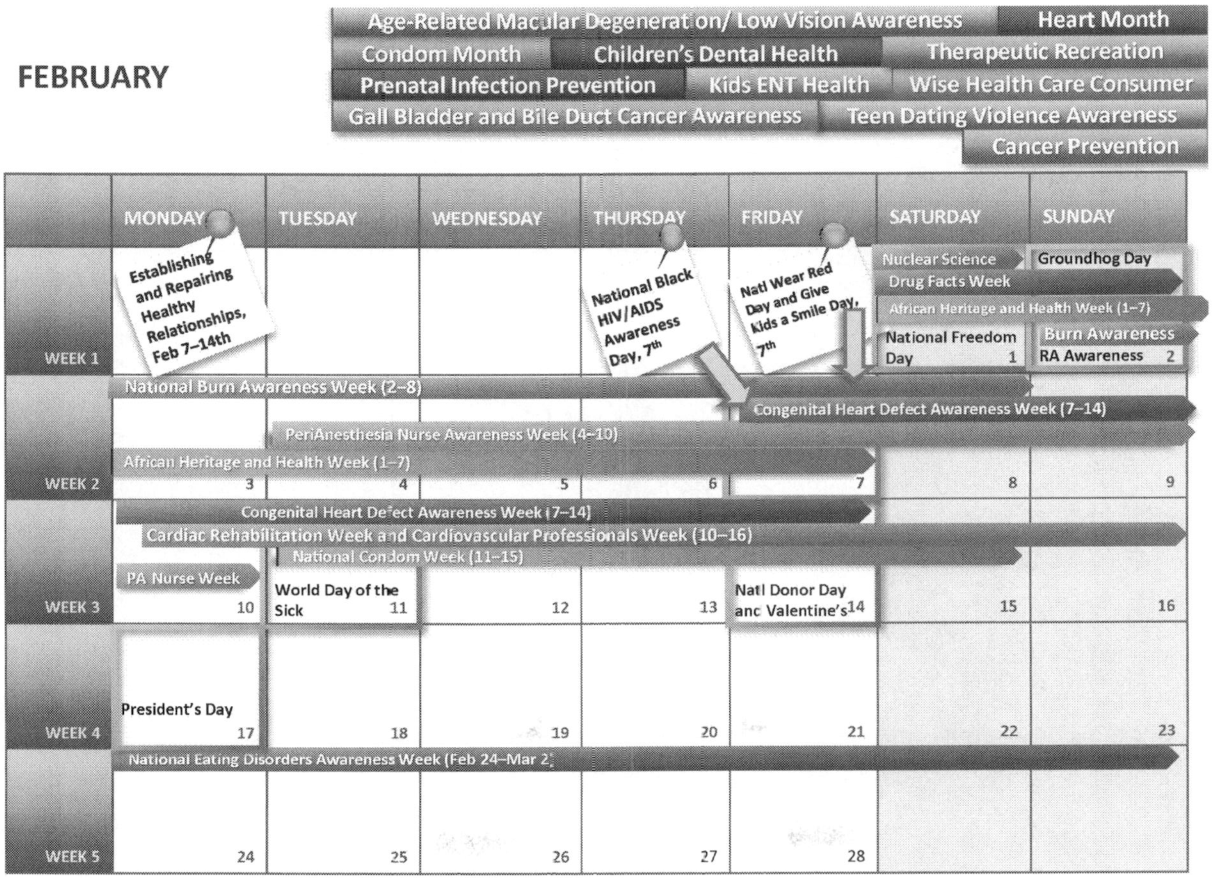

FEBRUARY
Age-Related Macular Degeneration/ Low Vision Awareness
Heart Month
Condom Month
Children's Dental Health
Therapeutic Recreation
Prenatal Infection Prevention
Kids ENT Health
Wise Health Care Consumer
Gall Bladder and Bile Duct Cancer Awareness
Teen Dating Violence Awareness
Cancer Prevention
MONDAY
TUESDAY
WEDNESDAY
THURSDAY
FRIDAY
SATURDAY
SUNDAY
WEEK 1
Establishing and Repairing Healthy Relationships, Feb 7–14th
National Black HIV/AIDS Awareness Day, 7th
Natl Wear Red Day and Give Kids a Smile Day, 7th
Nuclear Science
Drug Facts Week
Groundhog Day
African Heritage and Health Week (1–7)
National Freedom Day 1
Burn Awareness
RA Awareness 2
National Burn Awareness Week (2–8)
Congenital Heart Defect Awareness Week (7–14)
PeriAnesthesia Nurse Awareness Week (4–10)
African Heritage and Health Week (1–7)
WEEK 2
3
4
5
6
7
8
9
Congenital Heart Defect Awareness Week (7–14)
Cardiac Rehabilitation Week and Cardiovascular Professionals Week (10–16)
National Condom Week (11–15)
PA Nurse Week
WEEK 3
10
World Day of the Sick 11
12
13
Natl Donor Day and Valentine's 14
15
16
WEEK 4
President's Day 17
18
19
20
21
22
23
National Eating Disorders Awareness Week (Feb 24–Mar 2)
WEEK 5
24
25
26
27
28

Figure 5.2 Sample calendar of events

with the health situation, during a specific period of time; this would be the number of new cases during a specific period of time.

– Around 70,000 pedestrians are injured each year.

- Mortality. This refers to the number of deaths due to a cause.
  – In the US in 2010, the mortality rate of skin cancer was 9,154 per 100,000.

- Improvement over time. This would show how the nature of the problem has been reduced over time. With this, it may be suggested that these improvements are linked to the efforts that have been implemented. This can be framed to highlight the desire for more attention to the issue, or to illustrate that improvement has been relatively limited.
  – The number of drunk driving fatalities has been reduced by 49 percent between 1991 to 2011, from 6.3 to 3.2 per 100,000 population.

- Increased problems over time. This will illustrate how problems associated with a specific issue have increased over time, suggesting the need to take action to address it.
  – Prevalence associated with autism spectrum disorders have increased since the year 2000, going from 1 in 150 children diagnosed to 1 in 88 children diagnosed.

- Lack of change over time. This illustrates the fact that no changes have occurred, particularly when coupled with effort to affect such changes.
  – In spite of efforts to address the survival rate of people diagnosed with lung cancer, survival rates remain low.

- Consequences. This highlights the extent to which an issue of concern affects other issues.
  – College administrators believe that alcohol is involved with 25 percent of cases of students leaving college.

- Perceived results. This would measure how select groups of people might view the result of action or inaction on a particular issue.
  – The NHTSA estimates that motorcycle helmets reduce the likelihood of a crash fatality by 37 percent.
  – Mothers believe more effort is required to keep sons than daughters from experiencing injuries.

- Comparison. This compares one situation with another.
  – Lung cancer is the leading cancer killer in the United States, exceeding the number of cancer deaths among women over 25 years ago.

These types of data can be helpful in making a logical, rational argument for the selected approach being implemented. You can use these approaches individually, or in combination (e.g., combining prevalence rates and comparisons over time). You may also find other logical approaches, using data, to be helpful in making your case for a specific strategy or approach. **Creative epidemiology** (to be described shortly) may be used in a print material, as part of a campaign, within a workshop, on a public service announcement and elsewhere. This is an easy-to-understand and meaningful use of rates, ratios and percentages in health and safety communications. Similarly, an endorsement by a public health official may be useful within testimony to local officials, as part of a billboard, within a radio public service announcement or as part of a major speech.

By way of contrast, what it would be like to have an inventory which contained only a limited number of approaches? If all you had were data, you may then report the data to make your case. Similarly, if all you had was a range of stories, then you would likely tell the stories to influence your audience. If you had only cartoons, or only had tragic illustrations, then you would use these. Further, think about your audience; if you sought to reach people in a city, to illustrate your point with images of a farm or the plains of the Midwest would not resonate well with them, unless you were using these images as a contrast, an invitation or to make a specific point that benefited from their use.

As you think about determining what approach may be best for your campaign, talk, public service announcement or other communications effort, the main question focuses on a determination of what would be most likely to resonate well with your audience. You will want to think of what you want them to know, feel and do, and then look for examples that will fulfill this aim most effectively. Once you have a general sense of imagery, then seek out whatever data might be appropriate for it. Again, you want to be sure that your data is accurate and does not exaggerate the results. You want to refine this so it is brief and understandable. You will want to test it out with others in a similar grouping as your audience, to be sure that it meets your criteria. Ultimately, you are focusing on being persuasive with your approach and this is one of many tools that you can use to accomplish this.

Messages from the field

Using data to gain support for an important issue

Judy Rogg MSW and Stephanie Small MA, LMFT, Co-Founders, Erik's Cause

Data is an important ally for making a case. This is particularly true with "The Choking Game" (see www.erikscause.org). Many teachers, community leaders and parents hadn't heard of it and couldn't believe the stories. Judy's story of the death of her 12-year-old son, Erik, was, sadly, not an isolated situation. To bring about public awareness, we realized data was an important resource.

It is important to display data in a visually compelling format. Our journey with data started because we wanted to create an interactive map showing death/injury data. We built upon existing death/injury databases kept by other grass-root organizations and created our interactive map. We next created a map showing media articles, allowing for search by area, year and search terms. Then we started to track the growing number of "how to play" videos on YouTube—both the overall quantity as well as the number of views of several videos—to demonstrate the easy access kids have to these, in an effort to catch parents' attention visually.

The idea of gathering data came about from feedback we received when we applied for a federal grant to help develop knowledge about what works to make schools safe. Because very little statistical data on this activity existed, we submitted a large amount of anecdotal data (media reports) to support our proposal. Feedback suggested that in order to gain traction with public entities, additional statistical data was needed.

Our initial focus was on death data, but since so many of these deaths are misclassified as suicides, it would be years, if ever, to get corrected data. And tracking injuries would be even more daunting. We decided to step back and see where we could collect data. Our goal now is to get a question on existing student risk assessment surveys that will provide rich data about student knowledge of and participation in this activity.

While pursuing these larger data goals, we continue to focus on expanding the data we have already developed. See our current interactive data at www.erikscause.org/maps_data

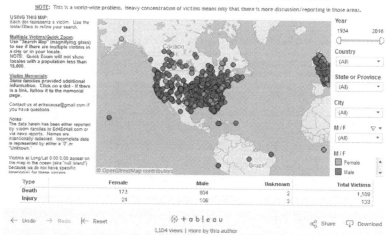

Choking Game Victims Across the Globe, The Tip of the Iceberg ...

This map represents only choking game deaths and injuries that have been reported by family, friends, or via media. Many deaths are misclassified as suicide, leaving families to suffer in silence. Our goal is to stop the spread of this epidemic with our non-graphic/skills-based prevention education so kids understand the dangers of this activity that they think is safe to play. The victims on this map demonstrate the need for such education as well as the need for further study and research.

Learn more at: www.erikscause.org ... Non-Graphic/Skills-Based Prevention Education

NOTE: This is a world-wide problem. Heavy concentration of victims means only that there is more discussion/reporting in those areas.

Type	Female	Male	Unknown	Total Victims
Death	173	934	2	1,109
Injury	24	106	3	133

←↩ Undo →↪ Redo |← Reset   ✿ +ableau   ⋘ Share ⊡ Download

1,104 views | more by this author

Pass Out Activities: Why is this an Epidemic?
Massive Numbers of "How To Play" Videos Your Kids Can Easily Find on YouTube*

This interactive chart shows thousands of "how to play" videos kids can easily access by searching just a few of the popular names for this deadly activity, and there are many more names that can be searched. (While some of these videos discuss the dangers, most do so while showing how it is played and can unintentionally pique curiosity. Some also refer to other risky behaviors that share the same name.) This search is only from YouTube; thousands of videos can also be easily found on Instagram, SnapChat, FaceBook, etc.

Kids can easily access these videos posted by others who think they are sharing a harmless fun "game." Without the balance of prevention education to teach them the dangers as well as how to say "no" to peer pressure, our kids are exposed to massive risk of injury or death.

Learn more at: www.erikscause.org ... Non-Graphic/Skills-Based Prevention Education

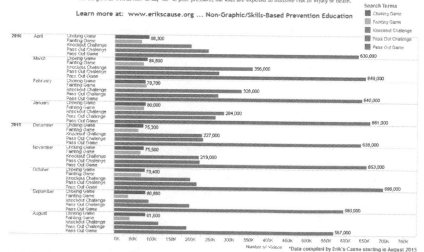

Number of Videos   *Data compiled by Erik's Cause starting in August 2015

Messages from the field

Mental Illness in the United States

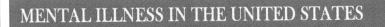

MENTAL ILLNESS IN THE UNITED STATES

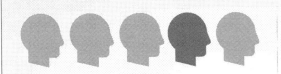

4.8% AGED 18-25

4.9% AGED 26-49

3.1% AGED 50 & OLDER

ABOUT 1 IN 5 ADULTS AGED 18 OR OLDER HAD A MENTAL ILLNESS

PERCENTAGE OF ADULTS WITH SERIOUS MENTAL ILLNESS IN THE PAST YEAR

✗SAMHSA

SOURCE:
Data, except as otherwise noted: Center for Behavioral Health Statistics and Quality (2015). Behavioral Health Trends in the United States: Results from the 2014 National Survey on Drug Use and Health. http://www.samhsa.gov/data/.

Overview of tools

An interesting challenge in health and safety communications is that one approach to reaching your audience will likely not be enough. Rather, multiple approaches are called for because the audience you seek to reach is not divided easily, based on what appeals to it. That is, you are not preparing an approach to only reach the logic-oriented individuals and another approach to reach those who are moved more by emotion. Your audience is mixed, with some respondents being motivated more by one approach and other respondents being more motivated by another approach. Second, individuals are not necessarily oriented to action based on a single approach, but by a blend of approaches. Thus, an individual may be moved by a story or example, but also want to know more about the data or rationale for undertaking a particular approach. Similarly, a person may hear the data and want to support an initiative, but find the personal example more compelling and memorable, and thus be the final factor that really makes a difference for them. The following sections describe useful **tools** for reaching the audience especially if multiple approaches are necessary.

Creative epidemiology

When you present data, this can be quite overwhelming, daunting and, in many cases, boring. It depends on the audience you seek to influence and the style and receptivity of those individuals. This is not to be disrespectful to the data or the hard work that has gone into its development, analysis and reporting. What it does mean is that many people need the data to influence their decisions, but they may not remember it.

Here's a classic example. The fact is that about 480,000 people in the United States die every year due to smoking. When you hear the number 480,000, what do you think? How many people is that? It's a lot. But what is it really? It's a number—a large number. But how can you make it more engaging, more memorable and more persuasive? You want to bring it alive. The way this can be done is to say, "The number of people who die every year in the United States due to smoking is the same as if two 747 jumbo jets crashed every day and everyone aboard died." You can make this more personal by reporting that two jets crashed today over Chicago, and two crashed tomorrow over Miami, and two the next day over Seattle and so forth. This creates a visual picture and presents the data in a way that is quite visual and visceral. Further, the presentation of this information in this manner typically has a result with the respondent of "Wow, that's a lot of people." In fact, it's the same number of people as 480,000, but it's just presented in a way that has the reaction you want. Clearly, this type of approach builds upon the "Logos, Pathos and Ethos" framework illustrated earlier, as the respondent "gets it" about the large number of deaths (logos), feels that this is too many people (pathos) and feels that more should be done to address it (ethos).

With "Creative Epidemiology," which some people familiarly refer to as "Social Math," the important aspect is that you are taking data that exists and restating it in a way that has a greater opportunity to have the desired impact that you seek. As a starting point, think about the definition of "creative": it involves thinking of new things, having originality, and being imaginative. And "epidemiology" is based on the study of epidemics and epidemic diseases. So what you are doing is, in brief, taking the data on health issues and transforming it in a way that is dramatic, touching, memorable and highly engaging.

The most important consideration with creative epidemiology is that you are taking the data and restating it in a way that is very visual and compelling. You are not exaggerating at all, but you are quite expressive with your approach. You will be brief and to the point. Further, you will be relevant to the audience that you are trying to reach. For example, if you are trying to make a point with a local audience, think about some example that will be relevant and visually accessible to them, such as a local school, park, highway, shopping mall, factory, residents, military base, industry or other factor. If you want to talk about the impact at the local level, your example may be linked to this local factor; for example, in addition to saying that the number of people who die every year from a certain disease is around 10,000, you may say, "this is the same as the number of people who would fit in our city's athletic arena which has 10,000 seats." To further localize it, you may say that the number of people who are treated in emergency rooms for burns every year is, in this community, equivalent to the number of youth in the local elementary school classrooms.

The use of creative epidemiology can be done in a variety of ways. You may do something with time images, such as "the amount of time spent … is equivalent to the …" This may be with cost equivalents, such as "If you smoke a pack of cigarettes a day, this is equivalent to six months of car payments" (if a pack of cigarettes costs $5 and a car payment is $300/month). If your audience is teens, you may say that the cigarette cost is equivalent to four iPads. The important thing is that your data is relevant to the audience, would have meaning for them and would be most likely to affect their behavior. It is also important that your data is relevant (for example, an iPad in 2016 costs $600, which may not be true in 2020 or 2025).

It is also important that your examples do not exaggerate. Tell the truth with the data, even if you under-report the extent of the problem. With the example of cigarette deaths, a 747 jumbo jet holds between 416 to 524 passengers. With 480,000 deaths, that computes to 1315 a day, clearly within the realm of two jets crashing. There is no point in saying "this is less than the number of deaths if three of the smaller size jumbo jets crashed each day" since, while accurate, this is highly improbable and would make the entire argument less believable. Further, with the capacity of jumbo jets increasing, such as the Airbus 380 with between 500 and 800 passengers, it is important to specify 747 for this example.

Your creative epidemiology approaches may incorporate proportions. This could be a factor such as the reporting on the extent to which a group may be affected by a specific health issue. For example, "the proportion of people who will be in a car crash sometime in their lifetime is represented by the number of people on the left side of this room."

Social marketing and social norms marketing

Social marketing is helpful for your efforts to achieve change. It is a process for influencing human behavior on a large scale, using marketing principles for the purpose of societal benefit rather than commercial profit.[1] Commercial marketers promote their product through a variety of means. You can learn a lot from these marketers while developing your own health and safety approaches. The main difference is that you are marketing a message and not a product. Of course, another difference is you are probably not operating under a comparable advertising budget! Still, you want to emphasize your message, be it healthier eating, relationship fulfillment, safe driving, immunization compliance or whatever. That is why you are relying on social marketing principles known as the four Ps: product, place, price and promotion in order to address the more urgent and complex social and public health issues of today.[2]

The product is your message. It is like you are "selling" a behavior or lifestyle choice (e.g., routine medical checkup, seeing the dentist semi-annually, having the car's safety system checked). The places for advertising and marketing health and safety messages are much the same as those for traditional commercial products—you seek locales that would be appropriate for reaching your audience. You will use channels and locations that are frequented by them. The difference, however, has to do with the budgets that typically do not accompany your community-based efforts. You will see how to address this in Chapter 9, which covers media issues and media relations. However, the essential piece with commercial products is that their advertisers typically pay for space, whether it is a billboard, an advertisement in a magazine or newspaper, or an ad on television or radio. So while the intent is the same (reaching your audience), the approaches typically differ because of lack of funding or resources. Of course, you can always take out ads, place billboards and do other types of commercial advertising as long as your budget permits this.

The price is the third aspect of social marketing. For the purpose of your selected approach, think about emotional, psychological, social and even physical prices the audience will have to pay.

- Going to the counseling center to get advice or support may have an emotional price—someone could feel like a failure for seeking help. While this behavior can actually be a strength, such as acknowledging personal limitations, it can be a factor that should be considered.
- The physical price may be tied into the access of a service, such as the location of a fitness facility or the ready availability of fresh, organic food. Wearing a safety belt may have a physical price of discomfort; a similar situation may exist with wearing a bike helmet.
- The social price of working out may be a loss of certain friends, whether because of the priority given to exercise or the reduced amount of time for social interactions.

So what is the importance of thinking about the price? When doing the marketing for a health or safety issue, it is vital to think about the audience you are trying to reach; consider which factors might be important to them and what obstacles, challenges, impressions or other 'prices' might be in their perspective. When you actively consider these, you can then be more aware of them and take specific action steps to address these in your marketing and advertising activities.

The last area within the traditional "four Ps of Social Marketing" is promotion. This is similar to what is found with commercial products, as you will be incorporating know-feel-do strategies to reach your audience. Again, the contrast with traditional marketing is that you typically won't have much of a budget to deal with this. You'll need to think of ways of marketing the lifestyle, or the health or safety effort, in ways that are appropriate to your audience and also within your budget. As you think of this, consider the use of social media (discussed in Chapter 12), to get your message out to the audience.

In addition to the standard social marketing approaches, five other "Ps" can be relevant to social marketing. These link to many of the underlying issues highlighted already in this section and resonate well with the other topics in this book.

- Publics: Your efforts with social marketing often must address several audiences. One way this is found is with the audiences that you seek with your message; you may want to reach youth and young adults, employers and workers, and drivers and pedestrians. While your messages may be a little different if you were only focused on one audience, your resources may not allow for multiple approaches; thus you blend your messages to reach several audiences at once. Another way this is found is when you are working with gatekeepers. A classic example is with materials you prepare for kids, but you are distributing them through the parents; your message must target and resonate with the kids, but be acceptable to the parents.
- Partnership: Social marketing can be particularly helpful when you work with other organizations and agencies to get your word out. If you are working on anti-smoking efforts, consider working with the local chapter of the American Lung Association or the American Heart Association, as well as with groups that work on fitness and quality of life. Your effort on your specific topic does not necessitate you working all alone on the topic; you may find greater reach, as well as synergy, and also endorsement, by working collaboratively with other groups.
- Policy: With your social marketing, it is not all about reaching out to the target audience to directly affect their behavior. Your efforts may also be linked to changing policies in the locale or region. Your efforts may be designed to, in fact, reach the policy makers so they have a different consideration of the standards by which your community lives. In Chapter 9, we will look in more detail at media advocacy and ways in which the media can be helpful in affecting policy change.
- Purse strings: As cited numerous times, the lack of a budget is a significant factor for your effort with health promotion. You typically have very limited resources and funding. Thus, your know-feel-do strategies are often more difficult to achieve and your reach may be limited. But you can—and have to be—more creative with your know-feel-do strategies to reach your audiences. You shouldn't let the lack of funding get in your way; it just requires that you use more energy and are more entrepreneurial in your approaches to your communication efforts. It's helpful to remember that you do have the "aura" of quality of life on your side, as you are promoting health; the uphill battle you face is one of lack of inertia and misunderstanding

of the importance of these issues, much of what is found in the theoretical grounding cited earlier in Chapter 4.

- Politics: The political context is a final consideration with social marketing. While many people don't want to address this, what is important is to understand this context of your health efforts. The political context has to do with what is current within your societal context. That is, years ago, it was not appropriate, politically, to talk about breast cancer and early detection. A forerunner of this was former First Lady Betty Ford who revealed her own situation and thus changed the landscape for others to address this. Similarly, to talk about drunk driving, or having a designated driver, was done but not to a widespread level. Mothers Against Drunk Driving (MADD) made significant headway with raising public awareness on this and thus the viability of legislation and public awareness about the importance of addressing this issue. The social context is the political landscape surrounding your issues. While some of what you promote may not be popular today, your efforts can be groundbreaking and affect change for tomorrow. Bringing in the Stages of Change Model, your know-feel-do strategies for your efforts may be relatively narrow today (as society overall or your audience may be in the "pre-contemplation" phase), but expanded tomorrow (as movement occurs toward "contemplation" or "decision").

Social norms marketing, or **social norming**, is a process that builds upon social marketing. What is different with this technique is that it takes the concept of "misperceptions" and strives both to correct these and to promote positive or healthy and safe behavior. The social norms marketing technique is based on the observation that many people have inaccurate perceptions of others' behavior. With alcohol abuse, for example, many college students believe that other students drink more than they actually do. What does that misperception do? It tends to drive students toward that behavior, particularly if the misperception results in beliefs that the majority of others are engaging in the behavior. In one sense, it is like "keeping up with the norms"; however, the actuality is that this aspirational behavior is based on a faulty view of reality.

Social norms marketing is based on the observation that, for many behaviors and attitudes, individuals misperceive what is, in fact, going on around them. It is also founded on the belief that many individuals will then choose to modify their behavior once they are aware of the actual facts (and acknowledging that they are misperceiving their environment). They may wish to "recalibrate" their behavior to be like the actual norm and to be consistent with current trends or cutting edge efforts, whether these are fashions or language or behavior. Or it may be that they don't want to be perceived, by others, as being different (e.g., healthier) or sticking out (e.g., being a trend-setter). Another consideration within social norming efforts is that individuals often stick together with others who are like them, who share similar beliefs and who enjoy similar things. With an example of heavy drinking, for example, individuals who drink heavily may hang out with those who also drink heavily; thus, they may believe that this type of behavior is common for others, further exacerbating their misperception of what the reality is. Plus, their own heavy drinking may be less than that of those around them. So when they hear new data about drinking patterns, the data must be solid and convincing if modifications of their heavy drinking pattern are to be expected.

Some research has found that individuals tend to over-estimate the negative behaviors of others and under-estimate the positive behaviors. Within the health context, this may translate to individuals over-estimating the number of people who drink or take drugs, who speed, who engage in unsafe sex or who eat in unhealthy ways. It would also translate to individuals under-estimating the number of people who drive safely, wear bike helmets, use safety belts, drink plenty of water, exercise and manage their stress well.

To correct misperceptions is not as simple as just stating "here are the facts." What you try to do is to provide the correct information and to do so in a way that is persuasive and convincing. Just as with other successful know-feel-do strategies, you are seeking to affect their decision-making by guiding them toward some specific outcome. The premise with social norming is that you offer the next step by, in essence, demonstrating that the majority of others are engaging in a behavior and that they, the individual being reached, "should join them." You are addressing some cognitive dissonance with them, but showing the audience the facts about the behavior and suggesting the desired behavioral or attitudinal path for them. In some ways, you are saying "your preconceived ideas are not correct; now that you have them corrected, perhaps you will be part of the majority."

As you prepare to gather data, you will be looking for issues that are consistent with the change in knowledge, attitudes or behavior that you are seeking. As a program planner, you may already have some insights about what seems to be "out of whack" for your audience (i.e., the misperceptions are high). So you should craft questions on issues that would support your project's goals, as well as the goals of the specific undertaking you are addressing. This means that you will be looking for data to support the desired course of action to which you aspire. Of course, the data will speak for itself; if the data does not show misperceptions that you expected, you may not be using that specific issue with your social norming. Further, you may wish to reassess your own perceptions about the issue—were you in error about the issue, or perhaps was your data collection not sufficient or appropriate to capture what you were seeking?

What is critical with social norms marketing is that you find areas where the behavior is already in the majority (see Figure 5.3). That is, you are looking for responses where there are at least 50 percent of the respondents who are already engaging in the desired, positive behavior. In that way, as you prepare the marketing

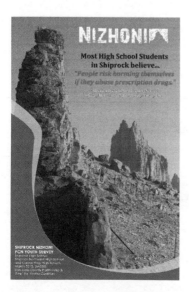
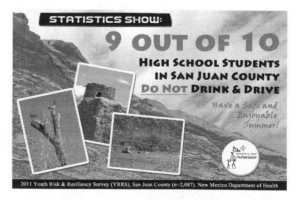

Figure 5.3 Social norming posters

strategy, you have the strength of "the majority" working on your behalf. It's not appropriate, with social norming, to find a behavior in which a minority of people participate; it wouldn't make sense to say "be part of a growing minority" or "be a trailblazer." That may very well be a viable strategy, but it is not this specific tool of social norms marketing.

You should also look for issues where the misperception rate is particularly high or problematic. For example, with research in one state, college students inaccurately believed that the use of ecstasy at least once a year was high (52 percent), where the reality was much lower (8 percent); that was an important difference to address. However, there would not be much point in correcting a difference that was not particularly dramatic (such as 52 percent perception versus 48 percent reality).

As you think about using this strategy, here are some thoughts that are important for this process. First, you need to start with good, solid data. The data must be gathered well, through a sound process and be suitable for sharing. This is vital in the social norming process, because typically you are challenging the perspectives and widely held views of others; since a typical respondent may not believe what the marketing is saying, they may look particularly close at the data and whether it is valid. You'll want to look closely at Chapter 6 on evaluation to gain skills for gathering sound data in a quality manner.

When you are gathering data, you will actually be looking at two things. First, you'll be looking at the reality of the issue you are addressing. Second, you'll be looking at the respondents' perceptions of others and how the respondent believes others are addressing the issue. Since you are looking for areas where the misperception rate is high, and where the issue fits into your overall goals, you will want to identify what data points are most helpful for you accomplishing your aims.

Messages from the field

The seven-step Montana Model of Positive Community Norms Communications

Jeff Linkenbach, Ed.D., The Montana Institute

The seven-step Montana Model of Positive Community Norms (PCN) Communications has been one of the most widely-used communications models in North America. It has evolved as a critical framework for promoting health and safety by identifying and correcting misperceptions of norms, and closing other critical gaps in knowledge, attitudes and behaviors. Misperceptions can impact behaviors at all levels of community systems connected as a social ecology. See www.montanainstitute.com.

By way of example, youth who perceive that the majority of their peers drink alcohol are more likely to drink themselves. Parents who believe most youth drink may be less likely to take protective actions with their own child. School leaders who believe most children drink may consider underage drinking a "rite of passage" and be unwilling to adopt appropriate policies. Law enforcement leaders who believe the community condones underage drinking may be less likely to strongly enforce underage drinking laws. A PCN communications campaign will seek to address the specific misperceptions of different audiences to support prevention efforts.

PCN communication campaigns intentionally focus on positive norms within the community. Some community leaders may be attached to old prevention practices, such as scare tactics, and thus it may be particularly challenging to get them on board with a new, positive approach. However, while those implementing fear appeals have good intentions, many groups (such as youth) often do not respond well to the "health terrorism" found in some anti-smoking, drinking or drug ads.

It takes approximately a year to design a PCN communication campaign and to get key stakeholders aligned and on board. The campaign itself can take several more years to implement. As prevention leaders learn how to implement a successful campaign, they will begin to see more opportunities to use PCN to energize and engage people in prevention activities.

The work of successfully implementing a positive community norms campaign can be daunting. Challenging misperceptions of norms is really about challenging people's core assumptions. And when we challenge people's core assumptions, they may become anxious and appear resistant. Development of these seven steps has continued to evolve with different projects and issues. While these steps are presented as if they are linear, many of them will overlap and, in fact, they will eventually loop back to the beginning in a cyclical process. Clearly, each community's journey is unique and there is still much to learn through ongoing research.

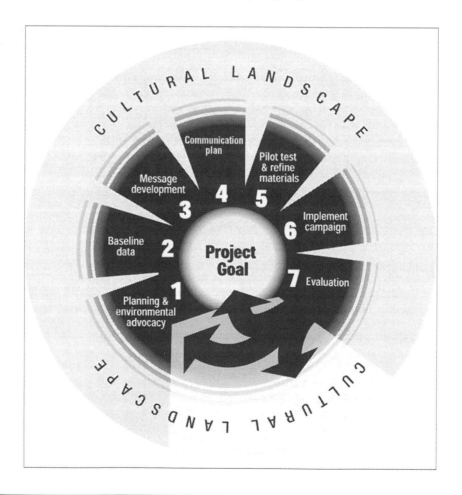

What are some of the elements you can examine with this process? The answer to this all depends on what you are seeking. This could be the quantity or frequency of individuals getting involved with a specific behavior (such as drug abuse or alcohol abuse). It could be how often someone engages in a health-oriented approach when faced with a situation; this may be bystander behavior or safety orientation. You may be looking at the respondents' attitudes about a behavior (such as buckling a safety belt or seeing a dentist twice a year); similarly, you may be looking at their behavioral intent, such as what they say they would do when encountering a specific situation. You may also be looking at some of the protective factors involved with various health and safety issues, and whether your target audience is aware of these, their attitudes regarding them and how likely they are to engage in these behaviors.

It is at this point that you start to pull together the marketing approach. This is where you determine which type of strategy is most appropriate for correcting the misperception. You may consider posters, fliers, brochures, other print advertising, public service announcements, workshops and more. Remember that this is part of an overall strategy, so this is one of the tools that you can incorporate in any of a variety of approaches. You may have a whole campaign that is organized around correcting misperceptions (for example, a whole series of "myths and misperceptions"). You may include the corrected misperceptions as part of the campaign and you may highlight various data points throughout the various communication approaches you choose to implement. So as you prepare the know-feel-do strategies such as posters or brochures, you will do these with the skills appropriate to that medium or strategy. The inclusion of social norming data is just a piece—and an important one when using this approach—of the communications approach you have selected.

Two final thoughts are appropriate for your know-feel-do strategies. First, for the data, it is important that you tell the truth. You want to be sure that you are not exaggerating any of the data. This is vital, since the audience already has misperceptions and will likely be skeptical of the data that is offered with your communications effort. You want to be sure that you do not exaggerate or misrepresent the findings. Second, you'll want to be sure to state the positive and desired outcome, since it is in the majority. You want to state the desired behavior as part of the statement with the misperception. With the ecstasy example, you will NOT say "This state's college students believe that 52 percent of their peers used ecstasy in the last year"; rather you WOULD say "92 percent of the state's college students have stayed away from the drug ecstasy over the last year." In brief, you are infusing the key words of what you want the audience to do "e.g., 'stayed away from the drug ecstasy'" in the message itself.

With social norms marketing, some other factors are important to remember. First, this process is not a silver or magic bullet; it is not a 'cure all' or panacea that will change individuals' minds about the behavior. It is not as if they suddenly say, "Wow, I was wrong, so I am going to change right now." Rather, it is part of an overall process of behavioral change which, as you know from your understanding of the theories underlying change with humans, is a tall order and a major challenge.

Another important factor, related to the previous one, is that this approach won't work for everyone. Of course, that is true for many different know-feel-do strategies; thus it is important to have a variety of approaches, and to use various theoretical foundations, in order to reach the different audiences that exist. There are some individuals who are so entrenched with their behavior, or who are not amenable to this persuasive strategy, for whom the social norming efforts have no effect.

A caution with social norms marketing is also important. This takes a lot of work! In order to do it well, you cannot just put together a poster that corrects some misperceptions. Rather, you need to think through what it is that you believe are misperceptions and identify those that may resonate well with your target audience. Then you need to gather data, very carefully, and examine it for those relevant issues for which the majority of people are already behaving in the desired manner. Following this, you start to build your message and approach, and then you'll need to pilot test the message and strategy. While the pilot testing process should be inherent in any approach you undertake with your communications effort, it is even more important here since you are blending marketing know-feel-do strategies with the social norming efforts.

Messages from the field

The Science of the Positive—cycle of transformation

Jeff Linkenbach, Ed.D., The Montana Institute

The Science of the Positive is the study of the ways in which positive factors impact culture and experience. It is based on the central assumption that the positive is real and is worth growing and its aim is to systematize the identification, measurement and growth of the positive—in ourselves, our families, our workplaces and our communities. This approach establishes a cyclical way to engage in health and safety communications across a variety of issues.

We are often distracted from the work of nurturing the positive by the difficulties we face and the problems we need to solve. The Science of the Positive reverses this problem-centered frame and focuses on reinforcing the healthy, positive, protective factors that already exist in each community. When we look at the world through this positive, hopeful lens, it has a profound impact on the questions we ask, the data we collect and the strategies we use to address challenges and transform our lives.

Four essential domains—Spirit, Science, Action and Return—make up the transformational process of the Science of the Positive.

- *Spirit* refers to the essence of a culture which is the positive, hopeful and energy-producing elements. All projects, campaigns, research projects and communications begin with spirit first.
- *Science* seeks to provide knowledge and understanding of what the world is and how it works. It refers to the systematic study and utilization of methods for empirically generating knowledge. Our science is constantly changing. Science can generate evidence-based approaches and best practices to direct actions.
- *Action* includes our behaviors, what we do, the steps we take. Actions manifest as practices, rituals, habits or campaign activities. In general, we are action oriented and often prefer to "jump" to this phase in our work instead of moving through the patience and rigor of Spirit first, then Science, to guide Actions. Our actions must be aligned with our deeper purpose in life to help us achieve the meaning we seek.
- *Return* is associated with rest, reflection, evaluation and taking time to turn knowledge into wisdom. Taking time with this domain includes studying elements of both change as well as transformation.

These domains, when fully engaged, work together to create a synergistic cycle of positive transformation. It is called the Science of the Positive because, like science itself, it is a system for discovery and innovation, involving a rigorous process that works across entire cultures. This process calls for amplifying the positive dimensions in every community and culture to address the suffering, pain and harm that are very real in our lives. One of its principal outcomes is to reduce that suffering in our families, in our communities and in our selves. See www.montanainstitute.com.

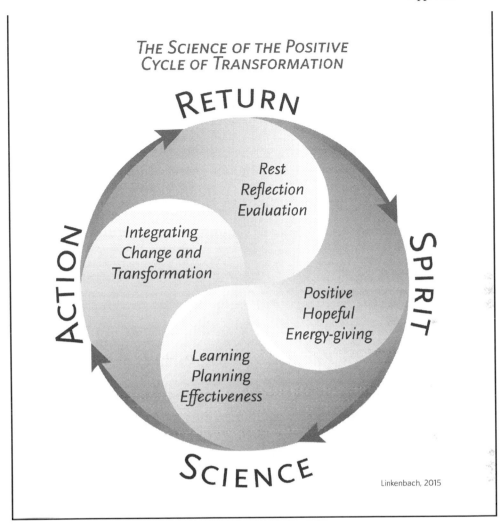

THE SCIENCE OF THE POSITIVE
CYCLE OF TRANSFORMATION

RETURN

Rest
Reflection
Evaluation

Integrating
Change and
Transformation

ACTION

SPIRIT

Positive
Hopeful
Energy-giving

Learning
Planning
Effectiveness

SCIENCE

Linkenbach, 2015

Positioning

Positioning is another tool for implementing or channeling your health and safety communication. **Positioning** means "what you do to the mind of the prospect."[3] Positioning dovetails nicely with marketing, although it is actually different from marketing. Positioning uses approaches that help propel the message above and beyond the numerous messages with which it competes. With positioning, the planner—you—is thinking of specific ways that can "relocate" the message into the mind of the potential recipient. In a grocery store, for example, products may be positioned (or placed) at eye level, or located at the checkout lines. In a department store, some items are located at the entry way, or in store windows, to catch your attention. For while preparing the health and safety messages, you are coupling the product (the health or safety behavior) with something else so that it is seen, or heard, more effectively than if you didn't do it. Of course, just as with social norms marketing, you are utilizing the range of marketing know-feel-do strategies to prepare your materials, such as art work, color, design, size and more. The positioning "tool" is another complement to your efforts and helps with your overall strategic approach.

Some specific ways of positioning your message would be to promote its placement as one of the following:

* First—the initial or first one that appeared.
* Largest selling—the most widespread or popular, whether based on numbers or areas reached.
* Longest-lasting—having been around the longest; survived the longest.
* Only—there is no competition.
* Price (high or low)—the higher price may suggest quality and greater effort; the lower price may be positioned to suggest value and cost-effectiveness.
* Speed—how quickly the effort can be learned, implemented, or used.
* Reverse an old idea—change of perspective or contrary to existing opinions or views; this could be based on new knowledge or emerging science.
* Repetition—a second or third or follow-on version or edition; part of a series.

As you incorporate positioning, here are some specific considerations for you as you prepare a communication approach:

* Make sure it is relevant and appropriate for the target audience.
* It may be particularly helpful to limit the target audience (e.g., women, older adults).
* Consider the setting (e.g., one frequented or used by the audience).
* Make it convenient (e.g., a linking to a setting where attention can be gained). For example, promote hand washing with an ad placed by a bathroom or sink.
* Have repetition—use an ad or phrase over and over.
* Consider the language; the choice of words can build upon something already familiar, like a tag line. Create, modify or "mock" a tag line.
* Link two topics or themes—for example, linking high tech to multitasking can be done with a video screen on a gas pump that is viewed when pumping gas.

Linking and pairing

Another helpful tool in channeling or implementing your approach is **linking and pairing**. Linkages or pairing occurs between what you are promoting and some other already-existing message that has had an impact on your intended audience. In a sense, it is like "framing" or "restating" your message into the context that already has some positive imagery or association in the minds of the audience. Just as it can be helpful to partner with other groups or organizations to get your message out, your health and communication efforts should consider ways of pairing your message with other elements. What linking and pairing does is to build on existing thoughts or perceptions existing in the minds of your audience. The process intentionally finds similarities to what already exists. In a sense, this process is "positioning" (see previous discussion) the health or safety effort within the mind of the audience; it is building associations with existing perceptions and knowledge. Such linkages and pairing can help your audience provide attention to your message, as well as to remember its key points (see Figure 5.4). Various ways of implementing this process are found in Table 5.4.

Table 5.4 Linking and pairing messages

Type	Approach	Example
Images	Age, success, health.	Have youthful look or impression of happiness.
Association	Create an image of a lifestyle or quality of life. Need to avoid negative associations.	White clothing and imagery to suggest purity.
Tie into existing timeline	Affiliate with an existing day, week month, available locally or nationally.	Have an event that is scheduled to coincide with existing awareness week. See the calendar of existing awareness days, weeks and months.
Seasonal	Holiday, season, time of year.	Associate images or events with July 4, Veterans Day, Memorial Day, St. Patricks Day.
Historical	Time with the anniversary of an event or the invention of some product.	Mark the date of what happened 10 years ago, 25 years ago, one century ago; this can be on the specific date or month or year.
Something new	A breakthrough or innovation.	Cite what is new with this approach or strategy; "new and improved."
Contrast	How this is different from other approaches or resources.	Demonstrate ways this effort has an entire different orientation; e.g., "top down" versus "bottom up."
Repeat and renewal	Do a rebranding or an update.	Go retro; i.e., "Remember the 1950s."
Celebratory	Note its location in development or delivery.	This is the first, the most recent, the 100th, the 1000th.
Endorsement	Garner support from a celebrity, public figure, leader with a title.	Cite the Chief of Police, head of the hospital's trauma services, a research expert.
Personal view	Include insights from someone linked to the type of issue cited.	Obtain testimonial from someone affected by an issue, someone who made a poor judgment (drunk driver) or someone who made a good judgment (designated driver).
Uniqueness with date	Look at the sequencing of the date.	Link to dates such as 3–3–33 or 12–13–14.
Relevance	Make it appropriate for the local or regional area.	Cite the relevance for the locality or state.
Comparisons	Find another county, namesake, or state for illustrative or visual comparisons.	Show that the number of people who are affected every year by a certain issue is equivalent to another, locally relevant number (e.g., population of a county).
Fun	Look for positive approaches and ways people might have positive feelings after seeing this.	Make the approach fun and enjoyable, such as why it is fun to recycle or exercise or eat fresh fruits and vegetables.
Provocative	Offer a compelling or interesting way of looking at an issue.	Suggest a new way of looking at things, such as what might be behind or underneath an issue (such as trauma).
Something unique	Look for any irony, controversy or twist.	Cite different points of view from audiences, such as how one group such as educators viewed an issue, which may be different from what is expected.
Link to demographics	Find differences based on demographics such as age, gender, education level, occupation, etc.	State how one group (e.g., men) are more likely to adopt a certain behavior than others (e.g., women).

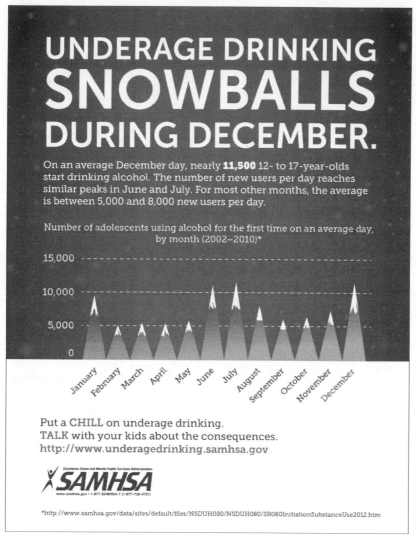

Figure 5.4 Poster using linkage tool

Additional tools

A variety of additional tools are available for getting your health and safety message to its target recipients.

1   Have a memorable acronym. With alcohol abuse, BRAD stands for Be Responsible About Drinking and is the name of a college student who died; BACCHUS stands for Boost Alcohol Consciousness Concerning the Health of University Students and was formed as a peer education approach for reducing alcohol abuse. MADD, Mothers Against Drunk Driving, was formed to fight drunk driving, particularly after the loss of a loved one. SADD, Students Against Drunk Driving (and then renamed Students Against Destructive Decisions), dovetailed from the MADD acronym and focused on high school students and healthy decisions about alcohol. RADD was another

one—Recording Artists Against Drunk Driving. Just keep in mind that several acronyms have lived past their prime so to speak with vague and possibly confusing meanings. For example, even back in 1985, HMO (health maintenance organization) was considered an outdated expression for pre-paid health care coverage.[4]

2 Have an easy-to-remember website or phone number. With the phone number, consider having a word that can be remembered. This can be helpful, particularly with a billboard that offers a location to gather additional information. A well-known example from the 1980s was 1–800 COCAINE (for help with cocaine use or addiction). When domain names for websites first became available, the National Clearinghouse on Alcohol and Drug Information got the site www.health.org, an easy-to-remember web address. There have been promising results in diabetes management for patients being familiar with and utilizing familiar telephone numbers representing proper self-care for the disease.[5]

3 Use QR (Quick Response) codes. This requires an app for the telephone and links the user directly to a website (see Figure 5.5). In this way, additional information can be provided without actually having it on a product. Further, the content on the website can change and be updated. In this way, someone accessing additional resources through use of a QR code can find the most current information, thus keeping more generic materials up to date and avoiding reprinting or continually worrying about whether it is up to date or not.

4 Link to local news. Most health topics are recurring at the national and local level. With careful attention, you can find ways of making the linkage with something that is in the news. In a parallel way, if a topic of importance to you is not highlighted in the news within a reasonable period of time, you can highlight that fact and raise questions about its omission (e.g., through a letter to the editor).

5 Include sponsorship or endorsement. Having the representation of a group or organization, particularly as a sponsor or co-sponsor of an initiative, helps lend credibility to your health message. Think about what might be relevant (e.g., a police chief linking to a traffic safety issue or a medical doctor linking to a health effort). You might also think about what might be a surprise, so that the reader may wonder why a particular organization or individual is linked to a specific health issue (e.g., a police chief commenting on a health effort, or a college administrator speaking out on a community issue).

The fifth step of the model for this book—found in Chapter 6 on review, revise and refine—emphasizes needs assessment and evaluation activities. With pilot testing, you will gain insights as you are testing out whether your work makes sense with the desired

Figure 5.5 QR code for CDC

audience. You might also be checking out which of several approaches might be best—is it a certain look with the brochure that makes sense? Which images look best? What catch-phrase wording best captures your spirit and will achieve your desired results?

Finally, these tools and resources are not meant to be all-inclusive. These are representative of many that are currently used. For example, the presence of QR codes would not have been included several years ago and is made more viable with the proliferation of smart phones incorporating technology to read these easily; however it appears to be fading in popularity. With the expansion of social media, as well as other approaches not yet popular or even developed, additions will undoubtedly be made in the years and decades to come. It will be important that you stay abreast of these, involving the appropriate methods that will be useful in best reaching your target audience. Also, it is most helpful if you engage your own creativity and ingenuity to prepare and implement your communication approaches.

Forward!

This chapter highlights numerous tools and resources helpful with the health and safety communications effort. This is like having a tool box with lots of resources available for your selection and use. This does not mean that you will use all of them—that would be a virtual impossibility! What this chapter is designed to do is to highlight many of the more commonly used approaches and to provide some examples about how these can be used for your various know–feel–do strategies.

As with various health and safety communications efforts, these tools and resources can be used across the various approaches, which will be described in much greater detail throughout Part Two of this book. These tools are not just for traditional approaches such as print materials or workshops; they are for use with each of the know–feel–do approaches, whether speeches or social media, public testimony or PSAs, or other approaches. The inclusion of these in this chapter is designed to acquaint you and enhance your ability to incorporate them as appropriate. You might think of this as a type of two-dimensional matrix: Tools on one dimension and Approaches on the other. Thus, when preparing an approach, think about the tools most helpful for incorporation to make the points you want to make with your identified audience.

A final point is that additional tools and resources exist and new ones will undoubtedly be developed in the years to come. The important factor is to remain up to date with their availability and potential for use. These can enhance your efforts and their effectiveness in achieving the impact you seek.

Notes

1 Smith, A. (2000). Social marketing: an evolving definition. *American Journal of Health Behavior*, 24, 11–17.
2 Lefebvre, R.C. (2013). *Social Marketing and Social Change: Strategies and Tools for Health, Well-being, and the Environment*. San Francisco, CA: Jossey-Bass.
3 Ries, A. and Trout, J. (1986). *Positioning: The Battle for Your Mind*. New York: McGraw Hill, Inc.
4 Luke, R.D. (1985). Anachronistic acronyms in health care: a comment. *Medical Care Research and Review*, 42(2), 157–162.
5 Krishna, S. and Austin Boren, S. (2008). Diabetes self-management care via cell phone: a systematic review. *Journal of Diabetes Science and Technology*, 2(3), 509–517.

6 Review, revise and refine

Step 5

Once implemented, an approach should be tested for effectiveness. The key question is whether the message had the intended impact on the audience. If the message was not effective, then the health and safety communicator should review the effort and consider revising it with the hope of refining it (see Figure 6.1). This explanation implies that you test the message following its delivery to the audience. In fact, you should test the effort before and during its implementation as well. This is called **pilot testing**. This chapter covers the important step of reviewing, revising and refining your health and safety communications during development and delivery. First, though, you should be familiarized with evaluation.

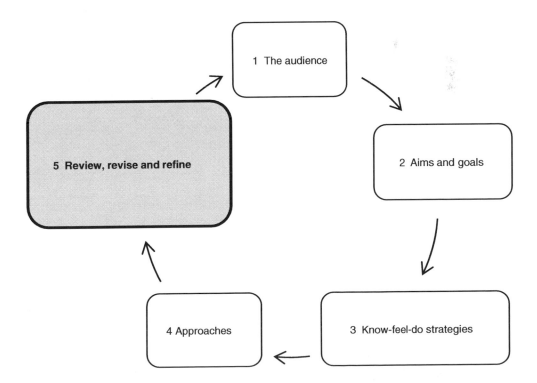

Figure 6.1 Review, revise and refine

Evaluation

Evaluation is comparative decision-making based on the perceived value of something.[1] Now that brief description might sound confusing, so it's helpful to review both parts of the definition. Comparative decision-making means comparing or contrasting one thing with another in order to decide what to do next. The perceived value of something refers to what you think is important about your health and safety communications effort.

Evaluation is recognized in Step 5 of the health and safety communications model. For the purpose of this book, it is referred to as review, revise and refine. If evaluation was not incorporated into your communication efforts, then what would be the result of these efforts? The probable answer is that your results would document that some effort or product was prepared, but that you would not know whether it is particularly effective or helpful. It may "look pretty" or "sound good," but whether it has the desired impact would be questionable. Your efforts may not hit the needs of the audience you seek to influence. But you just wouldn't know. So, without evaluation, the question of success or extent of impact would remain unanswered.

When many people think of evaluation, they have a negative impression. They may view evaluation as boring, difficult, irrelevant, inappropriate, inconclusive or unsound. To some, evaluation seems to interfere with the implementation of a communication approach or it might hinder the continuations of such an effort. To others, evaluation appears overwhelming, challenging and quite daunting. Individuals may feel that they do not have the skills to conduct an evaluation, or even to oversee that it gets done. On the other hand, some communicators are ready to dive right into their efforts without worrying how it is going to be "judged" at the end.

The key point to this chapter is to take out much of the "sting" often associated with evaluation. Material will highlight the importance of evaluation, specify ways of making it practical and provide practical tips and resources that can help you make evaluation a part of your communications. You can do this through a review, revise and refine process.

To get an initial flavor of evaluation, consider that evaluation can include any of the following assessment approaches, among others:

- A test of knowledge.
- Discussion groups.
- Interviews with experts.
- Observations of behavior.
- Telephone polling.
- Intercept interviews.
- An attitude assessment.
- A behavioral inventory.
- A focus group.
- Coding the occurrence of a situation or event.
- Comparisons with state or national results.
- Analysis by subgroup.

Why evaluate?

Before getting into the details about evaluation, it's helpful to reflect a bit about why evaluation is so important. Evaluation is vital to help improve your communication programs or strategies. It helps you and others maximize the quality results that are sought; it also helps the limited funding and resources to be utilized well.

Evaluation is an integral part of your communications effort, as well as with the actual planning and implementation of these efforts. If you didn't evaluate, you wouldn't know whether or not you were having the desired impact on the audience being targeted. Think about your health, for example—if you didn't have your blood tested, you wouldn't know that your cholesterol was too high; and if you didn't continue to monitor it, you wouldn't know whether or not your efforts to reduce it were working. Similarly, evaluation helps to determine whether or not you achieve your desired results and where you have room for improvement. Evaluation results can be used for comparisons—seeing how different materials affect the target audience differently, assessing how different workshop leaders have varying results, and determining the reach of the strategies used with a communications campaign.

Evaluation can be helpful not just for learning about the achievement of specific results, but also why this was the case. Evaluation can help understand why differences are or are not made. What is most helpful is to learn about the specific approaches or efforts that contributed to a program's success. This helps when thinking about the redesign of your program, strategy, communications effort or initiative, as you can take the results from the evaluation and determine which parts of the initiative worked well and which need improvement.

In addition to this, evaluation is helpful with funding decisions. Positive results achieved, and documented with the evaluation findings, can be most helpful in substantiating the value of a programmatic effort. Rather than reporting that "it seemed that people liked the campaign," it would be more helpful for the program planner to have specific results that demonstrated that the campaign resulted in a notable change in others' knowledge, attitudes, behavior, perceptions or other factor sought by the planners.

Related terminology

Evaluation is related to, yet distinct from, other data-related procedures operating within a health and safety communications effort. For instance, **assessment** is similar to evaluation but differs in the sense that it is merely the determination of the status of something—either part of or the entire health and safety communications effort. For example, you might want to learn more about your audience's areas of interest. You may want to learn about your audience's reactions to what you do, what they intend to do and what questions they may have. This requires you to determine the status of their interests, reactions, intentions and questions. Assessing some or all of your communication effort requires collecting data, whether this is measured quantitatively or qualitatively. Quantitative data are countable data whereas qualitative data are text or narrative in nature. Here are some examples:

- A knowledge test with correct answers: Quantitative.
- A question that asks respondents to select a specific choice: Quantitative.
- A question that asks respondents why they selected a specific choice: Qualitative.
- A group discussion on a topic or issue: Qualitative.
- Observing individual behavior or reactions to an event: Qualitative.
- Asking an open-ended question (such as, "What challenges do you face with ...?": Qualitative.

- Coding open-ended question responses into discrete categories and sub-categories: Quantitative (evolving from Qualitative).

Highlighted in the literature, professionals have recommended ways to use both quantitative[2] and qualitative[3] approaches while evaluating health communication efforts.

Measurement is another data-related mechanism. Think of measurement as assigning scores to data or placing data in categories. You will see examples of these two types of measured data in this chapter. Another data-related procedure is **statistics**— how measured data are analyzed for the purpose of reporting. For instance, items such as frequencies, averages, ranges and rates are actual statistics. Thus, in order to evaluate your health and safety communications effort, you will need to gather, score and analyze data. The data should represent some aspect of your health message (e.g., what you think is important in the message). You will then have to compare that aspect of your health message with some type of standard (e.g., what others think is important about the same message). After comparing and contrasting, you make some determination or decision about your health and safety communications effort. That could be that the message was effective and it should continue to be conveyed, or that the message was not sufficiently effective and needs revision.

There are various measurement tools that can be used (see Table 6.1). Each of these has advantages as well as disadvantages. No single tool is perfect for addressing the key question or questions you may have. Further, tools are often used to complement one another: for example, gathering some quantitative data with a survey and following up with focus groups to discuss participants' interpretations of some of the findings.

The point for emphasis here is that there is no "ideal" evaluation or evaluation strategy. Each evaluation approach has strengths as well as weaknesses. Since your aim with evaluation is primarily to monitor results, think about what information will best serve your purposes and what approaches might be most viable given the circumstances surrounding you and your communication efforts.

One other distinction has to do with **research**. Think of research as a disciplined effort to answer a question. While it is similar to evaluation, the distinction is that evaluation compares and contrasts something of importance against a standard in order to determine the next course of action.

Evaluation is vital in the successful development and delivery of health messages through approaches like campaigns, workshops, interviews and even printed material. Since the most important aspect of your communication is what you want the recipient to know, feel or do, then you will have to evaluate the message while it is being composed and channeled as well as after it has been received by the audience. Once you are clear about this, the actual structure of your evaluation can take shape. In fact, the more clear and focused you are with what you want to measure, analyze and compare, the easier it will be for you to craft the evaluation. Further, as you start to think about the evaluation of your effort, you may modify your desires about what you want to determine and decide. It is not uncommon to have grand aims—that "everyone will become aware of this issue" and "because of this campaign, there will be massive changes in behavior." The point is that your aims or vision go hand-in-hand with your evaluation. As you clarify your evaluation, you will likely refine and refocus your goal and objectives for the message.

Referring to the health and safety communications model, think about evaluation being performed throughout each of the steps. That is, merely tacking on evaluation at

Table 6.1 Measurement tools: advantages and disadvantages

Survey	**Advantages:** Easy to complete Can be completed quickly by respondent Simple to score Provides quantitative results Easy to keep anonymous Can compare with other data sources (e.g., national profiles) Can be scored by hand, by optical scoring or online Low-cost approach **Disadvantages:** May not capture respondents' feelings Some responses may not reflect accurately Questions may be interpreted in different ways For sub-analyses, requires professional skills May be viewed by respondent as intrusive or not useful Qualitative data requires work (entry, coding, analysis)
Online survey	**Advantages:** Easily included as part of existing national survey (add-on questions) Easy to incorporate questions into locally-developed survey Questions can be brief and limited in number Random list of individuals can be generated easily Data review is quick and easy to accomplish Easy to keep anonymous Low-cost approach **Disadvantages:** Respondents are less likely to complete if viewed as long or intrusive May need incentive to encourage participation May not capture respondents' feelings May be viewed by respondent as intrusive or not useful Qualitative data requires work (entry, coding, analysis)
Interview	**Advantages:** Provides rich insight Respondent can provide interpretation of results gathered elsewhere Person may speak honestly Respondent may feel honored to be interviewed Provides an opportunity to probe thoughts and perspectives **Disadvantages:** Requires skilled interviewer Respondent may not speak honestly, depending on trust Approach can take time Respondent may have limited time Challenges with coding and analyzing responses
Discussion	**Advantages:** Provides conversation on topics and issues Good insight and perspectives can be offered Can have give-and-take among participants Can be arranged fairly easily Can occur with intact groups (e.g., a team) Can be focused and brief Provides an opportunity to probe thoughts and perspectives **Disadvantages:** May provide less detailed and focused insight Respondents may refrain from speaking, and report only 'safe' responses

Continued

Table 6.1 Continued Measurement tools: advantages and disadvantages

Focus group	**Advantages:** Provides opportunity for excellent input Gain different perspectives Respondents can interpret findings gathered from other sources Small group can provide detailed attention to issue or topic Provides an opportunity to probe thoughts and perspectives **Disadvantages:** Requires skilled interviewer to manage process Respondents may limit comments because others are present Needs deliberative approach to select participants Requires an appropriate setting Approach can take time Limited to specific questions and issues May have difficulty recruiting participants Challenges with coding and analyzing responses
Observation	**Advantages:** Provides opportunity to observe activities and impact Can code behavior Provides rich data that is not commonly gathered **Disadvantages:** Requires skilled observer Needs clear coding sheet Data needs to be entered accurately Requires skilled analysis Approach can take time Need calibration to maintain consistency of ratings within and among observers Challenges with coding and analyzing responses

the end of the communications initiative has major limitations. Evaluation performed while you are planning and during your implementation of your health and safety communications approach is known as **formative evaluation**. It may include state-of-the art reviews, pretesting messages and materials, and phasing-in a campaign. Collectively, it is known as pilot testing. Evaluation directed at an individual step is known as **process evaluation**. For instance process evaluation during Step 1 would include making sure you understand the needs of the audience before proceeding with development of the message.

Evaluation performed after implementation of your program is called **summative evaluation**. Within summative evaluation are two broadly defined types of evaluation: **impact evaluation** and **outcome evaluation**. Impact evaluation is essentially a high level evaluation that assesses whether the message had desired short-term results such as changes in recipients' knowledge, beliefs and attitudes, or practices. Outcome evaluation addresses more long-term results. Attention is centered on participants' incorporation of lifestyles that are consistent with the intent of the health and safety message. These terms and their respective definitions have been standardized in the professional literature.[4]

Now that evaluation terminology has been defined, it is time to depict evaluation as a process of reviewing, revising and refining your health and safety communication effort. By reviewing, you will be determining if your conveyed message effectively had an impact on the intended audience. This is synonymous to performing a summative evaluation. Based on the results, you would be either satisfied with your effort or you would see the need to revise and refine it. But as you now know, evaluation can take place before or during the implementation of your approach. So as you develop and deliver the message, you can review to see if it is in need of any revision and refinement.

Review, revise and refine

As mentioned earlier, pilot testing is a good way to review your communication effort before or during its implementation (channeling). Some communicators rely on a **focus group** since it solicits input and feedback about the communication effort. This is a structured format with up to eight to ten individuals. They are shown the materials and know–feel–do strategies, and asked a series of questions about them. Depending on the tone developed with the individuals in the group, you'll want to decide how to make sure that individuals actually speak their mind and share their own opinions about the items. This can be facilitated with anonymous audience response systems (e.g., "click-ers") or personal reaction sheets with which individual reactions are gathered privately before any discussion occurs. In a focus group, participants will review the materials (e.g., poster, flier, brochure, PSA) and then be asked a series of questions, such as:

* What overall impressions do you have?
* What do you like and not like?
* What impression do you get with this strategy?
* Do you trust it and the source?
* What is it, specifically, that the program planners want you to know, feel or do?

Another technique is to engage others through a series of **concept reviews** in various phases of the project. Your participants in these would include representatives of your target audience as well as gatekeepers and other program personnel, in various phases of your effort. Your aim is to see what their reactions are to what is planned. They will be helpful in formulating the overall design, as well as in changing the general direction or specific direction of the planned activities. The concept review involves the audience that you seek to reach or affect with your effort. If you are designing materials for high school youth, then your pilot testing will involve them. If your materials are for those in the medical profession, then involve them. Similarly, if you are trying to reach a sub-population, such as female student–athletes on the college campus, or parents of pre-school children, then that is the group with whom you want to be involved for your review activities.

The concept review activities should be done at various phases of the project, as long as the allocated time for project development allows for this. First, you may want to do some assessment of your concept. For example, if you are planning a brochure, and envision it being distributed in a certain manner, then check out whether this is best from the perspectives of your audience as well as intermediaries and other key individuals. Second, you would benefit from testing the messages. Assess what the audience thinks about the message, how it resonates with them and what impact they think it would have on the specified target audience. Third, have samples of the types of images or illustrations that are envisioned reviewed to see if this style is appropriate; see how these are viewed by the target audience and affirm that they have a consistent "flavor" with the overall messages and outcomes sought. Finally, as you are nearing the final phases of your project development, you will want to plan more formalized assessment processes; these may involve a structured focus group to review the final products and will represent the specific pilot testing activities.

The specific ways in which you do these concept reviews will vary. At the earlier phases (concept and content development), you may have discussions and review of the items. This could be in an in-person format, or it may even be done electronically (whether on a conference call, or through an email review). As the development of the content gets refined, you may find yourself wondering which of several illustrations, styles or messages would be best. You may have some rough ideas and share these in a discussion group format with a group. For example, if you are working on a poster or billboard, you may have some imagery that you are proposing—and you may use existing ads to illustrate the type of approach you are envisioning, and ask your reviewers which would be most appropriate, and thus which should go through further development.

After implementation, you can review, revise and refine. This calls for determining the impact of the message. Essentially, you determine if your audience:

Knows

- Knows how to …
- Understands ways of …
- Knows the following facts …
- Is able to specify the difference between …
- Has a broader perspective about …

Feels

- Has greater empathy about …
- Accepts …
- Feels more …
- Identifies their own passion about …
- Has confidence with …

Does

- Is better equipped to articulate …
- Has a clearly defined mission for …
- Has the skills to …
- Is able to show others how to …

Useful measurement techniques for determining message impact are:

- a knowledge quiz;
- an instrument offered before and after a workshop;
- an attitudes self-assessment;
- observing behaviors or interactions;
- having a discussion group with a group leader;
- participating with an individualized, one-on-one interview;
- being in a focus group with eight to ten people around a specific topic;

- doing an online survey or self-assessment;
- keeping a log of specific behaviors, events or interactions;
- doing a series of telephone interviews with both quantitative and open-ended responses;
- comparing results of the data collection over time.

Messages from the field

Modifications with materials development

John McInerney, M.A, ICF International
Neyal Ammary-Risch, M.P.H., MCHES, National Eye Health Education Program,
National Eye Institute, National Institutes of Health

With people in the United States living longer, the growing prevalence of age-related eye diseases and vision loss are a growing public health concern. Currently, 4.2 million Americans age 40 and older are visually impaired. By 2030, when the last baby boomers turn 65, this number is projected to reach 7.2 million, with 5 million having low vision—a visual impairment not correctable by glasses, contacts, medication or surgery that interferes with activities of daily living. Vision rehabilitation can help people with vision loss to maximize their remaining vision and maintain their quality of life. The National Eye Health Education Program (NEHEP) of the National Eye Institute (NEI) at the National Institutes of Health (NIH) works to raise awareness about vision rehabilitation among healthcare providers and people with low vision and their friends, families and caregivers.

NEHEP, working closely with its support contractor ICF International, developed the Living With Low Vision booklet and complementary DVD to promote the benefits of vision rehabilitation. These materials showcase inspirational and uplifting stories of people living with low vision and the service providers who helped them. NEHEP worked with organizations that provide vision rehabilitation services to identify and film individuals with low vision performing a variety of activities of daily life. Interviews with each person and their family members, rehabilitation teachers and counselors captured the struggles and successes of overcoming a visual impairment. The use of personal narratives provided a first-hand account of how people with low vision can lead an active and independent life. The videos allow audiences to connect with these real-life stories more deeply, in a manner that cannot be conveyed solely through a printed narrative.

A draft version of the educational video was screened among vision rehabilitation professionals and people with low vision, who gave feedback that was analyzed and used to edit and finalize the video. Insight from this pretest led NEHEP to reduce the length of the video, rearrange the order of segments and add additional footage and audio descriptions.

The Living With Low Vision booklet—written using plain language and health literacy principles—was vetted with a select group of eye care providers and vision rehabilitation specialists before being finalized and printed. Screening the draft video among its intended audiences allowed NEHEP to gain valuable insight about the resource. This process allowed NEHEP to revise the video in a way that made it more relevant and impactful.

Following completion of the resources, NEHEP adapted the booklet and video for Spanish-speaking audiences. The literacy level, cultural appropriateness and design of the booklet were taken into account during translation and adaptation. Spanish-speaking eye care professionals, healthcare providers, public health specialists and low vision case managers reviewed the adapted resources and provided their recommendations. NEHEP revised the content of the booklet to improve the readability, based on their feedback. Profiles of two Hispanics/Latinos living with low vision were developed, along with a Spanish voiceover of the original video. To learn more about NEHEP low vision educational resources, visit www.nei.nih.gov/nehep/programs/lowvision/educational.

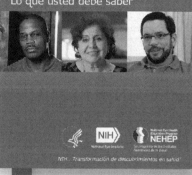

Cómo vivir con
Baja Visión:

Lo que usted debe saber

¿Cómo sé si tengo baja visión?

Hay algunos síntomas que puede notar si tiene baja visión. Marque los síntomas que usted tiene.

Aunque use anteojos o lentes de contacto le cuesta:

- ❏ Reconocer las caras de amigos y familiares.
- ❏ Cocinar.
- ❏ Coser.
- ❏ Hacer reparaciones en su casa.
- ❏ Escoger los colores de la ropa.
- ❏ Leer un libro.
- ❏ Ver las señales de tránsito.
- ❏ Identificar los nombres de las tiendas.

Aunque use anteojos o lentes de contacto, las luces:

- ❏ No le ayudan a ver claramente.
- ❏ Parecen más tenues de lo normal.

Si marcó alguno de estos síntomas puede ser que tenga pérdida de la visión o alguna enfermedad del ojo. Es importante que vaya de inmediato a su oculista para detectar cualquier problema a tiempo. Esto podría ayudar a salvar la visión que le queda.

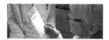

3

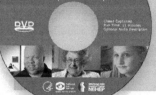

Living With
Low Vision:

Stories of Hope and Independence

DVD

Living With
Low Vision:

What you should know

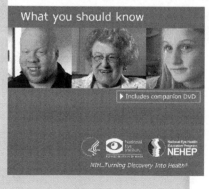

▶ Includes companion DVD

NIH...Turning Discovery Into Health®

How do I know if I have low vision?

Below are some signs of low vision. Even when wearing your glasses or contact lenses, do you still have difficulty with—

- Recognizing the faces of family and friends?
- Reading, cooking, sewing, or fixing things around the house?
- Selecting and matching the color of your clothes?
- Seeing clearly with the lights on or feeling like they are dimmer than normal?
- Reading traffic signs or the names of stores?

These could all be early warning signs of vision loss or eye disease. The sooner vision loss or eye disease is detected by an eye care professional, the greater your chances of keeping your remaining vision.

How do I know when to get an eye exam?

Visit your eye care professional regularly for a comprehensive dilated eye exam. However, if you notice changes to your eyes or eyesight, visit your eye care professional right away!

3

Messages from the field

Details do matter

Rena Needle, MPH Community Coordinator, Alexandria Childhood Obesity Action Network
Diana Karczmarczyk, PhD, MPH, MCHES, Chair, Alexandria Breastfeeding Promotion Committee

Due to the requirement that all businesses with 50 or more employees provide reasonable break time and a sanitary, private place for nursing mothers to express breast milk at work, training was offered to help employers support breastfeeding while reaping the benefits of a healthier workforce and fewer missed days due to their child being ill. Logistical considerations included having an identified room with signage to indicate when it is available and in use as well as educational information on breastfeeding. Posters were prepared and distributed to city employers to post in their lactation rooms. In drafting posters, the first poster was well received due to its image, layout and word choice, yet it had an image that was not clearly a woman and child. The second poster, while preferred, had a baby with a pacifier; however, that image of a pacifier is in direct conflict with one of the steps of a hospital to become Baby Friendly through the UNICEF/World Health Organization Baby Friendly Initiative. The process also served as a powerful reminder that, when developing health and safety communications materials, it is important to get feedback from a wide variety of stakeholders.

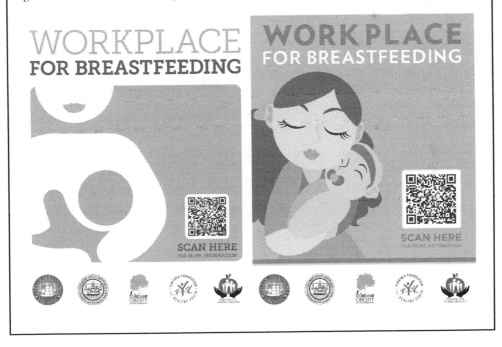

Conducting evaluation

There are various ways of conducting evaluation. A popular method of performing formative evaluation is systems analysis (or quality improvement). It focuses on improving the work processes associated with composing and channeling health messages—making sure the health and safety communications model step–work is efficient and effective. Systems analysis is particularly useful during the implementation of the message. Evaluation can also involve the blending of information or results from various sources, known as **triangulation**. For example, you may gather some quantitative data from surveys and use it as a foundation for qualitative approaches with focus groups or discussions.

A popular means of conducting summative evaluation is goal–outcome. It centers on determining how your health message and associated know-feel-do strategies related to what you want the audience to know, feel and do. When you think about evaluation, you will benefit from doing so within the context of a communication initiative's goals and objectives. Goals are broad statements of intent of what you want to see accomplished. The goals are fairly general and are expected to last over a period of time. To accomplish the goals, objectives are established. **Objectives** are prepared to support goals; each goal has multiple objectives. The objectives are statements of desired outcomes, with a specific audience, and are very helpful in establishing the evaluation. The objectives specify the resulting "condition" and what qualifies as "success," a process quite helpful as you move to establish measures with the evaluation. Objectives have four criteria: the audience, the time period, the condition sought (e.g., for success) and the level of that condition that "qualifies" for success.

Whether formative or summative, evaluation is not a "tag-on" or something thought about at the end or at the last minute of a health and safety communications production. Evaluation helps you decide which communication approach to use as well as how to coordinate or blend one approach with another. Evaluating allows you to determine not only if the message was successful but also how to maintain or improve the message in future efforts of this kind.

Messages from the field

Strategic communications planning for accountability and impact

Mark Weber, M.B.A., Public Affairs, U.S. Department of Health and Human Services

All too often, "launch, leave and hope" is the approach taken with digital and print communications designed with the best intentions. At the U.S. Department of Health and Human Services (HHS), a strategic communications planning tool was developed to focus program and communications staff on proactively setting goals and measuring impact of communications products. The new online tool walks HHS staff through (1) defining a *goal* (what do you want to accomplish with this product or campaign?), (2) setting specific target *outcomes* reflecting that goal (presented against an estimate of the total number in the target audience that might be affected by a particular product or campaign), (3) devising *metrics* for measuring progress towards those outcomes, (4) gathering *data* relevant to those metrics and (5) *reporting* on results. A specific project focused on misuse of prescription drugs that helped to shape the principles used in the strategic communications planning tool was implemented by the Substance Abuse and Mental Health Services Administration. Messages about proper disposal of prescription medications were targeted to patients picking up prescriptions most often misused in the states with the highest rates of misuse. Over a five month period, over 15.5 million proper disposal messages were printed at the point of purchase. Based on market research assumptions, over 7.1 million patients were reached and 85 percent (6.1 million) read some or all of the information they received with their prescription. Of those who read the materials, 80 percent (4.9 million) found the content useful, 48 percent (2.9 million) kept the materials for future reference, and of those who kept the materials 26 percent (760,000) shared the content with at least one other person. With outcomes identified and measured, program and communications staff members have the ability to create products that demonstrate impact, improve overall performance of communications products over time and provide the basis for new products and services.

Forward!

In conclusion, thinking about evaluation can be daunting. Evaluation can be overwhelming and complicated. Evaluation can be complex and difficult. However, evaluation doesn't have to be any of these things. What is important is for you to recall your role—you are a health communicator and you want and need to attend to the fact that evaluation does occur.

You do not need to be the coordinator of all the evaluation efforts and you may not necessarily be the one who has to do it. What is important for your role is to make sure that evaluation does occur and that it is done in a way that is helpful to the health and safety communications effort.

While there may be circumstances where you will actually be doing the evaluation, because of limited funding or staffing, consider who can provide assistance to you. Think about where you can gain some additional perspectives and insights about the most appropriate way to know what you want to know and to learn what you want to learn. Recall that your evaluation does not need to be perfect—it just needs to be helpful and targeted for your needs and purposes.

Finally, try not to get discouraged. You are working with a challenging issue—behavior change with health and safety issues. Your challenge, or your opportunity, is to make some movement as much as possible. This will not be an overnight success; take pride in the small successes that you do accomplish, as long as you can document that they occur! Thus, make sure your evaluation is prepared in such a way that accomplishes these measurements. The evaluation can be helpful in documenting your accomplishments, as well as identifying needs in the future. You can use evaluation findings to prepare for additional resources, to identify new directions and to substantiate needs and progress.

If you remember your desire to make a difference, and that you want to be engaged with quality projects and outcomes, then you have made the most significant step. Integral for those needs, and the focus of this chapter, is that you also will want, and need, quality evaluation.

Notes

1 Knott, T.D. (1987). View point: response to the research agenda evaluation model. *American Journal of Health Promotion*, 1(4), 53–55.
2 Abbatangelo-Gray, J., Galen, E., Cole, J.G.E. and Kennedy, M.G. (2007). Guidance for evaluating mass communication health initiatives: summary of an expert panel discussion. *Evaluation & the Health Professions*, 30(3), 229–253.
3 Bolam, B., Mclean, C., Pennington, A. and Gillies, P. (2006). Using new media to build social capital for health: a qualitative process evaluation study of participation in the CityNet Project. *Journal of Health Psychology*, 11(2), 297–308.
4 Jemelka, R.P. and Borich, G.D. (1979). Traditional and emerging definitions of educational evaluation. *Evaluation Review*, 3(2), 263–276.

Part II

Health and safety communications approaches

7 Campaigns

Overview

A campaign is an approach often used with health and safety communications. This approach involves multiple know-feel-do strategies, is widely distributed and requires a substantive amount of planning. While in some ways it is the same as a political campaign, about which most people are all too familiar, in most ways it is quite different. Campaigns for health and safety issues are typically on a much more stringent budget and have a very different kind of "sales pitch." The campaigns with which you may be involved, around a health initiative, are all about a singular issue or set of related issues. Of the common approaches in health and safety communications, you will see how the campaign is a composite of several other approaches.

In looking at campaigns, you might think of something that is short-lived and focused. Or, it may be something that extends over the years, as the need for addressing the topic may never end. The campaign may actually ebb and flow, with a long-term initiative that gets activated more substantively during certain times of the year or seasons.

Whether the campaign is about forest fires (with Smokey the Bear), or pediatric dental care, or drunk driving or the "Clean Up Hawaii" campaign, the important foundation is that these initiatives have the potential for really making a difference. They are extensive in scope, operate using a range of know-feel-do strategies and seek to reach their audience through a variety of complementary approaches.

This chapter goes into detail about what constitutes a campaign, what various elements can be included, how to plan one and the incorporation of a kick-off event. You should feel more comfortable working with the development and implementation of a campaign following your study of the chapter's contents.

What is a campaign?

A campaign is an orchestrated initiative around a specific health or safety topic, designed to reach a specific audience through a range of approaches. A campaign is typically targeted within a given time period, so the focus on an issue is concentrated with its message. What a campaign does is to have dedication to a specific issue that incorporates a range of venues or approaches.

Here are some quick examples:

- The National Institute of Health offers "The Heart Truth" campaign, focusing on lowering your risk of heart disease. Orchestrated during February, the campaign includes

tips, a video with testimonials, a risk assessment, a speaker's kit and video, materials for physicians and nurses and more: www.nhlbi.nih.gov/health/educational/hearttruth/
- The Centers for Disease Control and Prevention has the "Let's Stop HIV Together" campaign, promoting awareness about HIV and its impact, and seeking to address stigma. This campaign includes posters, brochures, palm cards, banners, fact sheets, video public service announcements and more: www.cdc.gov/actagainstaids/campaigns/lsht/
- AT&T sponsors the "It Can Wait" campaign, with an aim of reducing texting and driving behavior. The campaign incorporates individuals taking the pledge never to text and drive, uses social media, includes a video public service announcement, offers mobile apps, has news, data and personal stories, and incorporates an activation kit and a texting and driving simulator: www.itcanwait.com/all

These examples provide a sampling of ways of going about having a campaign and some of the elements included in a campaign. The general tenor of a campaign is to have a specific, dedicated period of time. These are often linked to a topical awareness day, week or month, generally the same time year after year. Linkage to these events can provide an excellent starting point for anchoring a campaign and for including a kick-off event. Depending on your local needs, you may wish to schedule your campaign at the same time as the national or regional campaign; similarly, you may wish to schedule it at an entirely different time.

These examples of illustrative campaigns demonstrate the variety of approaches offered with a campaign. Said differently, a public service announcement, when used alone, is not a campaign. Similarly, a brochure series is not, alone, a campaign. A campaign, by definition, includes a variety of approaches on a single topic area. This is important because a campaign attempts to reach one or more groups of individuals using a range of approaches.

Think about a single audience as a starting point. While you may have designed a brochure or two to address your topic with this audience, it is unwise to assume that all members of your audience will be reading brochures; some members of this audience may be more likely to listen to the radio and others are active with the internet or with social media. And others may be viewing television and its public service announcements. Further, by having your message communicated using multiple channels, you are likely to reinforce your own message, thus increasing the dosage received by the audience and ultimately the impact of the communications effort. The fact that you have a billboard with a campaign message, and complement it with a radio or television public service announcement, and then have some fliers with the same message, all serve to reinforce one another. You can imagine someone seeing one of these communication approaches and having a "soft" memory of it; then, when hearing or seeing it again with a different approach, they may react with a thought "I've seen that somewhere before." That's exactly what a campaign is and what you want to have happen. One approach reinforces another approach.

Another rationale for the campaign is with reaching different audiences. Cited elsewhere in this book was the importance of thinking about intermediaries when targeting an audience with your communications effort. As noted, the focus was upon the intermediaries as gatekeepers; your message must be acceptable to them if it is to get communicated to the ultimate audience. For example, if part of your campaign involves materials that you want to get distributed to school teachers, your efforts will typically go through the school principal; if s/he does not approve them, the teachers will not get your message through that venue. In a campaign, not only is this consideration valid, but also important is the aim of having the intermediary or gatekeeper involved as an audience, too. With the school example, you may have certain messages to communicate to the teacher; you may have other, complementary messages appropriate for a different target audience, the school principal. This example was found with the healthy heart campaign cited earlier, with specific materials designed for the medical professionals.

Messages from the field

Children's oral health

Ad Council

To help improve children's oral health habits, the Ad Council and The Partnership for Healthy Mouths, Healthy Lives developed a public service advertising campaign. Grey Group and Wing joined the team as the pro bono advertising agencies. The campaign aims to educate parents and caregivers about good oral health habits and motivate them to get their children to brush their teeth for two minutes, twice a day. The long-term campaign goal is to improve children's dental health, so they can develop into healthy adults. The campaign directs parents to the website 2min2x.org, which provides tips for parents and caregivers on how they can teach their children good habits.

From the start, we knew that many children were not practicing good oral health habits and that many parents were not prioritizing this issue at home. We opted to speak directly to the parents and caregivers who would have the most influence on their children's habits. We took a multi-prong research approach in order to explore the current perceptions of oral care benefits and to better understand the barriers and challenges that parents face in getting their children to develop and practice better habits. Through research, we learned that parents know that their children should be brushing their teeth; however, they lacked understanding of the long-term consequences their children could experience due to poor oral habits. This lack of knowledge coupled with busy lifestyles causes parents not to prioritize oral health care on the list of daily parenting responsibilities. We discovered that parents generally supply their children with the proper tools for good care (e.g. toothbrush, floss), but they rarely monitor how long or how well their children are brushing their teeth or flossing. We decided to focus the campaign strategy on making the task urgent yet easy. Ultimately, the campaign attempts to move parents away from the idea that oral care habits in their home are "good enough" to making it a top priority. Thus, our main campaign idea became telling parents that by having their kids brush two minutes, twice a day, they will prevent their child from suffering unnecessary dental disease, pain and potential tooth loss.

The advertising uses the notion that kids spend a lot of time doing all sorts of ridiculous things, from dressing up the family pet to watching silly TV programs, so they have the time to spend two minutes brushing their teeth, twice a day. The notion that taking care of teeth is actually quick and easy resonated with parents, who often feel strapped for time on a daily basis. The call to action for their child to brush two minutes twice per day made oral care seem manageable and the benefit of avoiding pain for their child was clear.

We developed an engaging website (and mobile platforms) in English and Spanish which offer free, two minute videos featuring notable characters from children's shows and networks from partners such as Sesame Street, Cartoon Network and My Kazoo! The videos are designed to entertain children while they brush their teeth for the full two minutes. The site also includes helpful information about the fundamentals of oral care—brushing, flossing and visiting a dentist.

Following the initial campaign launch, we continued to develop new content beyond traditional PSAs that could reach parents and caregivers through different platforms. A mobile text messaging program for parents provides children's oral health tips to subscribers. A mobile application called Toothsavers has a virtual brushing game for children and includes a fun two minute instructional video for the child to watch while brushing, as well as a running tally of how often the child brushes. We created English and Spanish language brochures, DVDs and stickers for dental offices. And, the campaign has been instrumental in creating a new national in-school oral health education program with Scholastic that aims to reach lower income and minority children and their families.

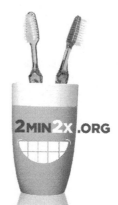

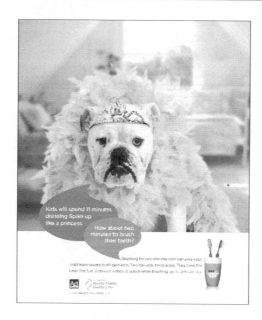

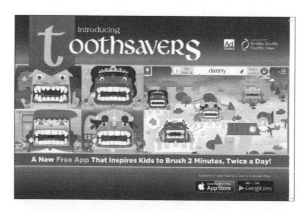

Messages from the field

Diabetes and healthy eyes toolkit

Marcela Aguilar, M.H.S.; ICF International
Neyal Ammary-Risch, M.P.H., MCHES; National Eye Health Education Program, National Eye Institute, National Institutes of Health

Diabetes affects more than 29 million people in the United States and another 86 million people are estimated to have prediabetes. People with diabetes are at risk for diabetic eye disease, including diabetic retinopathy, the leading cause of vision loss and blindness in working age adults. Visual impairment and blindness can have a negative impact on employment, mobility and overall quality of life. Hispanics/Latinos experience disproportionate prevalence rates of diabetes and diabetic eye disease. Recent National Eye Institute (NEI) statistics show there has been a 150 percent increase in diabetic retinopathy cases among Hispanics/Latinos in the past decade and cases are expected to double by 2030.

The Diabetes and Healthy Eyes Toolkit was developed by the National Eye Health Education Program (NEHEP) of NEI at the National Institutes of Health (NIH), with assistance from its support contractor, ICF International. The purpose of the toolkit is to address health disparities by providing materials for populations at highest risk for vision loss due to diabetic eye disease. The toolkit, which can be used to enhance diabetes education programs or as a stand-alone resource, provides culturally and linguistically appropriate materials and tools to inform people how diabetes affects the eyes, the importance of comprehensive dilated eye exams and how people can protect their sight from diabetic eye disease.

This educational resource was created specifically with community health workers (CHWs) and health educators in mind. CHWs are typically members of the community whose primary functions are to provide health education and help people understand and access the healthcare system. NEHEP carried out a rigorous development process that included obtaining feedback from medical experts, program managers, CHWs and community members. Pretesting ensured the materials were scientifically sound, appealing and understood by CHWs and their intended audiences.

The toolkit features a flipchart with colorful graphics and a comprehensive facilitator's guide. Other support materials included in the toolkit are a booklet, magnet and poster with educational messages. The toolkit is available in both English and Spanish and CHWs can use it with small groups of people in community settings or during diabetes self-management classes.

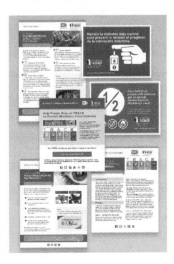

To build capacity in promoting eye health messages at the community level, NEHEP also developed a workshop to train CHWs to use the toolkit. The 90-minute workshop is based on adult pedagogy and uses participatory methods to introduce participants to eye health and to the toolkit. Participants also use group exercises to explore toolkit resources and practice using the materials. An online training course that uses animations, interactive features and quizzes complements in-person workshops and teaches participants about the anatomy of the eye, the effects of diabetes on vision and the importance of getting a dilated eye exam.

As of January 2016, more than 800 CHWs and other health educators have been trained to use the toolkit. The results of these workshops have been measured through pre- and posttests and evaluation forms, which show increased levels of knowledge, high levels of satisfaction with the training and toolkit, and applicability of the content to local communities. To learn more about the toolkit, visit www.nei.nih.gov/diabetestoolkit.

Messages from the field

Make SMART Choices campaign

David Arnold, BACCHUS Initiatives of NASPA

National Collegiate Alcohol Awareness Week (NCAAW) has been a successful method for raising awareness of alcohol abuse and impaired driving concerns at colleges and universities for decades. In 2012, the BACCHUS Network created a NCAAW campaign that capitalized on the multi-environmental exposure as a method for communicating related alcohol and impaired driving prevention messages. This campaign, #makeSMARTchoices, orchestrated its messaging around the SMART acronym: Set limits, Make a plan, Act to help others, Respect the choices of healthy peers, Talk to a friend. These messages formed an appropriate educational message for non-drinkers and heavy drinkers alike, capitalizing on the harm reduction and bystander intervention behaviors common in collegiate alcohol abuse prevention.

The campaign design included an interactive and adaptable model toolkit for campus implementation, pre-designed social media messages and physical media to communicate health promotion messages. Campus prevention professionals were provided with the theoretical and practical perspectives on building a local campaign that configured with the larger national effort. Pre-designed social media messages shared quick facts and know-feel-do strategies for reducing risk at strategic intervals for national exposure through BACCHUS and partner social media outlets, but also for local institutional communication and online social environment peer group distribution. Finally, physical media helped communicate the campaign's educational components and reinforced the messages that students were receiving from prevention staff and as part of social media.

The engagement of student peer educators as campaign distributors (both in physical space and as part of online social environments) was pivotal to the success of the #makeSMARTchoices campaign. Peer engagement is a strategy that was outlined as part of the campaign toolkit. Because of the capacity of peer educators to serve as role models within multiple peer groups, this holistic strategy added a further opportunity for the health messages to be communicated.

Coupling in-person and virtual health and safety communications messaging from a national campaign was very successful in this campaign implementation surrounding alcohol abuse and impaired driving awareness.

Core campaign elements

The important aspect with a campaign is that a variety of approaches are used, all organized around a central theme or issue. Within that, the campaign will typically have a common "look" and "feel," even if the campaign involves reaching out to a variety of audiences.

Several know–feel–do strategies can be used to accomplish this consistency. One approach is to have a logo or image; this can permeate the entire campaign, whether it is at the end of a television public service announcement, at the bottom of a fact sheet or incorporated into a brochure.

Another way of having a consistent feel is with a slogan. For aspects of the campaign that are not visual, this can be particularly valuable. Consider one of the classics in the impaired driving movement "Friends Don't Let Friends Drive Drunk"; this phrase is included throughout the materials promoted by the National Highway Traffic Safety Administration, as well as by others committed to reducing alcohol-related fatalities and injuries.

Materials in the campaign can have a consistent look, whether that is through the use of a color schema, slogan, imagery, spokespersons or graphical appeal. These, too, can permeate the materials of the campaign, as individuals may then start to associate different color combinations with a specific cause. For example, this has been done with colored ribbons representing various causes. Consider the following:

- pink for breast cancer awareness;
- purple for Alzheimer's disease, ADHD and pancreatic cancer;
- light blue for prostate cancer, men's health and thyroid disease;
- lavender for cancer awareness (all kinds) and epilepsy;
- red for AIDS and HIV and cardiovascular disease;
- brown for anti-tobacco.

These listings represent a starting point, as some diseases are identified with several different colors and most colors have multiple topics associated with them.

Not too many years ago, prior to having resources and materials posted on the web, a very different approach was used to conduct a campaign. While this approach can still be found, its utilization is much lower due to printing and postage costs, and limited budgets and other funding; the widespread use of the internet has been helpful in replacing this more traditional, print-based approach. Nonetheless, a review of these can be illustrative for a conceptual overview of campaigns and their contents.

The earlier "standard" approach for doing a campaign relied heavily on the intermediary and on preparing a campaign kit for his/her use. The kit would arrive through the mail and would include the materials necessary for a campaign. Typically, this kit would include a cover letter, fact sheet, question and answer sheet, brochures, radio public service announcements, press release, clip art, poster or flier series, evaluation form, sample materials and order form for more materials. The design of this approach was for the intermediary to review the campaign materials and then make or order copies to distribute to the appropriate audience. Here are some illustrations:

- A school principal receives a kit about bus safety. Some of the information is designed for bus drivers, some materials are prepared for crossing guards, some resources are for teachers, some information is for the parents and some materials are for the students themselves. The principal orders some of the items (e.g., stickers for students and special buttons for the crossing guards) and makes copies of other items for distribution to the specific audience.

- A health educator receives a communications kit on handwashing. This kit's cover letter explains the various resources included in the kit, such as fliers that can be distributed in the local jurisdiction and public service announcements that can be sent to the local radio stations. In addition, a flash drive is included with PDF files of brochures, fact sheets, informational fliers, research studies, resource links and additional resources; these can all be copied as needed for use throughout the community.
- A local sheriff receives a kit about aggressive driving. This includes a fact sheet with current statistics, a sample brochure, fliers ready for distribution, a press release and a script for radio public service announcements. The brochure is prepared with two versions: one is ready to be copied and the other has a section blank where the sheriff's contact information can be inserted. Similarly, the press release and radio PSAs have sections where the sheriff or local spokesperson can insert names and local contact information. Also included in the kit is a CD or flash drive, or link to a website, where the adaptable version of these resources is included.

The contents of a campaign are localized based on the scope and direction of its planners. No single master plan works across all campaigns. What is common is the general thread or look that unifies the entire initiative. The specific content can be as large or small as is deemed appropriate; many of the specific content items are identified in the following section.

Messages from the field

Emergency preparedness

Ad Council

The goal of the Ready Campaign was to educate and empower Americans to prepare for and respond to emergencies (natural and man-made), ultimately increase the level of basic preparedness across the nation. The target was parents with kids living at home (primary)/Hispanic parents (secondary). The basis of the campaign is three-fold: 1) parents are locked in their ways and cemented in their complacency; 2) they prefer not to dwell on the negative and don't believe "it" will happen to them; and 3) if something does happen, they believe they will find a way to cope on the fly.

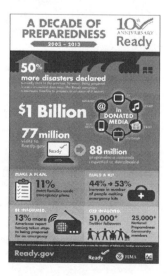

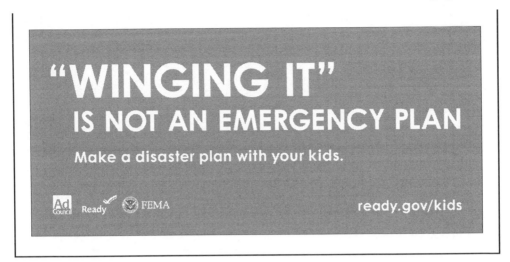

Potential contents of a campaign

For a campaign, any of a variety of elements can be included. As with other health and safety communications efforts, the specifics regarding what you might include will vary based on your audience, their preferences, your available resources and how much you want to provide. It's easy to get carried away and provide lots of information in your campaign; on the other hand, it's more appropriate to be focused and deliberate with your efforts.

One thing you might consider with a campaign is to be very narrow and targeted, particularly if this is the first one conducted in your jurisdiction and/or with this audience on this topic. If, for example, you determine that you want to have 25 different items, this means creating and pilot testing 25 items; if, however, you determine that having eight different items would be sufficient, that narrows significantly what you need to prepare. Thus, particularly for the first year of a campaign, you might want to be very narrow, as that would limit what you need to prepare. For future years, you might use some of the same materials, you might update other materials and then you might add some new resources into the campaign kit. Some of the approaches won't be dated and can be reused over and over for future campaigns with no intensive programmatic development effort.

What follows is a summary of the types of things that you may consider for inclusion in a campaign. Just as with preparing for a workshop (see Chapter 11), you undoubtedly won't be using all of these; you'll select what you think are most appropriate and relevant given your audience and also given the scope of resources you have available to prepare and implement these items. Further details on many of these are found in other sections of this book (e.g., press release information is found in the media chapter (Chapter 9), and brochures and posters are found in the printed materials chapter (Chapter 8)).

Introductory materials

- Cover or welcome letter. This is a letter or information page that provides an overview of the campaign and its intent. This can include information on how to use the campaign elements, a brief statement of need with statistics and a testimonial statement documenting the need for this effort.

- How to use the campaign materials. This summarizes the contents of the campaign kit, as well as ways in which the campaign can be implemented. It can include where to get more information or materials, as well as ways of getting others involved with the campaign.
- Press release. This announces the beginning of the campaign. The press release is usually in a generic format, with areas where locally specific information, quotes and contact information are provided.
- Order form. This provides a way for the campaign coordinator to order additional resource items included in the kit; some of these may be at no cost and others may be for a fee. This can be a way for the sponsoring organization to gain greater awareness about its presence, as well as to bolster its income somewhat. For example, some sponsoring organizations may have quantities of T-shirts, booklets, fliers, stickers and other products available for purchase; these may also be adaptable with local information, such as a website or phone number, also imprinted on the product.

Messages from the field

Promoting healthy lifestyles with the Move It Movement

Cartoon Network

The Move It Movement Tour travels around the country showcasing different sports and fitness activities. It provides a chance for children and young people to try new sports and an opportunity to showcase healthy food and nutrition information. The Move It Movement represents the evolution of Cartoon Network's Get Animated initiative to battle against childhood obesity through daily recess, education and active after-school involvement. The platform goal is to get youth to participate in at least 60 minutes of daily physical activity. Through the Move It Movement, the Cartoon Network works with the President's Council on Fitness, Sport & Nutrition to promote youth and family registration and participation— both in-school and at after-school facilities—in the Presidential Active Lifestyle Award. This initiative empowers kids with relevant messages, unique experiences and impactful tools to live a balanced, healthy lifestyle. Presented in a themed, exciting and fun outdoor environment, the Move It Movement tour features multiple activity and learning stations, incorporating core partner organizations: President's Council on Fitness, Let's Move, NBA, NFL, PGA, and Boys & Girls Clubs of America.

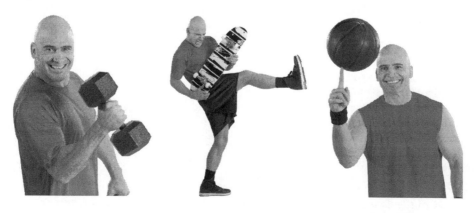

Content background materials

- Fact sheet. This provides basic statistics and information about the topic. It should be as current as possible. It may include changes over time with relevant issues, documenting progress or lack of progress; data will demonstrate a need for the campaign. This can be updated on a regular basis for recurring campaigns. Fact sheets can be very straightforward, or can be done in a more creative, artistic format.
- Research summary. This can complement a fact sheet, with annotated summaries of research conducted about the topic or issue. This should also include full documentation of relevant research and sources.
- Expert statements. This represents quotes from experts on the topic, including researchers, practitioners and specialists. Their organizational affiliation as well as what makes them an expert is helpful.
- Endorsements. The need for and importance of the campaign may be endorsed by individuals who believe in the strategy or resource, or who have been personally affected by it. These may be individuals with strong name recognition, or whose title or organizational affiliation may draw greater attention and credibility by the audience.
- Testimonials. These can be from individuals who are personally affected by the issue included in the campaign. They may also be from someone who has reviewed the campaign materials and wants to illustrate how helpful it would be to utilize the approach included with the campaign.
- Clip art. This is actual art work that is used with the campaign. It should be high resolution so it can be used in various formats utilized by the local campaign planners.
- Charts, graphs and tables. Information can be presented in a visual format that illustrates the nature of the issue, know–feel–do strategies that may be considered, trends over time and various information. This can be epidemiological or otherwise illustrative of key points undergirding the campaign and its need.
- Additional resources. This may include information helpful for the program planners as they seek further information or background on the topic. This may be organizations or agencies, reports, print materials, video resources, websites or other helpful information.
- News reports and articles. Complementing the resources listing, it may be helpful to include reprints of articles or news reports. This can help document the depth of understanding of the issue. This may also include annotated summaries of professional journal articles published on the topic.
- Evaluation. This evaluation would be useful for the groups implementing the campaign, so they can be informed about what went well and what might be improved with future iterations of this or other campaign initiatives.

Audience specific resources

- Tips sheet. This incorporates specific know–feel–do strategies that can be adopted by the audience identified. If the campaign involves multiple audiences, different tips sheets will be prepared.

Messages from the field

Texting and driving prevention campaign

National Highway Traffic Safety Administration and the Ad Council

The Texting and Driving Prevention Campaign was chosen for a few high-profile partnerships in 2015–2016. The campaign collaborated with BuzzFeed to create two custom social posts about the dangers of Texting and Driving. The posts were titled:

- 11 Amazing Moments When You Felt Like The Smartest Person In The World
- 12 Things We Judge Other People On But Definitely Do Ourselves

Both posts utilized popular internet memes and GIFs to send the campaign message that "nobody is special enough to text and drive" using humorous comparisons that people experience in their daily lives. The campaign also collaborated with the incredibly popular mobile phone platform Snapchat to create a customized filter for the app that encouraged users to take the pledge not to Snap and drive. Launched in April 2016 for Distracted Driving Month, the filter allowed Snapchat users to promote the campaign's tagline Stop Texts Stop Wrecks in both personal and public messages to their friends, thereby increasing awareness about the dangers of distracted driving.

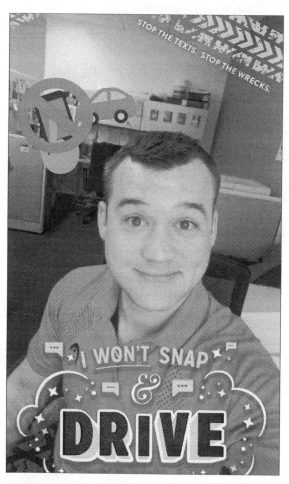

- Brochure. This provides a nice synopsis of the issue and may include rationale, data, tips, know–feel–do strategies, testimonials and graphics. Different brochures for complementary topics, and for different audiences, may be appropriate within the campaign. These can be prepared as ready to go, or as adaptable with local contact information, resources and data.
- Fliers. These can be prepared in a ready-to-implement or modifiable format, suitable for posting on bulletin boards. The campaign may have fliers with an overall, similar look with different messages that complement one another; there may also be different fliers for different audiences.
- Poster. Larger than fliers, the posters can blend the overall campaign theme together, illustrating the involvement of numerous audiences; different versions may also be appropriate.
- How to get involved. This can be a summary of specific know–feel–do strategies that the audience(s) would find appropriate. This could include individual, group, family or community know–feel–do strategies. It may include specific offerings suitable for the sponsoring agency or individuals.
- How to or skills enhancement guide. This illustrates specific ways of implementing the proposed initiative; consider the proper installation of a child safety seat or ways of conducting a breast or testicular self-exam.
- Video segments. Prepared scenarios can complement the case studies, as well as document the need for or solutions contributing to addressing the issue.

Messages from the field

"9 people you become when you're drunk" poster campaign

Ashlee Carter, M.S., Associate Director, Dean of Students Office, Seton Hall University

In an effort to lower high-risk drinking and substance abuse behaviors amongst students, the Department of Student Life at Seton Hall University implemented a nine-week poster campaign that highlighted nine, not-so-glamorous, personalities of people who have heavily consumed alcohol. The messages that were displayed on the posters were humorous, yet thought provoking, in an effort to educate students on knowing their limits when it comes to drinking alcohol. The campaign also corresponded with a large-scale on-campus event that was scheduled for the ninth week of the campaign. In contrast to the eight initial posters prepared in black and white, the final and ninth poster of the campaign was prepared in color and highlighted behavior related to that event specifically.

The large-scale event that was taking place on campus was GrooveBoston, a massive-scale production and dance party driven by electronic dance music. As with any large-scale on-campus event, there is often a high-risk behavior culture associated with it, something to be addressed, in part, with this campaign. Staff reported success with this campaign, which also coincided with other campus initiatives that highlighted the negative effects of high-risk drinking and substance abuse, when the number of medical transports was cut down by almost 60 percent. While this success cannot definitively be attributed to the poster campaign alone, messages portrayed in the posters did have an impact on students' decision-making.

9 People You Become When You're Drunk...

#1 "Chatty Kathy"

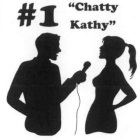

You want to become best friends with everyone in the room by harassing them with your voice. Those humiliating, supposed-to-be-private things you wouldn't ever dream of letting another person know, why not talk about them at high volume so everyone at the party can hear?

Know Your Limits.

SETON HALL UNIVERSITY Office of Community Development. 973.761.9076. University Center, 2nd Floor.

---

9 People You Become When You're Drunk...

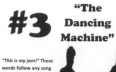

#2 "The Cry Baby"

"He just looked at his phone instead of looking at me."

"Do you hate me? Because it seems like you hate me. Ugh, never mind, I shouldn't have said anything. But do you?"

"The bromance I share with my frat brother is too beautiful for words."

All valid reasons to let the water-works flow, right? Or just a good way to make yourself look like a hot mess.

Know Your Limits.

SETON HALL UNIVERSITY Office of Community Development. 973.761.9076. University Center, 2nd Floor.

---

9 People You Become When You're Drunk...

#3 "The Dancing Machine"

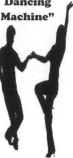

"This is my jam!" These words follow any song that comes on, whether it's "I Will Always Love You" or "The Cupid Shuffle." You've just become Michael Jackson's stand-in, and have no shame in erratically moving your body while spectators are busy uploading your awesome dance moves to YouTube™. Miley ain't got nothin' on you!

Know Your Limits.

SETON HALL UNIVERSITY Office of Community Development. 973.761.9076. University Center, 2nd Floor.

---

9 People You Become When You're Drunk...

#4 "The Ultimate Cage Fighter"

"She said what?!" "He did what?!" It doesn't matter. It's time to misconstrue everything you THINK you heard and take it as a personal attack. It doesn't matter if it's not worth arguing over. It doesn't matter if that person is 3x your size. Thanks for ruining the night.

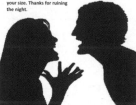

Know Your Limits.

SETON HALL UNIVERSITY Office of Community Development. 973.761.9076. University Center, 2nd Floor.

---

9 People You Become When You're Drunk...

#5 "The Magician"

Abracadabra! You can now make everything disappear! You lost your phone, wallet, purse, jacket, keys, money...even your pants. Houdini would be impressed.

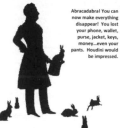

Know Your Limits.

SETON HALL UNIVERSITY Office of Community Development. 973.761.9076. University Center, 2nd Floor.

---

9 People You Become When You're Drunk...

#6 "Starvin' Marvin"

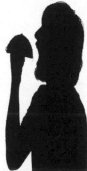

Eating all things deep-fried and dripping with grease is now the goal of the night. That 60 minute cab ride to White Castle becomes essential to living. You just might die if you don't get 3 burritos and 2 slices of pizza into your system. Fitting into your skinny jeans or maintaining your six pack is no longer a priority.

Know Your Limits.

SETON HALL UNIVERSITY Office of Community Development. 973.761.9076. University Center, 2nd Floor.

---

9 People You Become When You're Drunk...

#7 "Richie Rich"

You're drinking? I'm buying! I'll buy a round for everyone! Next 30 rack is on me! Oops! So much for having money for books...or food...or money for Spring Break....or just maintaining any kind of social life.

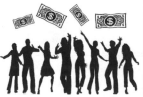

Know Your Limits.

SETON HALL UNIVERSITY Office of Community Development. 973.761.9076. University Center, 2nd Floor.

---

9 People You Become When You're Drunk...

#8 "The Karaoke Queen"

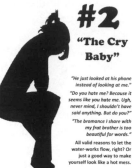

Move over Aretha Franklin! No one has pipes like you after 6 shots. The dog from across the street is starting to howl, but that's okay, because you are totally impressing that hot guy that lives down the hall.

Know Your Limits.

SETON HALL UNIVERSITY Office of Community Development. 973.761.9076. University Center, 2nd Floor.

---

9 People You Become When You're Drunk...

"The Person Not Getting in to GrooveBoston"

#9

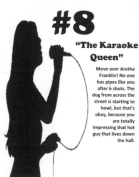

So you thought it would be an awesome idea to pre-game before heading to GrooveBoston. Except you drank too much, and couldn't even compose yourself while you were in line. Now you're in trouble, and missing out on the event of the year. Good job.

Know Your Limits.

SETON HALL UNIVERSITY Office of Community Development. 973.761.9076. University Center, 2nd Floor.

#RAGERESPONSIBLY

Messages from the field

Caregiver assistance

AARP and Ad Council

AARP identified a need for resources and support for those providing care to older loved ones. While this group isn't the core of AARP's membership base, AARP sought to position themselves as a valuable resource on this topic. An online community was created where caregivers can connect with experts and other caregivers to access resources unique to their challenges. The objective of this was two-fold: 1. *Self-identification*: To raise awareness among boomer women that the help they are providing an older adult is caregiving; and 2. *Resources available*: To raise awareness among caregivers that there are resources available to help them and their loved ones. The target audience was women aged 40–60, who are taking care of an older loved one. The specific call to action was to connect these women with resources, as well as other caregivers for tips, tools and support. This campaign included online community forums, live chats and a SMS messaging program. The campaign promoted a wealth of informative content regarding health, finances and emotional issues as they pertain to caregiving, including tools such as a care provider locator, long-term care calculator, as well as personal testimonials.

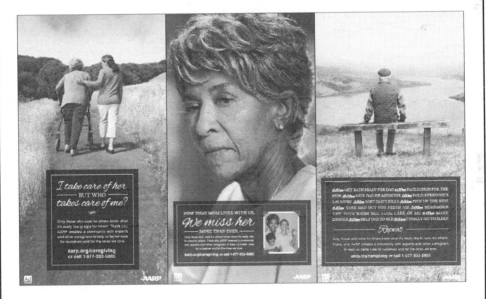

The Thanks Project allowed families and friends of caregivers to recognize the caregivers in their lives for all of the work they do and "thank" them via the campaign microsite. The microsite hosted a visual tapestry of the submitted "thanks," which came in the form of a note, picture or video. There was a strong social component, as all the media was submitted through Facebook, Twitter, Instagram and YouTube. The platform showcased the support and gratitude for the 40 million caregivers across the country.

THERE ARE MORE THAN 42 MILLION CAREGIVERS IN THE U.S. WE'D LOVE TO THANK THEM ALL.

ThanksProject.org

- Question and answer sheet. This includes typical questions of relevance or interest to the target audience. This may also be framed as a "myths and truths" sheet.
- Test/quiz. This is an approach that can help the respondent assess the extent to which they have knowledge about the topic; it may also assess a respondent's attitudes or perceptions about others. For items with correct answers, the reasoning for what makes it correct or incorrect can be shared. For any of these, typical responses or a summary of others' scores may be helpful.
- Self-assessment. Similar to a quiz, this focuses on an assessment about a respondent's own susceptibility or potential need for engaging in the know–feel–do strategies identified within the campaign.
- Bookmarks. Quick reminders of a more permanent nature can be prepared with the use of a bookmark. This can be an inspirational quote, facts, tips, website and other reminders that link to the campaign. Also, a series of bookmarks can be offered, linking together various aspects of the campaign; these may be prepared as a series so the overall campaign message is reinforced in different ways.
- "Bill of Rights." Framing the issues of the campaign into a type of "Bill of Rights" can help organize the issues in a memorable way. It can also be helpful in emphasizing a sense of personal responsibility and opportunity for engagement with the campaign's messages.
- Calendar. This can be prepared as a print or online version. Key dates associated with the campaign's theme can be included, with facts and quotes inserted throughout the calendar. Some campaign calendars have recipes incorporated and others have tips or even coupons that can be redeemed.
- Youth-oriented elements. Games, coloring pages, quizzes, crossword puzzles and other youth-specific know–feel–do strategies can be included. These age-appropriate efforts can illustrate how the topic is valuable for various age groups.
- Activity sampler. This may include ways in which an individual, family, a group or organization, a community or other affiliation group may address the issue in locally appropriate ways.
- Contact and resource information. This includes agency addresses and telephone numbers, additional resources, helpful websites and other information for follow-up.
- Sample letters. This approach can be used for individuals or groups to speak up within the local community. It can include letters to the editor as well as letters to elected or appointed officials.
- Sample agreements or pledges. This can be the basis for an agreement between parties about proposed, desired behavior. Whether a pledge to be tobacco-free, to not text and drive, or to monitor water, fruit and vegetable intake, this can stimulate people to action.
- Checklist. This can include things to do that would help accomplish the aims of the sponsoring organization. It can be focused on individuals, families, groups or larger settings.

Application resources

- Conversation starters. These may be helpful with select audiences, such as between parents and youth, mentors and mentees, supervisors and supervisees, peers, fellow employees, community members or others.
- Case study. Similar to conversation starters, a case study can provide a scenario that raises key issues relevant to the campaign and offers a foundation for solution-finding by members of the target audience. It may also include key questions or issues to address by discussants.

- Radio public service announcements (PSA). Radio public service announcements can be prepared in print or audio format. With print, the narrative would be read by the radio announcer. Localized quotes from key officials could be inserted. If pre-recorded, the PSA could include actual voices from experts or noteworthy individuals, as well as sounds useful in calling attention to the issue (e.g., background noises such as the ocean waves, city traffic, airplane jet engines or children crying).
- Television public service announcements. These would actually be prepared for airing and could be used locally. These may have a segment usable at the beginning or conclusion where local contact information could be appended.
- Movie announcements. In video or slide format, the content could be similar to the television PSA, with local contact or resource information appended as deemed appropriate. These are often played when guests are arriving at the theater, prior to the feature film. Typically, they are silent, with audio announcements included immediately prior to the film (whether before or after the film clips of upcoming movies).
- Newsletter inserts. This involves content that could be included in local print materials, whether a newsletter, organizational flier, faith community bulletin or other resource. This may include narrative as well as visual content.
- Sample workshop. A workshop's materials (slides, handouts) as well as background content can be prepared so local personnel could be trained to implement this to others in their work, community or family setting.
- Talking points. These can be useful when sharing information with others in community or business meetings, media interviews or general conversation.
- Best practices. Specific summaries of what other organizations are doing to address this issue can be helpful; these may be individualized efforts, or more broadly-defined comprehensive approaches. Insights from their implementation can be useful to encourage local personnel to adapt or adopt their approaches.

Messages from the field

Lead the Break Instagram

Foundation for Advancing Alcohol Responsibility

The purpose of the initiative was to highlight the "reality" of Spring Break to media, parents and students. The campaign also encouraged students to enjoy Spring Break responsibly and productively. Reaching 8,000 college student leaders and advisors on 330 campuses, the Instagram contest showcased the different productive and creative activities students engaged in during Spring Break. Throughout the contest, students submitted nearly 1,000 photos through their Instagram account using the hash tag #LeadtheBreak to show how they were making a positive difference during the Spring Break. Three students received prizes for their creative submissions which encouraged their peers to have a safe and responsible Spring Break.

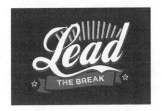

As noted, each of these know–feel–do strategies could be included as part of the campaign. It is rather overwhelming to consider implementing all of the know–feel–do strategies identified; these are provided as a way of thinking more broadly about what might be included in your own campaign. As you prepare your materials, you are constrained only by your imagination and your resources, whether financial or personnel. With the use of the internet and web–based repositories, you can be well-equipped to prepare a variety of resource materials for your campaign.

Planning a campaign

As with any health and safety communications effort, appropriate and thorough planning is essential for the ultimate success of the initiative. Whether you have a role of conceptualizing the campaign, gathering various components, identifying writers or artists, assembling materials, organizing the evaluation or doing some other aspect of campaign preparation or implementation, you have a tremendous responsibility. You also have a great opportunity to spread the word about your issue and make a difference.

Since the campaign is defined as having multiple components over a limited period of time, the overall consideration has to do with your vision of the campaign and its logistics. Consider whether you will link your campaign to an existing topical month, week or day, as cited earlier in this chapter. Also consider whether you will be looking for an existing campaign and implementing it within your area of purview. As an alternative, you may be creating a campaign, adapting one or working as an advisor or consultant with campaign planners. In any of these situations, the considerations cited here can be helpful for preparation and development purposes. Some basic campaign approaches blending these considerations are summarized below; these serve as a foundational point, and adaptations and refinements for your own organization's purposes are most appropriate.

General considerations

In preparing the campaign, one of the starting points is what you consider to be the breadth of the campaign. What is the time period over which it is to be prepared? What is your budget, both in terms of actual dollars as well as personnel time? Who is your ultimate audience and who are intermediaries? Are there times of the year when it might be most appropriate to implement the campaign, such as already-existing awareness weeks or months with which you could link your efforts?

As you consider this overall scope, you can actually implement a campaign with limited funding and resources. You may envision a campaign that dovetails with a national or state initiative and incorporate some of their publicly-available materials (with appropriate attribution, of course). Sometimes these state and federal agencies prepare these materials in print-adaptable format, so you can add your own contact information and local resources to them, prior to distribution or posting. It may be as simple as adding your organization's contact information, including name, website, telephone number and perhaps address to a place provided on the materials master; similarly, sometimes radio or television public service announcements have an opportunity provided at the end for your organization to add relevant locally appropriate information.

Messages from the field

Use of on-air campaigns for youth

Cartoon Network

Spot the Block was an educational campaign launched by Cartoon Network and the Food and Drug Administration to encourage youth ages 9 to 13 to look for and use the Nutrition Facts to make healthy food choices. The Cartoon Network's Get Animated initiative, implemented about a decade ago, was a place where kids could Get Active, Get Healthy and Get Involved with the world's best cartoons. Get Animated empowered kids to take action with information and programs on TV, on the web and in the community.

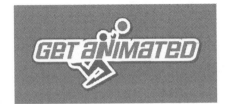 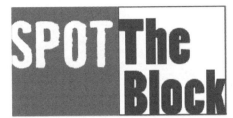

With limited funding and with the widespread use of the internet, you may decide it is appropriate to have your campaign entirely lodged on a website; this could be a dedicated website, just for the campaign, and it could also be a portion of or highlighted within your organization's existing website. The content could include those items you deem appropriate for inclusion, such as a "cover letter" or welcome statement from a key official, facts and graphics, testimonials, PSAs, printable fact sheets, background papers, additional resources for background information and more. Envisioned in this manner, there may actually be no print or postage budget.

Another way of expanding your reach as well as your credibility is to engage one or more partners. Sometimes individuals or groups can be "silent partners" where they share their mailing list or ideas. Partners may be involved to lend their name to your campaign, but not provide any effort. Another organization could also be a full partner, with much more active involvement, technical assistance, graphic design resources, funding, ideas, collaboration and more. This can be very helpful with your initiative, as it can virtually extend your staffing, resources and potential impact, with no major loss to your aim of getting the word out and achieving your desired results.

This same approach could be adapted, with some items printed and distributed. You may envision a campaign that has a quarter page flier that gets inserted within an already-existing mailing (e.g., electric power or telephone bill) or other publication, advertisement in a local paper or your own mailing. Depending on who are identified as key intermediaries, you may have a select mailing that could include a cover letter, brochure and information card, and your primary aim may be to point the recipient to the website for further resources.

A final thought is that your campaign may target more than one audience. You may decide that you need different messages for different audiences, all within the larger construct of the campaign's goals and objectives. For example, you may work through the intermediary of a school principal, yet have materials specifically designed for and appropriate for teachers, counselors, parents and kids.

Develop a campaign

From a basic perspective, consider the fact that you may develop a campaign from scratch. You have a vision of a local need and audience that you and your colleagues believe would benefit from a targeted initiative—your campaign. So with the repertoire of various know-feel-do strategies identified earlier in this chapter, consider what might constitute an appropriate and feasible campaign for you and your organization. Whether you actually host everything on the internet, have a campaign with print materials only or incorporate a blend of these approaches will depend on your overall vision and your budgetary and resource availability.

Implement a campaign received

Another approach for implementing a campaign is that you may be the recipient of a set of campaign materials you receive or find. From a print perspective, you may receive a packet of campaign materials, encouraging you or your organization to implement it. In that sense, you have been identified as an "intermediary," where you might typically think of others as an intermediary. Upon receipt of these materials, you may find that these are "ready to go," with press releases already written and ready to be adapted with local data and contact information. Sometimes, these materials will attempt to engage you as a local distributor or intermediary; you then would distribute the materials to your local audience, whether that is a direct distribution to the identified types of recipients, or sent through whomever you identify as the appropriate local intermediaries.

Adapt a campaign

Blending the receipt of a campaign and the development of a campaign, you may decide that you want to adapt an existing campaign for your local needs or organization's purposes. What may occur is that you see a campaign (or even a set of materials that is not currently constituted as a campaign) that you believe would be appropriate for you and your organization's purposes. You may use this as a foundation, such as a "trigger" for local discussion about how you and your organization might adapt that for your purposes. You may determine that this existing approach is just what you need, so you would then contact its sponsors to determine what can be adapted and how to cite the appropriate permissions. You may wish to use only certain portions of it and then decide ways of preparing what else would be appropriate for your local implementation. Of course, you need to be careful of any copyright factors, such as the materials, images, slogans, logos and resources associated with other campaign sponsors. When in doubt, it is important that you seek appropriate permission for using or adapting existing know-feel-do strategies.

Serve on a planning group

You may not be implementing a campaign personally or organizationally, but you may be part of a group planning a local or statewide campaign. Your role may be one of representing your organization, your region or a particular perspective or point of view. In this type of situation, your awareness of the wide range of types of approaches that could be included in a campaign will be most helpful. You can also be a valuable asset through your awareness of appropriate planning know-feel-do strategies and audiences, such as the needs of and interests associated with the target audience. You can be a helpful contributor through the broad awareness and skills you can share for more effective design, messaging and orchestration of the larger campaign.

Messages from the field

Collaboration makes a difference

Tom Flamm, IAFF Burn Coordinator, International Association of Fire Fighters

"It can happen in a flash with a splash." This is the warning of the National Scald Prevention Campaign, a multi-organizational initiative designed to raise awareness about the dangers of scalding, particularly among children and older adults. Concerned about the close to 70,000 scald burn injuries each year associated with consumer household appliances and products (e.g. stoves, coffee makers, tableware, cookware, bathtubs), five national organizations joined forces to develop an educational campaign on the risks of scalding and the simple steps to prevent liquid and steam burns in and around homes.

   The organizations—International Association of Fire Fighters (IAFF) Charitable Foundation Burn Fund, American Burn Association Burn Prevention Committee, Federation of Burn Foundations, International Association of Fire Chiefs, and Safe Kids—had worked together before on other initiatives related to burn prevention and safety. Funding from the Federal Emergency Management Agency (FEMA) to the IAFF allowed the five organizations to work together to develop the informative website http://flashsplash.org, a key tool to help spread scald prevention awareness in local communities.

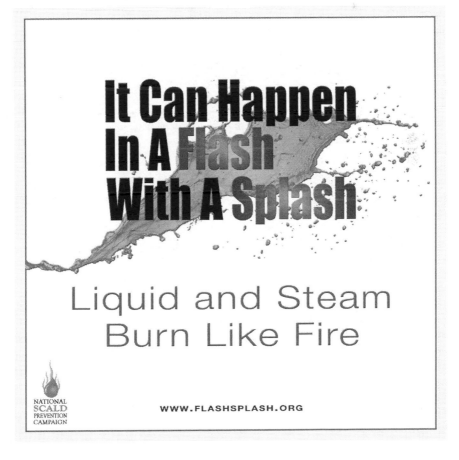

Collaborative relationships were the roots that allowed the National Scald Prevention Campaign to grow and flourish. The lessons learned included:

- *Have the right people around the table.* In addition to subject matter experts and FEMA representatives, the five organizations reached beyond traditional medical communities and invited representatives involved with prevention and child/youth safety. The 40-member Task Force was comprised of professionals committed to the cause and willing to "roll up their sleeves" to get work done.
- *Create structures that facilitate action.* By utilizing smaller work groups to guide the process, the Task Force worked collaboratively and reached consensus on most issues. A Steering Committee (16–20 people) was formed to maintain focus and move the process forward; every six months, the Steering Committee met, reviewed interim work products and provided input. In addition to these meetings, an Executive Team of eight individuals helped to keep the ball rolling. The Executive Team communicated frequently and met quarterly. The full Task Force met at the beginning of the campaign and three years later, at a final wrap-up meeting. Other structures helped to advance decision-making and action: (1) bringing in a facilitator for larger meetings, (2) using regular email communication among all members and (3) creating a mock website so members could give valuable feedback before the website's launch.
- *Build on past successes.* The Task Force didn't try to reinvent the wheel. Utilizing the subject matter experts and good, existing resources from Task Force member organizations, the Campaign reworked the information to be user-friendly, updated it to reflect new risks posed by technological and societal changes (e.g., microwaves) and placed it all on a "one-stop (information) shopping" website.
- *Ensure that the initiative continues.* While the website was launched in summer 2015, the National Scald Prevention Campaign carries on. The Executive Team stressed the importance of avoiding the common trap of developing a useful product only to have it sit on a shelf unused. The national partners continue to use and refer to the website, its fact sheets, infographics and the tool kit in their education campaigns. Many of the national organizations publicize the website during the annual National Burn Awareness Week (the first full week in February). As a result, local members utilize the website to access information, social media and PSAs and tailor them for education campaigns in their own communities.

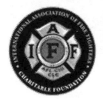 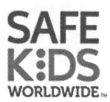 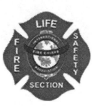 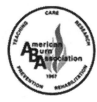

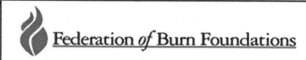

A campaign launch or kick–off event

While not essential, a campaign may begin with a launch or kick–off event. This can be done in a face-to-face, live format, or it can be done in a virtual manner. This is an opportunity to announce the start of the campaign, providing an opportunity for media coverage of the event.

An advantage of having a kick-off event or launch is that it provides another opportunity to communicate your message or theme. This launch can be a part of the campaign itself, as it can provide an anchor for the activities that follow. As highlighted with the chapter on media relations, having the attention of the media can be most helpful in distributing your message. By earning the coverage, the program sponsors gain additional, free distribution of their campaign. Greater public awareness of your organization, as well as the campaign itself, can accompany the kick-off event.

A kick-off event can be particularly timely if coordinated in conjunction with already-existing awareness months, weeks or days. For example, your organization may decide to announce its campaign about not smoking when linked to the Great American Smokeout; you may wish to link your prescription drug awareness initiative with the Talk About Prescriptions Month. This may also be a time when you release the results associated with a major study.

The kick-off event doesn't have to be a stand-alone press conference, such as you may have envisioned. It can actually be organized in a more creative manner. Consider the following:

- Have the event at the start of or middle of a sporting event.
- Offer this at a popular location, such as a shopping mall.
- Organize the event to coincide with a particular time of day and/or day of the week.
- Schedule this at the same time as another event, such as a parade or festival.
- Arrange a location that has topic relevance to your campaign, such as a recreation center for a fitness initiative, a grocery store for a nutrition-based campaign or a bicycle trail for a bike helmet program.
- Plan this for a setting that has photographic power; think about media coverage and what might spark coverage by them and interest by their audience, such as having a backdrop of the U.S. Capitol or Statehouse, a community center or police headquarters, a park entrance or an abandoned building.
- Make it audience-appropriate: for example, have a youth center for a teen-focused effort, a retirement community for a campaign focused on older adults or a college campus student union for a student flu immunization program.
- Make it setting-appropriate; for example, include a local park for a neighborhood event, a highway rest area for an aggressive driving program or a food store or restaurant for a nutrition-oriented topic.

As you plan a kick-off event, consider this with a celebratory type of flavor. You are excited about the start of the campaign and want to communicate more widely the availability of the resource and messages.

Finally, the kick-off event should be viewed as a type of event that can proceed with or without the media present. Typically, you would want the media to be present, as this dramatically expands the opportunity for your reach and wider dissemination of your message. However, it is important to realize that, while you want the media present, and the media may commit to being present, last minute changes with media priorities do happen, so you should be content with proceeding without their presence. In any situation, you may consider gathering your own media footage—capture some of the festivities on your own, post this in a visual way on your project website and distribute it through various channels, including social media, to various stakeholders, followers and others who might be interested.

If you do decide that you want to have the media present, you should consider several know–feel–do strategies that would maximize the opportunity that they would be present. More detail is provided about the overall media context in Chapter 9.

- Develop an appropriate angle or way of framing your event that builds upon what would make your campaign, and thus the kick-off event, worthy of media coverage. Use some of the ways identified in the general know–feel–do strategies chapter (Chapter 4) that help frame this event.
- Utilize media relations skills and/or personnel to determine what days and times might be most appropriate from the perspective of the media. If you can identify times that do not conflict with some pre-existing commitments of the media, that can be most helpful.
- Notify the media with enough lead time to garner their presence. Also, provide reminders several days before, as well as the day before, the kick-off event.

Messages from the field

End Impaired Driving campaign

Foundation for Advancing Alcohol Responsibility

The objective of the #EndImpairedDriving campaign is to raise awareness about impaired driving, highlight these dangerous and preventable behaviors, encourage all drivers to focus their attention on the task of driving when behind the wheel, and model good behaviors for the next generation of drivers.

The initiative was a call to action from the Administrator of the National Highway Traffic Safety Administration (NHTSA), Dr. Mark Rosekind, when he said "An impaired driver is a dangerous driver. We need to be focused on the 'four D's'—drunk, drugged, distracted and drowsy." Responsibility.org responded to this challenge and commissioned a national survey to learn more; results found that more than eight out of ten Americans identify distractions (texting, talking on phone, eating, etc.) and alcohol as the leading impairments to a driver's ability to safely operate a motor vehicle. Armed with increased knowledge, Responsibility.org took a leadership role in developing and testing public service announcement (PSA) concepts and messages. The feedback revealed that having a positive tone and uplifting message that communicates the importance of making positive choices when driving would get people involved in the effort to stop impaired driving. The result is the "End Impaired Driving" video which stresses the importance of personal responsibility and the modeling of proper driving behaviors.

Knowing that traffic safety organizations often compare one form of impairment against another—i.e. distracted driving riskier than drowsy driving—but that these comparisons often overlook the fact that some impairments happen simultaneously, Responsibility.org shared its research findings with traffic safety and health advocacy organizations to build and promote a collaborative effort to end all forms of impaired driving. Ultimately 22 organizations joined together, for the first time, to announce this new initiative to end impaired driving in December 2015.

The cornerstone of the campaign is a PSA, which can be found at www.EndImpairedDriving.org. The site encourages individuals to share an advocacy message to #EndImpairedDriving. As the PSA says, "in a perfect world, impaired driving wouldn't exist."

To extend the impact and reach among the Hispanic population, Responsibility.org and its partners launched a Spanish language version of the PSA as well as other resources to help Spanish-speaking audiences understand the risk of impaired driving and what they can do to avoid engaging in dangerous driving behaviors.

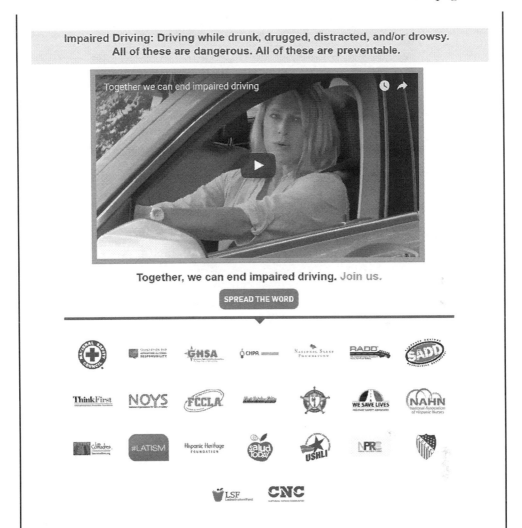

- Prepare background information (media kits) that includes relevant information that they can use. Some of this will be the same as with the campaign materials (such as fact sheets); other content will be unique for this kit (such as a press release, testimonials and contact information for experts).
- Locate the kick–off event in a location that may be of particular interest to the media. While appropriate locations are identified above, and linked to the topic, audience or setting, consider a kick–off event that may provide a visual backdrop that would be of interest to, and potential impact for, the media.
- Conduct follow-up with the media following the kick–off event. This can help address any questions as well as to show interest in the media for their participation and potential coverage of the event as well as for the campaign as a whole.

Forward!

In summary, campaigns may, initially, seem daunting as an undertaking. Certainly, they can be just that, as they can incorporate numerous know–feel–do strategies, as well as have a significant amount of product creation, development, implementation and follow–through. Further, a campaign may incorporate a kick–off event to celebrate the beginning of the breadth of activities and know–feel–do strategies.

On the other hand, a campaign can be very straightforward. It's actually putting together many of the individualized events and approaches found throughout the realm of health and safety communications. The focus of a campaign is narrow, within a time period. If you think about getting the word out about your topic or initiative, scheduling a campaign can actually provide you a focal point in terms of scheduling and calendaring, so that you can focus your energy into that time period. Having a campaign can be helpful for garnering additional media attention, something that can go beyond the announcement that you have a brochure available, or that your agency is conducting a workshop in the coming week. A campaign sounds, and is, much broader with approaches, yet narrow with timing.

The challenge with a campaign is to make sure that your efforts are well planned. As noted, consider the audience you seek to reach and what know–feel–do strategies may be most appropriate for them. Consider potential partners who can lend their name, credibility, mailing lists and other resources to the effort. Most importantly, keep the campaign tight; if this is your first one on a topic, keep it narrow with respect to the number of materials needed to be developed, so that it is done with quality and focus. Then, after all the planning is done, savor the process and enjoy the experience!

8 Print materials

Overview

One of the primary approaches for health and safety communications involves the use of print materials. This incorporates a wide range of approaches, but always engages printed words and imagery. Brochures, posters, fliers and billboards are evident examples. Some smaller items, such as fact sheets, question and answer pages, resource documents, bookmarks, door hangers, business cards and numerous other print items serve as complementary know-feel-do strategies within this framework.

As with many of the other topics in this book, the attention to print materials is provided with an applied orientation so that you can accomplish your identified aims. As with the other chapters in this Approaches section (Part II), the focus is on many of the practical ways of bringing together the range of elements from the Model section (Part I) of this book.

Some caveats are relevant at the outset. First, the preparation of print materials will be designed to maximize the achievement of your identified goals. Second, and consistent with earlier attention to preparing communications efforts, all of the tools, theories and other foundations are not going to be used in a single item or set of items. You will identify those elements that are most appropriate for your purposes. Third, no single best approach is anticipated or identified. The attention in this chapter is upon broad-based and specific considerations for you as you prepare your materials. As you design a brochure, for example, you will be pulling together various elements from your growing repertoire of know-feel-do strategies and resources, to maximize the results you want to achieve. Could this have been done a different way? Absolutely. Would others design a brochure with a totally different look? Sure. Within that context, the focus here is upon specific elements that will be helpful in maximizing, not guaranteeing, the impact that you seek.

This chapter provides attention to the most commonly used print approaches. If you were to look at a product catalog, you would see hundreds of print materials, with logos and slogans, websites and QR codes, images and more printed on them. Whether it is a pencil, an eraser, a mug, a refrigerator magnet, a T-shirt, a notepad or some other product, these are all considered to be "print materials." Obviously, some are more detailed than others (contrast a brochure with a bookmark or a billboard).

The initial example in this chapter is with the preparation of a brochure, which can be seen as a prototype for publications. While most of the publications are more succinct, some publications will be longer (like a booklet). The specific insights and recommendations incorporated in the review of a brochure's construction will serve as a type of template or foundation for the other publication approaches cited.

As you prepare any of these print materials, you should rely on the health and safety communications model described in Chapter 1. This foundational work is critical to the quality and ultimate success of your materials development. In short, you need to be clear what you want from the reader of your materials—what is it, specifically, that you want them to know, feel or do? You will want to think clearly about what content you want included. That is, to get the reader to the desired endpoint, specify the key content elements that are necessary to achieve this result. A follow-on planning activity is to determine what types of materials or approaches will be helpful in getting your audience to this desired endpoint. This is where you review the general and specific tools from previous chapters—will you want statistics? Testimonials? Graphics? Pictures? References? This gives you an overall framework from which to work. As you start to generate the specific design, whether for a brochure, flier, poster, booklet or other print material, you will want to be checking with others (such as members of the target audience) to gather their reactions to what you are planning and how you are designing it. You may show them several choices, to gather their input and suggestions. This formative process is helpful in ensuring that you are on the right track.

With this background, attention to specific approaches will be addressed in the following chapter sections. These various sections that follow provide guidance about ways of preparing the different kinds of materials.

Brochures

For the purpose of this guidebook, a **brochure** is single-page, folded leaflet. Preparing a brochure is like preparing a cake. That is, you want the cake to taste good, look great and be as healthy as it can be. With a brochure, you want it to accomplish some purpose, be visually attractive and have the content and graphic appeal that works best for your audience. Also, and as no surprise to you, there is no one, single best cake; different tastes and styles exist. The same is true for a brochure; if you and numerous other individuals prepared different brochures on the same topic for the same audience, and were given the same background information, you would very likely come up with quite different designs. No single one is best; some may be more effective in meeting some of the desired aims of the initiative and others may be more effective in meeting other aims. Creating a brochure, just as with preparing other communications efforts, is an art and a craft; you blend a sound process with your skills and your imagination to create what you hope and expect will be a quality effort.

In thinking about preparing a brochure, a good place to start is with a standard, tri-fold brochure. There are brochures with other shapes and styles, but your starting place for an initial brochure is with this six-panel resource. A simple, straightforward approach is to use an existing template; this almost makes it too easy, as it provides a standard look and can guide you to include key elements, such as a title, imagery, sponsors and various content items. With Microsoft Publisher, for example, you can select the specific template and work on the content for each of the panels. You select an overall look and color, and then prepare the specific content for this as you go along.

With this type of template, the important thing is that you let the computer program do what it is that you want to do. That is, if you really want a reverse image (e.g., white lettering showing through a colored template), then make sure the computer program does that for you. If you want images that are slanted in style, or that overlap one another, make sure that this is what you get. The important thing is to not settle for something that is easy or convenient, but to become proficient enough so that the computer program is doing what you want it to do. The best way to accomplish this is with practice and experience; some guidance through training, mentoring, online help or self-guided instruction can be helpful in achieving this.

As you design your brochure, think about each of the six panels individually and collectively. The cover is perhaps the most important part of the brochure; this will catch the potential user's attention and generate interest in even picking up the brochure, or looking inside it. You want to be sure it is visually appealing and is inviting to potential readers, to make them want to read the brochure. Generally, keep the cover fairly simple, attractive, appealing and straightforward. It may include a photo or graphic design, a few large words, some smaller (subtitle) words and perhaps the sponsor. You may include a leading question on the cover, or it could be the topic only. You may incorporate a topic in a cute way and then use a subtitle to state clearly what it is all about (examples could be "Going Up in Smoke: Facts of Tobacco Use" or "Why Weight? Diet and Your Health"). In short, you want the cover to be both clear about the brochure's topic and inviting (see Figures 8.1 and 8.2).

Typically, the contact information, website, phone number and such information is included on the back panel. While this is sometimes found on the cover, this isn't necessary or appropriate, as it tends to clutter this page. Someone looking for this type of information will generally find it at the end of the publication (on this back panel). Also on the back panel are additional resources, sponsors, disclaimers if needed, web links and other supporting information.

Four panels remain for content with the brochure. This is where you have the opportunity to make your case for your issue or topic. For ease of description consider the inside page as three adjoining panels, to be discussed in greater detail. The remaining panel is the one that is visible when you open the cover; this is available for content of a type of 'stand-alone' nature. For this single panel, you want to be consistent with what is inside on the three adjoining panels (as the reader will see the left panel next to this stand-alone panel when the brochure is opened). You might consider something like a summary statement of the brochure's key points, next steps, tips, common questions and answers, myths and truths, a brief quiz, a summary of helpful resources, conversation starters or something else that can "hold its own" in the context of the brochure.

Now, the emphasis is on the entire inside of the brochure. These three panels should fit together well. Since readers typically start reading material from left to right, any flow of your content should move the reader from the first panel on the left, to the center and then to the right. Sometimes you may have an orderly flow and sometimes there is no flow or logic as you have distinct, independent elements being communicated. The reader will see these three panels as a whole, so they must appear virtually seamless. As a starting place, include three parts of your overall message within these three panels. If you have five parts, decide how you will break these up; it is important to keep together the similar items (i.e., all similar items are together on the same panel, without spillover to the next panel). You might decide to have one of the parts on the stand-alone panel; the challenge is that the reader sometimes sees that panel first and sometimes sees the inside left panel first.

As you start to design this, you'll likely be moving things around so you obtain the desired look and feel that you want. You'll want to have the content that holds together with itself maintained in the same section of the brochure. Thus, if part of your brochure is providing an "A, B, C" approach for some issue, you can put each one of these on

General mockup of fliers
(Using 8½" × 11" paper)

TRI-FOLD BROCHURE (6 panels of material)

Inside panel	**Back panel**	**Brochure cover**
Includes stand-alone content, such as FAQs, myths and truths, testimonial, quick facts.	Could have additional information such as helpful resources	Attention-getting, inviting
		Few words
	Organization name	May have organization sponsor
	Contact information (address, telephone number)	
	Website	
	Email address	
	Possibly QR code	

Fold along dotted lines into thirds

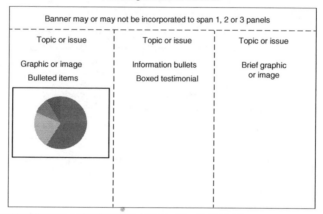

Banner may or may not be incorporated to span 1, 2 or 3 panels

Topic or issue	Topic or issue	Topic or issue
Graphic or image	Information bullets	Brief graphic or image
Bulleted items	Boxed testimonial	

BI-FOLD BROCHURE (4 panels of material)

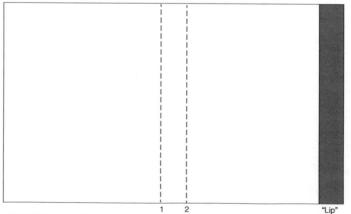

1   2   "Lip"

Fold the paper on line 1 to include a "lip" (which may include some wording visible whether the brochure is open or closed). Fold the paper on line 2 for a brochure with no lip.

Figure 8.1 General mockup of fliers

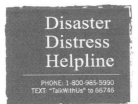

Disaster Distress Helpline

PHONE: 1-800-985-5990
TEXT: "TalkWithUs" to 66746

☎ **Call us:**
1-800-985-5990

✎ **Text:**
'TalkWithUs' to 66746

✎ **Visit:**
http://disasterdistress.samhsa.gov

Like us on Facebook:
http://facebook.com/distresshelpline

Follow us on Twitter (@distressline):
http://twitter.com/distressline

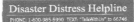

Disaster Distress Helpline
PHONE: 1-800-985-5990 TEXT: "TalkWithUs" to 66746

*Call 1-800-985-5990
or text 'TalkWithUs' to 66746*
to get help and support
for any distress that you or someone
you care about may be feeling
related to any disaster.

The *Helpline* and *Text Service* are:

- Available 24 hours a day,
  7 days a week, year-round
- Free (standard data/text messaging
  rates may apply for the texting service)
- Answered by trained crisis counselors.

TTY for Deaf / Hearing Impaired:
1-800-846-8517

Spanish-speakers:
Text "Hablanos" to 66746

Administered by the Substance Abuse and Mental Health Services Administration (SAMHSA) of the U.S. Dept. of Health and Human Services (HHS).

✖**SAMHSA**
www.samhsa.gov • 1-877-SAMHSA-7 (1-877-726-4727)

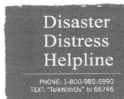

Disaster Distress Helpline

PHONE: 1-800-985-5990
TEXT: "TalkWithUs" to 66746

If you or someone you know is struggling after a disaster, you are not alone.

"Ever since the tornado, I haven't been able to get a full night's sleep ..."

"I can't get the sounds of the gunshots out of my mind..."

"Things haven't been the same since my shop was flooded ..."

Talk With Us!

Disaster Distress Helpline
PHONE: 1-800-985-5990 TEXT: "TalkWithUs" to 66746

Disasters have the potential to cause *emotional distress*.

Some are more at risk than others:

- Survivors living or working in the impacted areas (youth & adults)
- Loved ones of victims
- First Responders, Rescue & Recovery Workers.

Stress, anxiety, and depression are common reactions after a disaster.

Warning signs of distress may include:

- Sleeping too much or too little
- Stomachaches or headaches
- Anger, feeling edgy or lashing out at others
- Overwhelming sadness
- Worrying a lot of the time; feeling guilty but not sure why
- Feeling like you have to keep busy
- Lack of energy or always feeling tired
- Drinking alcohol, smoking or using tobacco more than usual, using illegal drugs
- Eating too much or too little
- Not connecting with others
- Feeling like you won't ever be happy again.

TIPS FOR COPING WITH STRESS AFTER A DISASTER:

Take care of yourself. Try to eat healthy, avoid using alcohol and drugs, and get some exercise when you can- even a walk around the block can make a difference.

Reach out to friends and family. Talk to someone you trust about how you are doing.

Talk to your children. They may feel scared, angry, sad, worried, and confused. Let them know it's okay to talk about what's on their mind. Limit their watching of TV news reports about the disaster. Help children and teens maintain normal routines to the extent possible. Role model healthy coping.

Get enough 'good' sleep. Some people have trouble falling asleep after a disaster, others keep waking up during the night.

If you have trouble sleeping:

- Only go to bed when you are ready to sleep

- Don't watch TV or use your cell phone or laptop computer while you're in bed

- Avoid eating (especially sugar) or drinking caffeine or alcohol at least one hour before going to bed

- If you wake up and can't fall back to sleep, try writing in a journal or on a sheet of paper what's on your mind.

Take care of pets or get outside into nature when it's safe. Nature and animals can help us to feel better when we are down. See if you can volunteer at a local animal shelter- they may need help after a disaster. Once it's safe to return to public parks or natural areas, find a quiet spot to sit in or go for a hike.

Know when to ask for help. Signs of stress can be normal, short-term reactions to any of life's unexpected events- not only after surviving a disaster, but also after a death in the family, the loss of a job, or a breakup.

It's important to pay attention to what's going on with you or with someone you care about, because what may seem like "everyday stress" can actually be:

- Depression (including having thoughts of suicide)
- Anxiety
- Alcohol or Drug Abuse.

If you or someone you know may be depressed, suffering from overwhelming feelings of anxiety, or possibly abusing alcohol or drugs ...

Call 1-800-985-5990 or text 'TalkWithUs' to 66746.

You Are Not Alone.

Figure 8.2 Sample flier

separate panels. If you have more content beyond these three items, you could put all three together on one panel. Of course, if there is much more content for one of these, such as "A," you might have "A" on one panel and "B" and "C" on another. This is all based on your overall content and your aim to appear as orderly as possible.

With the design of the brochure, balance the content and any visuals or graphics. You want to be sure that the look is inviting, pleasant and encourages the user to read the entire document. You should have section headings and subheadings, using bold or italics with larger font size to clearly indicate what the sections and subsections are. Similarly, you want to have a balance of words and any graphics; too many images can detract from the content and too much content can be overwhelming. It's helpful to have a blend of these approaches so your messages are clearly communicated and done so in an attractive manner.

Brochure tips:

- Have a consistent look and feel throughout the brochure. The images and graphics should match the font and should be appropriate for your topic and audience.
- Make sure your visuals work well for your audience; they should not be too simplistic nor too complicated.
- The font should be appropriate for your topic; there are times you want an elegant font, other times you will want a fun font and others still where you need a more serious look.
- You may mix fonts, but make sure this mixture works well.
- The font size should be large enough to be legible, but not too large.
- The font should be easily legible and appropriate for the topic and audience; also, larger fonts are desired for older and younger audiences.
- Make sure there is plenty of white space (but not too much white space); the content should not be too crowded.
- Consider a range of styles, such as paragraphs, boxed narrative, bullet points, numbered items, clip art, photos, graphics and more.
- Use borders to your advantage; you may have a simple (bold line or dotted line) border around a section or box or illustration; you may also have a more festive look for these.
- The design should pay attention to the folding of the brochure; your inside panels should attend to the natural fold lines or creases with the brochure.

As you work with preparing the brochure, again, you want the computer to "work for you," and to have the look that you are trying to achieve. You might consider preparing different versions of this, whether with different color combinations, different fonts, different levels of graphic content, or substituting paragraphs of narrative with bulleted points. As you work with others to review your drafts, you'll get further input and guidance about what might be most appropriate.

In preparing the brochure, be sure that it appears credible, something that can be done in several ways. First, clearly identify the sponsor of the publication; if you are preparing this for an organization or agency, make sure its name, address, website, phone number and logo are clearly included. It can also be done by having references (e.g., on the back panel). You may also include quotes from experts (such as a doctor for health and safety issues, or a traffic safety specialist for motor vehicle topics). Consider having other websites that you believe would provide additional helpful information, as well as credible national or state organizations or agencies.

Another aspect that is important is to make sure that the spelling and grammar are accurate. You want a clean look, so that words or sections of the narrative do not disappear or get cut off. It's helpful to have someone else look at drafts of your materials as you prepare it. Similarly, as you prepare the materials, many computer programs automatically incorporate hyphenation; with this feature, the program may hyphenate most words in a short paragraph, something that can be quite distracting to the reader. Thus, consider turning off that feature, changing words to reduce hyphens from occurring or forcing the spacing when a hyphen is not needed. Of course, with any change you make, new areas of concern can occur, so continue to double-check your work.

A final thought about the brochure incorporates the frustration that many health specialists have with communicating about their topic. They, and you, are typically quite passionate about their area of specialization; you will know a lot of content, have many facts and will want to incorporate as many of them as possible. However, you are limited to a specified amount of space; this finite space is such that everything that you want to include will not fit. Or, if the content does fit, it may be so small in size, or jam-packed with content, that it is actually unattractive and unusable, and thus ineffective in meeting your needs. Just acknowledge this balance, and emphasize the key points for your audience. You may refer the reader to your organization's website for more information, and you may also point out other helpful resources and places where they can go. Further, consider the use of a QR code, as introduced in Chapter 5; with this QR code, a reader can link directly to a website and receive more information. Not only does the presence of this code suggest permanence and credibility, but it also provides you with the opportunity to continually update information and provide the latest in resources on the topic being addressed. You may decide to incorporate the QR code on your brochure, with a message that says "come back each month for the latest information on this topic"; in this way, you can have a permanent web location accessed by a reader using the QR code and then update the information. This can encourage them to keep coming back to the website, simply to see what is new, which thus helps reinforce your message and enhances the opportunity for you to achieve your desired goals.

Some logistical tips about printing:

- As you design the material, consider how it will be printed. If you have color that goes up to the edge, make sure the printing capability you access is able to accommodate this. You may have a color that you want to definitely go up to the edge; that may require you to print on paper that is larger than the content and then cut the paper. Of course, this can add costs to the production.
- With color, you can include different intensities of a color, so these complement one another. This may be done with borders, or with different aspects (box, panel, section) of the brochure; you can use the "transparency" feature in the computer program, which adjusts the level of intensity. Having the same basic color, and different intensities, allows for cost-savings when printing because this requires different screening and not different ink.
- To get some of the effect of color, you might have your brochure printed on some colored paper; whether this is a basic color (e.g., blue, green, yellow) or a brighter color (such as a neon look); this can be quite a cost-saving.
- If you do print in black and white, then consider the shading process, using various gray tones. This can give the impression of more gradation than the straightforward solid black ink.

- Another thought about color is how you will make copies and the financial and physical resources you have available. This is also related to the size of the printing job that you will be undertaking. It's helpful to do some cost analysis of this, based on your needs and your distribution plans. If you are printing large quantities, you'll undoubtedly want to involve a professional printer. For smaller quantities, you may find it easier and much cheaper to do the printing using a single color printer rather than having copies made from an original. With the decreasing cost of printers, two-sided printing of a color brochure can be relatively inexpensive.
- A final thought about printing is with the selection of paper. You might find it helpful to use paper that is other than the standard white copier paper; consider heavier paper stock (index paper), knowing that it can be more challenging to fold in a crisp manner. Also consider glossy paper, which can sharpen the image on the brochure.

The last area to consider with a brochure is to move beyond the traditional tri-fold brochure with six panels, printed on paper that is the standard size of 8½" × 11". A variation on the traditional six-panel brochure is with the layout of the inside panel. The discussion thus far in this chapter is with six separate panels. However, the layout of the inside three panels can be modified. First, look at the entire inside panels (the 8½" × 11" sheet) as a template within which you can work. One thing to do is to have a banner that goes across the entire top of the inside panels, while the rest of the inside maintains the three distinct panels. Another is to have a banner cover two of the panels. You can also blend the panels, so that you have one larger panel (perhaps covering the first and second panels inside) and have the third panel maintain its original shape. You may also have boxes of information, some of which float across the fold lines and others which don't; similarly, you may have boxes that are not perpendicular; these may be offset, one from another. Any range of approaches can be used here, which simply require you to use your imagination and then guide the computer support services to generate the look that you want to have for your materials.

Here are some other specific tips that extend the nature of and creativity for the product you prepare:

- Prepare the brochure as a self-mailer. This would have the back panel prepared with a return mailing address and a panel for affixing mailing information and postage, and then seal them shut. This process eliminates the need for an envelope and getting them stuffed for mailing.
- Use a legal sheet of paper—8½" × 14"—or some other specialty size. You can still do a tri-fold brochure; while the end product won't fit into a standard mailing envelope, it can be very useful.
- With legal paper, you can now consider preparing a brochure with eight panels rather than six, resulting in a different folding process.
- Consider, with the 8½" × 11" paper, folding it only once. This would then be a bi-fold brochure, a four-panel brochure (cover, two inside panels, back). This negates the "stand-alone" panel.
- With this single-fold, four-panel brochure, incorporate a lip on the right side; this means folding the paper off-center to allow words (vertical format) or imagery to appear. Remember that this would be visible with the cover of the brochure, although it is actually printed on the inside, right panel.

- Consider having the brochure with a landscape orientation when opening it. Since brochures are typically vertical, you may flip the brochure, and have the bottom be 8½", and then have the brochure open upwards. Just as with the previous example, you could have a lip on the bottom, with words or images that are visible from the cover but also visible when opening the brochure.

In overview, the preparation of a brochure is an excellent starting place for each of the other print publications with which you may become involved. This is seen as a type of focal point for thinking about health and safety communications. Brochures are commonplace and, with practice, become relatively straightforward to do. They do require a lot of detailed work and refinement, but that also gives you the opportunity to refine and revise and incorporate what you believe to be helpful and appropriate.

You can have fun experimenting with various looks and content, to see what works best in achieving your specified aims with your identified target audience. As you become more and more familiar with communications approaches, you will notice and be increasingly attentive to know–feel–do strategies used for any of a range of products or topics; you will find approaches that you think work, as well as those that you think could be improved upon significantly. Your exposure and experience, as well as your innovative approaches and commitment to achieving your goals more effectively, will sustain you through this process of materials development.

Pamphlets and booklets

Dovetailing the brochure is a straightforward expansion of this process—a pamphlet or booklet. While a **pamphlet** can also refer to a brochure (which would be a small pamphlet), the intent in this section is to look at a publication that is longer than the brochure. This would be a multiple-page publication that is compiled and put together (e.g., with a booklet stapler or binding machine). A pamphlet usually focuses on a single topic or issue.

The pamphlet or booklet is intended to provide much more detail on the specific topic. Often these can be viewed as briefing papers, white papers, background documentation, how–to guides, handbooks and more. While some of the same principles and know–feel–do strategies identified for the brochure apply, the main distinction surrounds its length and how the content gets accommodated. With the brochure, you are limited to a finite amount of space; you have one piece of paper to open with six panels (or four or eight panels) within which to condense the necessary information. You are being efficient with your use of words, the overall quick view is important and you want to be both brief and complete. That is often a challenge, as you may want to say so much more, but don't have the space in which to do that.

With the booklet, the overall length will be determined based on various factors: what level of detail and content is needed for the audience and your purposes, how much there is to say, what length you envision as appropriate (not too little and not too much), your budget, your distribution plans and the overall look that you desire. With the booklet, the format will depend on your audience and your purposes; you will find booklets that have a lot of white space; this helps break up the narrative in a visually attractive way.

Just as with the brochure, the booklet may be prepared with different size considerations. If you want the booklet to be the size of a regular sheet of paper (8½" × 11"), then use 11" × 17" paper and fold it in half. You may similarly use the 8½" × 11" paper and fold it in half, resulting in a booklet that is 5½" × 8½". Or, with an 8½" × 14" paper, your booklet would be 7" × 8½". Knowing how you plan to use the booklet, and the nature of the content to be included, will all factor into your specific design considerations (see Figure 8.3).

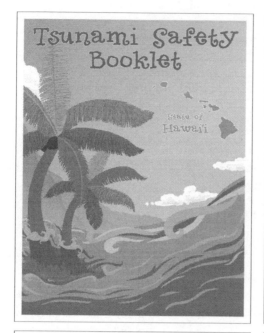

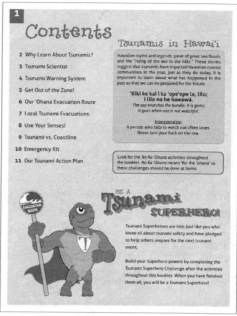

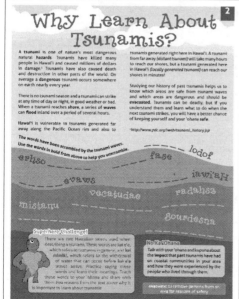

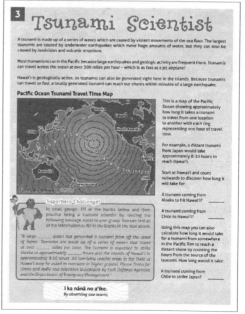

Figure 8.3 Booklet designed for kids (4 of 12 pages)

Here are some specific design factors that can be helpful for a booklet:

- Have text on every page, typically presented in paragraph format.
- Include wide vertical margins on the left and/or the right side of each page of the booklet.
- Include a key sentence or pull-out quote for each page; this may be embedded within the paragraph or it may be in the margins.
- Have clear pagination as well as section and/or sub-section headers.
- Incorporate visuals to help with the look of the publication. These can be graphs, tables, charts, pictures, images.
- Use graphic design elements to make the pages visually attractive and hold together.
- Include summary segments, whether it is an outline at the beginning or a summary and next steps segment at the end of a section.
- Use color and shading.
- Have consistent approaches within sections.
- Include a front and back cover using index stock paper, or something more substantive than the remainder of the booklet.

Putting together the booklet can be done in several different ways, depending to a large extent upon the size and thickness of the publication. With something that is eight panels (two pieces of paper, both sides, with a half page for each panel), 12 panels, 16 panels and often more, you can use a specialty stapler, which is basically a stapler with a long arm. This is called a booklet stapler or a long reach stapler and allows you to staple the publication along the center "spine"; you would typically use two or three staples to hold it together firmly.

Another way of preparing the booklet is to use a binding machine; this can be done with a GBC brand machine, which punches about 20 horizontal holes in each page and uses a plastic spine to hold the pages together. You can also have a coil used for the binding, something known as a VeloBind, and other processes. Some of these can involve equipment that you can have in your office, and others may be more suitable for having a professional in an office supply store or printing shop do on your behalf. Just as with the brochure, it depends on how many you will be making and how often you will be doing it. For example, you may want to have just a dozen booklets prepared for a specific purpose; if you owned a binding machine, you could assemble these in your own office setting, thus minimizing costs as well as allowing for last minute changes to the content of the product.

What binding does to a publication, such as a brochure or booklet, is to make it much more professional looking. You could easily print something on 8½" × 11" paper and staple it in the upper left hand corner; however, having a spine or a different format with a staple, and a cover with thicker paper, communicate greater professionalism. If you have your own binding machine, in particular, you might find it helpful to prepare individual documents with binding; this may be something like a briefing book, some background information, a series of tables and charts, or other documents that you are using with a workshop, a public presentation or a briefing with a key official or executive. You can design your own cover for these publications, helpful for your purposes as well as for gaining the support of those with whom you are communicating; again, printing these on more substantive paper, such as card stock, can more easily suggest more permanent, credible and important content. This type of packaging communicates to others a type of professionalism that just isn't done as well when those same materials are included loosely in a folder or a three-ring binder.

Fliers and posters

As you think about other types of print materials, consider having a **flier** or a **poster**, or a series of these items. Both a flier and a poster comprise a single sheet of paper. The basic difference between these two publications is that fliers are much smaller in format, while posters are larger. You might generally think of a flier as 8½" × 11" and as something that might get posted on a bulletin board. Posters might be 20" × 30", or 24" × 40", or some other size. The specifics will depend on your overall planning design and how you envision getting these distributed.

Messages from the field

Flier: Spot the Block

Cartoon Network

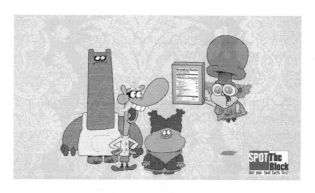

The concept with a flier or poster is generally that of a one-time view for an individual flier per person. As you think about the placement of the flier or poster, think about having the same flier or similar fliers posted in multiple locations throughout an area. If it's on college campus, consider the student union, residence halls, library, dining halls, recreation centers, academic buildings and kiosks. If it's for a community, consider locations such as the library, recreation center, government buildings, public bulletin boards in coffee shops, stores, bus stops, telephone poles, trash cans and other appropriate settings for reaching the potential audience you seek.

Be sure that your locations are those that are allowed; to do otherwise may result in consequences that are not advantageous to the sponsoring organization, including a reputation as a group that does inappropriate things. Some locales require advance permission, even with an approval stamp, before a flier or poster can be posted. Further, some allow for posting only for a specified period of time. Thus, if you choose to do this, you may need to replace the poster or flier on a regular basis.

As you design the flier or poster, many of the same design factors found with brochure preparation are important. What is different is that you are attempting to communicate your message in a clear and concise manner in space that is even more constrained.

For fliers in particular, it's important to think about the concept of "positioning" outlined earlier in Chapter 5. The simple way of thinking about this is "What will help your flier stand out from the dozens or more other fliers around it?" This could be the color (you might use a neon color, if most others are not neon; or you might use a photo or graphic image, if that helps it to stand out).

It could also be the placement of the flier—like at eye level. Or, it could be that you post several of these together and these might be arranged in some format such as six in a circle, or nine in an "X" format. If you have several versions of the flier, arrange them together. You may use words in a particularly large font, or a font that is unique when compared with other fliers typically found in that setting. Much of this is true for posters, too, except that they would be of the size that having several together probably just wouldn't work out well.

Other more non-traditional settings exist for posters and fliers. You may be familiar with these in restrooms. Sometimes, a poster or flier will be placed above a paper towel machine or hand drier, or even above the sink on the mirror itself; this would probably be about the importance of washing your hands thoroughly. These may be placed on the inside of the door to the toilet stall, or above the urinal. These still need to be attractive, but because of their placement they don't need to attract the attention of the reader in the same way; they can thus be a bit more content heavy.

One strategy often used with posters is having the content incorporated in an info-graphic. This approach conveys a significant amount of content; it also provides the opportunity for the poster to include varied content issues and even visuals that can be sub-divided into numerous distinct posters, each with focused content.

Messages from the field

Poster: Alcohol Awareness Month infographic

Foundation for Advancing Alcohol Responsibility

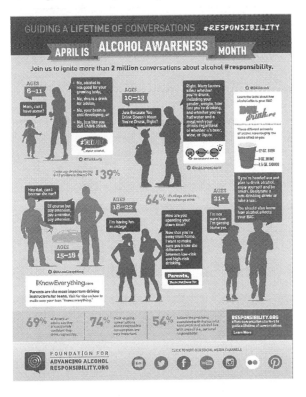

Here are some suggestions that may help with specific formatting of a poster or flier:

- Be eye-catching. Make sure that something catches the attention of the person. Typically, the setting for these fliers or posters is in places where a person is walking by; thus you want to have something that "grabs" them and draws them to read your poster.
- The primary message must be clear. What is it, specifically, that you want the viewer to "know, feel or do?" If it is advertising an event, fine. If it is designed to motivate a person to action, or to suggest a new behavior, these are fine, too. Just be clear.
- Incorporate colors that appeal to your target audience. Further, use these in a way that works within your budget and the way in which these materials will be prepared.
- Consider black ink on colored paper and various shades of gray. This is important if your budget is limited. You might use two colors and use shading for each of the colors to give the impression of a greater breadth of colors.
- Make sure the layout works well together. That includes the images, the fonts, the size of the text, the overall formatting and the look. This should all be consistent within itself.
- Be sure that the sponsoring organization or agency is included. This helps establish credibility of the resource.
- Include appropriate contact information; this includes website, telephone number, location or other relevant information. It will be helpful for this phone number or website to be something that they can remember fairly easily, if this is something they are expected to access later. With the phone number, consider a word or acronym that relates to your topic or issue; also, you might use more digits with the number than the seven necessary for a phone number (after the 800 or area code exchange) so you can have a complete word or phrase.
- You might include a QR code on this; even though the audience is typically a mobile one, if the poster or flier was attractive enough to get them to stop, it may also be intriguing or of interest for them to want to gather additional information.
- Some fliers will include a set of response cards or "tear-off" tab at the bottom; this is so a person interested in the topic or event can have the contact information so follow-up can be easily accomplished.
- Have varying size fonts, with the largest ones being the primary points and smaller fonts being secondary or tertiary points. You might box various items to set them aside or highlight them.
- Incorporate bullets with items of a similar nature, such as key elements, things to remember, specific content items or other like-spirited items.
- Use graphics that help make your point. These can be photos of people or things or settings; they can be clip art or cartoon-type images. They can also be circles and lines and borders and various shapes and colors.

Messages from the field

Wellness print media campaigns

Linda Hancock, Ph.D., Virginia Commonwealth University

A media guru once said, "When everyone else zigs, you should zag." With that in mind, over the past decade, as many types of campus outreach have gone digital, VCU's Wellness Resource Center has found through both process research via mall intercept surveys and through large annual random campus online surveys, that the "Stall Seat Journal" (SSJ) is the most effective way to reach the campus population of 32,000 students and 15,000 faculty and staff.

The *Stall Seat Journal*, as the name implies, is placed on the back of the bathroom stalls or over urinals. It is published monthly with 1200 copies posted across campus and in residence halls. Market saturation studies consistently reveal that only 5–10 percent of students have *never* seen an SSJ, 20 percent skim the headlines, 20 percent read more than half and over half of students read the entire edition (with 20 percent reading it multiple times). Because of its location, the amount of copy in each 11 x 17 poster can be larger than in hallway posters. This allows more space to educate about health concepts, social norms and campus resources.

The *Stall Seat Journal*'s primary purpose has always been to use campus wide data and to publicize the truth about alcohol use and other health behaviors on campus. To avoid "push-back" from an alcohol only focused campaign, the SSJ addresses a plethora of health and safety issues relevant to college students.

The two examples shown here show the synergy between the usual monthly Stall Seat Journal and "The Real Ram's Campaign." The concept is that "Real Rams take charge of their health." The campus mascot is presented as Party Ram, Study Ram, Savvy Sexy Ram or Fit Ram, and social norms statistics from the campus wide survey as well as funny statistics, collected through web polls or clicker polls, are used to engage students in reading about health norms. Examples include "Most students drink alcohol 5 or fewer times per month" and "Most students have 0–1 sex partners per year." The newest ram is "Caring Ram" which is part of VCU's bystander education campaign and works synergistically with the explanation in the Stall Seat Journal teaching how to overcome the bystander effect. There is also a social media element to the campaign #VeryCaringU, utilized in both posters.

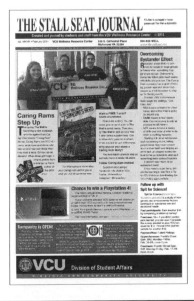
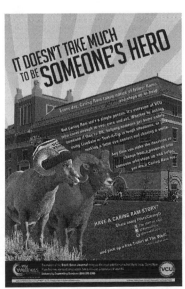

Just as with the brochure, there is no single best approach for preparing a poster or flier. Multiple people creating a flier or poster on a specific topic, with a specific audience, will have varying looks and content. This will be based on their underlying theories and desired outcomes. It will also be based on their specific design interests and what they believe will have the greatest likelihood of having the impact desired. So any number of approaches will certainly be viable. Consider trying out various approaches or looks for your design and content—and, as with any of the health and safety communications approaches, test out these concepts and looks with members of the specified target audience to see what their reactions are.

Messages from the field

Poster: Underage Drinking Prevention infographic

Substance Abuse and Mental Health Services Administration

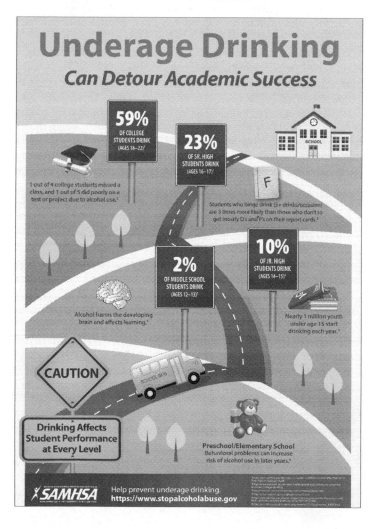

Billboards

Billboards are another print resource, although one that you undoubtedly will be using specialists to prepare. You may be involved with the design, but not the actual publication and posting of these. However, many of the key points identified with posters and fliers will apply to billboards, with a couple of caveats.

First, billboards are typically designed for different types of settings. One of these is next to a highway where the traffic is moving quickly. Another is near a highway or road where traffic may often be stalled or is moving much more slowly. A further is on the side of a building, often frequented by pedestrians as well as motorists.

Second, the general guidelines for preparing billboards will be based on the type of setting. With the high speed traffic setting, it is much more vitally important that the content is very simple, easily understood and not distracting. While the audience may be the passenger in a vehicle, it also can include the driver. You want to be informative and to point the reader of the billboard to a logical next step. If there is a phone number or website that you want the reader to remember, it must be very simple. Remember, the viewing time for billboards typically is very short, and if you are trying to affect a driver, anything to remember must be quite simple. Thus, the number of words included on a billboard will, by necessity, be limited.

In the more urban or slower traffic setting, these general standards can be relaxed a bit. The assumption is that the reader has a bit more time to absorb what is on the billboard, as there may be stopped traffic. Again, it is important to not distract the driver, so the standard about having an easily remembered website or phone number still applies. The number of words and complexity of the billboard can be a bit more enhanced than is found with the setting of the fast-moving highway.

Finally, in the environment that is used primarily by pedestrians, more words can be included. This is not meant as a license to have complicated and wordy billboards; you still want it to be visually attractive and clear, and to engage the reader. You want to attract viewers' attention and then provide them with something that achieves your desired outcomes. You may include a quote, a memorable statistic or question, some images and one or more action steps.

With any of these billboards, it is important that you design it in a way that accomplishes your aim in the most efficient manner possible. You also want to be sure that it is viewed as credible, so including the name and/or logo of the sponsoring organization(s) or group(s) is helpful for accomplishing this.

Complementary print materials

This final section of this chapter highlights many additional types of print materials. This provides an introduction to some of the types of approaches that might be considered. As with other health and safety communications approaches, these are designed to be used in a targeted manner. Many or all of these may be appropriate for inclusion as part of a campaign. Overall, each of these can be prepared as a stand-alone item, which may or may not be part of campaign materials. Your budget and resources may be limited and you might only want or need to prepare the resource for a specific purpose. The intent with this chapter section is to suggest these as possible one-time, periodic or supportive materials that best address your needs. Further, the intent is to generate some creativity in your thinking, as you might think of additional ways in which print materials can be designed and distributed.

Messages from the field

Pinterest board on healthy living

Foundation for Advancing Alcohol Responsibility

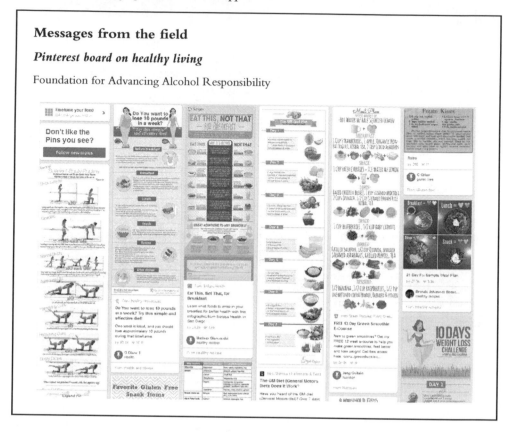

Print materials can be placed in various settings; you've seen them on entry doors for businesses or other buildings, on grocery carts, on gas pumps, on trash cans, on the side of buildings, on the sides or backs of buses, on the top of taxi cabs, on bus shelters, on benches, and more. There may be some places where you haven't seen advertising yet, but that can easily change.

Central to the development of these materials is a good understanding of your audience. As you think about a specific complementary item for printing, you'll want to know what might resonate with them. For example, with an increasingly digital audience, will they have use for a bookmark? Or, for what audiences would a coloring book be most appropriate? Alternatively, you might implement one of these approaches precisely because it is not currently common among the audience. So think clearly about your audience and your aims, and proceed with developing these products.

Further, you'll want to think about your audience and what would be appropriate for them as you identify locations for print materials. What might they use? What could you provide, that could be used for a specific purpose of theirs, yet meeting your purpose? For example, you might prepare something that is attractive and that your audience may want to use as a type of refrigerator magnet (this may be a series of tips or reminders on a specific topic); you might prepare the resource and suggest that they actually prepare the resource in this way, and then show them how to make it viable as a refrigerator magnet by gluing it to magnetic material. This can save you the expense of fully preparing these magnets.

Some general guidelines for these complementary print materials include the following:

- Make the item as visually attractive and functional as possible. The "look" you provide should represent your group or organization well. Remember this item may be the first or only visual image the viewer has of your group, so make sure it communicates an impression you are proud of.
- The item won't necessarily follow all the detailed guidelines found with the more extensive publications, simply because of space limitations.
- It is important that the organization's name and/or logo are clearly displayed on the product. It is also helpful to have contact information, such as a phone number and/or website.
- These can be great places to incorporate a QR code. Since space is limited, the content you offer will be focused. Additional information can be provided through the website linked with the QR code; further, the website content or feature page can be updated as needed.

Here are brief descriptions of numerous print materials that can be considered for use. These may be stand-alone items prepared for your purposes; these also serve as a repertoire of items that can be used, as appropriate, within campaigns (see Chapter 7).

- Bookmark. A bookmark provides brief information about a topic and can be of various sizes. It can be laminated and may include a ribbon or tail. Consider having a bookmark series (someone might collect them all), or different bookmarks on different areas of emphasis within your topic.
- Fact sheet. A fact sheet can be helpful in summarizing important data and research and might also include testimonials. These can be prepared simply, as bulleted or boxed points. They can also be done in a more artistic manner, with angled boxes, different fonts and varying colors. These provide a good opportunity for documenting the research and scientific grounding for your effort and include references, resources, documentation and websites.
- Myths and truths. This is a helpful way of highlighting what is often misunderstood or not known about your topic area. It can be prepared as simply as "Myth" followed by "Truth"; it can be posed as a question ("What is this—myth or truth?"). Be sure to be very clear what the truth is and cite the source so the reader can seek additional information if desired.
- Questions and answers. This can be a helpful approach, particularly with your understanding of the needs of your audience. You can pose typical questions (e.g., "How do I approach my daughter about …?" or "What's the best way to …?"). These can incorporate brief or more detailed responses, depending upon the parameters surrounding the document. These can also be prepared as a series (e.g., one question at a time, with a new question each week). The entire series of questions can be compiled and stored on a website or distributed as a larger package. Additional resource information can also be provided.
- Quiz. This provides the user an opportunity to test knowledge about the topic area. Make sure the correct answers are provided in a convenient way (upside down at the bottom of the page, on another page or on a website); it's also helpful to have the rationale for the correct response provided, so the reader can learn about the reasoning or "why" for the correct response, thus maximizing retention of the content.

- Door hanger. Much like a hotel "Do Not Disturb" sign, the door hanger can be used to communicate key messages. This might be used on a room door, but could also be placed in other settings, such as a shower head pipe, a rear view mirror or a refrigerator door. If used in a shower, it would be useful to have this laminated.
- Magnet. A magnet can be affixed to a metallic item, such as the side of a refrigerator, microwave, toolbox or other metal object. This can have some brief information or a visual image that reminds the viewer about some health or safety issue.
- Activity book. This can provide the user with various ways of implementing the specified health issue. Often helpful for those with responsibilities for a group of people (such as a teacher, a youth group coordinator or a recreation center organizer), this resource can suggest specific ways of helping their audience understand important points with the topic. It may include discussion topics, controversies, issues, little known facts, skill-building sessions, interactive activities, role playing, practice events and much more. It can also include some visuals, whether photographs or drawings.
- Idea sampler. Similar to an activity book, the idea sampler includes ways in which a community group might seek to address the specific health or safety topic. This may include policy initiatives, media know-feel-do strategies, workshop topics, events, sponsorships, letter writing, mentoring, training opportunities and more.
- Stickers. These are small items that communicate a key message very simply, such as the "I Voted" stickers often distributed at polling places. These can vary in content and can be linked to the achievement of a milestone or just for general public awareness.
- "Bill of Rights." Just as with the Bill of Rights referring to the first ten amendments to the U.S. Constitution, your topic may find itself amenable to a similar approach. This can be a non-smoker's bill of rights, a driver's bill of rights, a bicyclist's bill of rights, a community's bill of rights and so on.
- News reports, articles and resources. It may be helpful to distribute copies of selected news clippings or articles. Depending on your purpose, you may wish to distribute entire articles, provided this is acceptable under copyright laws. You may also wish to prepare a brief abstract of selected articles that will be helpful to your audience; be sure to include the full reference so someone can read the entire document if desired.
- Newsletter. The newsletter is a nice blend of various types of information. If this is a periodic resource, have a consistent format (main features or columns) with new content or themes in subsequent editions. The newsletter can include items such as a feature store or topic, myths and truths, frequently asked questions, resources, tips, know-feel-do strategies and more. While prepared as print format, they can easily be stored as a PDF document on a website, as well as prepared in electronic format. Depending on the scope of the reach for this, consider a newsletter that has a generic format for most of its content, but localized content for a portion of it; in that way, a national publication can have regional or local content relevant for the specific user.
- Sample scenarios. This can provide some real-life situations that a person might encounter. These can be framed as a "What if …" or "What to do when…" thus providing the reader with a sense of ways of handling a situation. The discussion following the situation can provide insights surrounding the most healthy and safe approaches, as well as the rationale for that decision. With these, it is also helpful to offer additional references and resources.
- Crossword puzzle. This approach can be a way of illustrating key words or concepts with the health or safety approach. While it can be used as a stand-alone approach, it might also be a feature in a newsletter. This can be geared to the specific age group of individuals to whom the initiative is targeted.

- Coloring book. Having the outline of a drawing on a health topic can be an interesting way of getting youth, in particular, engaged in the topic. The same drawing can be used with different age groups of youth, and results can be gathered by age group; noteworthy are differences in coloring style and ability based on the age group. Further, these completed drawings can be reviewed with a specific one (or one for each identified age group) being selected as a "winner"; the ones selected could be posted in a public location, or even printed in a local newspaper or newsletter.
- Calendar. This provides a way of preparing a variety of messages on your topic, with changing areas of emphasis for each time period covered (e.g., month or quarter). You can have visual images or photographs included that are attractive, so the calendar is used. The content can be part of these images or photographs, but can also be embedded in the calendar itself (e.g., on a tab or section of each month's days).
- Table tent. Typically for placement on restaurant tables, these can provide information about your health topic. Your messages can encompass the entire table tent, or it may be one segment of it with the remainder of the item including some advertising or other promotional approach. The format of this can be one-sided printing that is folded (thus having two sides when it is displayed), or even three sided or four sided.

Forward!

This chapter highlights a wide variety of print materials, from the very traditional to some more cutting edge approaches. Does this encompass all the approaches valid for print approaches? Clearly not. These are commonly used know-feel-do strategies and many, many more could be identified. Also, as highlighted primarily with the complementary print approaches found in the last section of this chapter, many of these can be blended one with another. Further, many of these can be blended within digital media approaches, whether through listservs or websites, Facebook or Instagram, or other platforms. The important thing is that these serve as a foundation or type of "idea tickler" for your consideration as you prepare materials that will work for your communications efforts.

As society evolves toward being more and more digital, a final issue is that there remains a place for print publications that are actually printed and distributed in paper format. Are brochures obsolete? No, they are still used for various purposes, perhaps not as often as a decade or so ago, but still valid. Are posters outdated? No, and for the same reason. As you prepare these, however, realize that it is also important to have a digital presence, such as having your materials available on a website. Your primary approach may, in fact, be digital, but you may wish to have print copies available.

The concept of preparing materials with the general print know-feel-do strategies approach is a helpful starting place. Then, as with all communication efforts, the specific approaches to be used will be based on the various factors of knowing your target audience and its needs and what it accesses, as well as your own organization's budget and resources. Having this variety of approaches as part of your "tool kit" can be helpful for the range of communication efforts in which you engage.

9 Working with the media

Overview

The media plays a tremendous role in society. Simply put, the media provides current news and information, it offers commentary from various points of view, it serves as a watchdog, it offers advertising and it informs the public; certainly, the media does much more than this. Through its efforts, it can help shape the culture.

It is within this context that you want to be as familiar as possible with the media, so you can engage it as a resource for your health and safety communications efforts. Since the media plays a large role with whomever your audience may be, it is important that you acknowledge this, understand something about how it works and learn how you can use the media to support and help promote your efforts.

This chapter provides some insights into the general construct of "the media," so you can identify ways of enhancing your efforts with or without their involvement. By having this insight, you will be better equipped to articulate your message. The **media** is considered the main means of mass communication through use of various traditional approaches, such as newspapers, magazines, radio and television.

The focus of this chapter is on a "non-profit" approach to the media being involved with your health and safety communications effort. That is, there are always opportunities for you or your organization to have your voice heard: you may take out an advertisement by purchasing time on the air (whether radio or television) or taking out an ad in a newspaper or magazine. The focus of this chapter is not upon that approach; rather the emphasis is upon identifying ways in which the media will cover your story and communicate your message, because, you hope, the media will find that your message is also of value to them. This chapter is about you earning media coverage, whether through their initial initiative or by you "asking" for the coverage; in any event, it is up to the media source to determine whether your health and safety communications effort has value for them and is newsworthy or worthwhile for them to address.

Understanding the media

Within the media, you will find a range of venues that are national in focus and those that are more local. For example, you'll find the national news stations, such as NBC, CBS, Fox, ABC and CNN; indeed more stations do exist. Also with the initial five of these, you will find local affiliates, with local news bureaus. Similarly, you will find newspapers that are national in scope (*USA Today*), but also those that are locally prepared but have a national flavor (such as the *New York Times*, the *Washington Post* and the *Los Angeles*

Tribune). Then there are those that are strictly local, including local news and having a local audience. Similarly, you will find there are magazines with a national, regional or local emphasis. The same is true for radio shows; some are prepared locally and distributed to select markets nationally, some are national and others remain entirely at the local level.

Beyond these traditional media approaches, other venues or areas considered to be media are emerging. You might consider webinars to be subsumed under media; similarly, a blog or a social networking approach may be media focused. These are increasing in number and scope and are highlighted in Chapter 12.

Attention here is not on entertainment, sports, fashion or other specialty topics (and this is true whether it is television, radio, newspapers or magazines). Rather, attention is on the media with which you have an opportunity to communicate your message. This includes news media as well as other discussion opportunities, talk shows, columns or related approaches. The primary emphasis in this chapter is upon the media as an entity whereby you can communicate your health or safety message in an effective and appropriate way.

The final thought with respect to the media has to do with its general structure. In short, media outlets and their success or viability are based on profits and/or ratings. Even the non-profit, public-oriented stations (such as public radio or public television) have to pay for staff and equipment, as well as other expenses. The standard media outlets are driven to a large extent by profit (or at a minimum, breaking even); that in turn is driven by ratings. These two elements—profit and ratings—have a symbiotic relationship, whereby higher ratings can bring higher charges for air time (e.g., advertising) and higher quality programming. If a show's ratings are high, that means that there are more viewers or listeners, which then means that there is greater value attached to advertising in that particular medium or market. This issue of profit and ratings will come to bear, as you learn more about ways of getting your health or safety message communicated effectively and appropriately in this setting.

What the media likes

Within this context of the media, what are some of the things that the media likes, and by inference what does it not like? Of course, this will vary by setting, as you have undoubtedly encountered different "flavors" or styles of media as you have become engaged with different sources. Knowing the preferences of different media approaches, whether in print or on air, will make a difference with how you become engaged with media personnel.

From an overall perspective, media like those stories that have appeal to the audiences they serve. Building on the theme of profits and ratings, the audience for different media approaches will vary, depending on their defined mission. If you consider a magazine dealing with a specific sport, it will have a targeted audience different from that for a magazine dealing with cooking (although there might be some overlap). Similarly, a media outlet or broadcaster may have a particular point of view (you've undoubtedly heard clear differences of opinion, and even the facts, on the same topic from radio commentators who are more conservative, as contrasted with those who are more liberal). That doesn't mean that your voice may not be heard, but rather that you may find different levels of receptivity to what you have to say with different media outlets. The point is that you may have a specific viewpoint that you'd like to get communicated, and it may find greater receptivity in one venue when compared to another venue.

A related perspective on this is that media outlets typically "know their audience," as they will seek to incorporate content that is, in their opinion, most salient and appropriate for their audience. Just as the model for health and safety communication stresses the need for you to know your audience, the media is faced with the same set of priorities. It is your job, as a health communicator, to know the media outlet's audience in order to know which ones are most appropriate for you to communicate your message. For example, you may know that the average age of viewers for a particular station is over 50, thus making it inappropriate for a communications initiative about teen pregnancy prevention (unless you seek to reach intermediaries or parents or grandparents).

Within this context, the media source will like stories that have appeal to their specific audience. They will prefer a story that will create higher ratings and larger audiences. For your health or safety initiative, you will want to present it, through the various approaches identified in this chapter (and more), in ways that maximize this appeal. This may mean rethinking your message or reframing it so it has clear appeal to the media's decision-makers.

Another factor that is helpful is a story that illustrates or stimulates debate, controversy, conflict and different points of view. This can be a factor that helps a media source want to sponsor an article or discussion. There are numerous controversies within the arena of health and safety; this is a way you can position your issue or story in a way that becomes more newsworthy from the media's perspective.

The media typically likes something that is new or fresh. This can be ground-breaking science, a new perspective on an issue, a different way of thinking about the topic, a blending of different approaches or some other strategy that is intriguing or interesting for their audience. Media sources are typically not interested in an old story, particularly if there is nothing especially new or different with what you are suggesting. The media typically doesn't want to report on something that has already been reported, unless there is a different twist or orientation for it. They want something that has some new or interesting perspectives, so that they stand out from other media sources. Consider the issue of their ratings and how your story, if it is covered, will be perceived by their potential audience. Some personal, human interest perspective can also be helpful in providing a news slant that is attractive to the media source; this could be revisiting a store from a month earlier, or a year ago, and following up on the individual(s) cited in that story to see what is different, or new, with them. Thus, as you organize your thoughts about your issue for communication, think about what might be viewed as "new" or "different" or "fresh" rather than the "same old, same old"; the latter certainly would not be picked up by the media, so it must be avoided. Blending some of this with earlier content in this book on specific tools and resources, the tool of linking and pairing (Chapter 5) is something that can be helpful as you present your approach for consideration by the media.

Another element essential for working with the media is to be sure your information is accurate. You want to be certain that you provide specific, detailed information to the extent that the media would like. You want to provide as full an accounting of the data as possible and not exaggerate. While the media may condense what you offer for the outlets they deem appropriate, you want to provide clear and truthful information; it should be accurate and complete. If the media sponsor chooses to not report on some part of what you think is important, you want to determine if that is misleading or inappropriate. Generally, the media has limited space or time and strives to boil down a story to the key elements, from their perspective. If you are not satisfied, you may then complain, or you may choose to not engage with them in the future; however you handle this after the incomplete reporting is up to you. What is important is that, when you engage initially with the media, you are accurate and complete.

Finally, the media likes prompt responses. While you may prefer to wait to respond, thinking about whether to get involved and carefully crafting your response (or getting approval to submit a response), the opportunity to be connected with the media source may pass you by. If you do choose to be engaged with the media, then it is important to do so in a timely manner. Very often, media sources have their own limited resources and work on a timeline. While some media efforts are built over a period of weeks or months (e.g., preparing the background information for a story), others are done in a matter of hours or days. Thus, if you are contacted by the media and you want to be involved, respond promptly. Also, since media personnel are typically over-extended with too many issues or stories to cover, you want to be sure you are efficient with use of their time; thus, make sure that you have your key points outlined ahead of time and have resources ready to share promptly.

The important concept here is that the media is looking for ways to enhance their own readership, their ratings and their profit. To do so, they want to cover things that help them accomplish their mission. Remember that different media sources have different priorities, as well as different orientations. So you want to be persistent with your efforts to get coverage in the media source.

Also, realize that one media source will often be looking at other media sources to find ways that the issue can be addressed by them. Thus, to have an article in a local paper may be just fine, as it could have a broader reach by being picked up by a national news source and distributed widely. The local article may also be seen by a national newspaper, or magazine, which then wants to go deeper with the topic; in that case, you may be contacted for further information. Also, it may not be you who gets contacted, but the fact that you (or your organization) had some coverage at the local level may stimulate coverage of the issue on a larger scale. In a similar way, coverage in a local or national newspaper may result in a television station, talk show, discussion panel or other media outlet deciding that they want to cover the issue, within their parameters of media reach. You never know where the media interaction that you have can take you or your issue; the important thing is that you feel grounded with your interaction with the media. Further, should you want to be gaining media coverage for your effort, you should always be "ready to go!"

Media relations

The concept of "media relations" encompasses the overall activities that you have with professionals in the media. **Media relations** is working with the media to inform the public of your organization's important communications in a positive, consistent and credible manner. The emphasis here is primarily on the proactive side of the media. It's about you thinking how you can get the media involved in your issue or cause, so they will want to cover it. It's about being continuously vigilant with your efforts to engage the media with your activity, so that they will respond to your requests or will initiate contact with you at the appropriate time. It's about building relationships and nurturing these.

With the media, your aim is to get them to provide coverage for your topic or issue. You want to get the media involved with supporting your efforts, whether it is through preparing a news article, writing a feature story, sponsoring a public service announcement you provide, printing an article you wrote, offering their opinion through an editorial, sponsoring an event or some other approach. This requires that they know about you and your effort; it also means that they must trust and respect you and your organization as viable resources.

One way of building quality relations with the media is to involve media specialists or public relations specialists, if your organization is of the size and nature to have one. Some organizations may just be too small to be able to afford this type of specialty role; others may not prioritize this type of media or public relations specialist. Through this chapter, the emphasis is on preparing you to work directly or indirectly with the media; in either case, it is helpful for you to understand the various factors associated with getting your issue covered by the media. If your organization has a media specialist, then you may rely upon the individual(s) in that division to handle this; your organization may also have a policy that only those specialists will talk directly with the media. All of the specific circumstances depend on your situation and your resources. In any event, the considerations throughout this chapter are helpful to maximize a positive interaction with and support by the media.

If you are in an organization that has media personnel to serve as a liaison with the various media sources, it is incumbent upon you to build your relationship with those specialists. They are the ones with the expertise to know what may be newsworthy and with whom. They will know how and when to prepare media releases, who should be contacted and when to do so. There are times that a media source is looking for a content expert or a person with specialized knowledge on a specific topic, to help provide background information or examples for an article or show on which they are working; you may be contacted by your media specialist (your representative) to see if you are willing and available to provide this resource to the media person. In a similar way, your organization's media specialist may be seeking ways to communicate your message, and that of your organization, to the media; they will continually "pitch" the message to the media and try to generate interest. All of this means that you must develop awareness on the part of your media specialist about your interest in and availability for having direct conversations with the media.

As this occurs, whether with an intermediary or on your own, you may find that you are contacted about topics or a part of your issue for which you believe that you are not the expert, you are not up–to–date or current with the latest information, or you are not the most appropriate resource to interact with the media. It is important that you are honest with this. You may state (to your media specialist or directly to the media source) your concerns about your limitations; they may decide that your perspective is, indeed, what they want, or that they find it helpful. What you are doing by being honest is building the longer-term relationship. This can serve you well as future opportunities arise for obtaining coverage for a topic or issue.

Another consideration with media relations is to be timely in your responses. Again, whether it is with a media specialist in your organization, or directly with the media sources, be prompt with returning calls or inquiries. Media personnel are very typically on a deadline, often having only a matter of hours to complete their article. You also want to be efficient with the information and resources you send them; you may have a single follow-up call, but not multiple calls, as that suggests that you were not fully prepared.

With the media source, there is always negotiation with some of the logistics. If you demonstrate your interest in and ability to cooperate with their parameters, you may gain greater respect for getting your voice heard now, as well as in the future. For example, if you are asked to participate in a television or radio interview, you may find that it requires some juggling in your schedule or location to accommodate it. If you are traveling and not available for a television studio or camera appearance, consider calling in using an internet broadcast connection (e.g., Skype) or from a land line, and ensure that your location is quiet. If it's voice only, you may have a photo displayed on air (as if you were a foreign correspondent); this can be obtained from a website where your photo is available. What this requires is your flexibility and adaptability to be included, through knowing and respecting the constraints of the media and also seeking to maximize your exposure and your reach.

In building media relations, you want to be respectful of the media personnel's decision to not cover an issue or event. Recalling what is important to the media, you may want to frame your issue within the context of what might "sell" from their vantage point. You don't want to badger a media contact, as that certainly won't be helpful in building a longer-term relationship with them. You may, and probably will, strongly believe that your story is important; while that is your perspective, it may not be shared widely, or at least by the media. It is incumbent upon you to be persuasive about why this issue should be covered; again, using the tools identified earlier can help frame your point of view.

With your interaction with the media and promoting quality media relations, try to think about the longer-term relationship you want to develop with the media. You may want to have coverage of your event in the more immediate future. However, if this does not seem viable from the perspective of your media specialist or the media personnel directly, consider deferring your request until another, more appropriate time. You may find that it can be more "newsworthy" when linked to something external, such as an awareness week or day; further, and sadly, there may be a tragedy at the local or national level with which you can link your initiative.

You may be in an organization that does not have a media specialist; this is very often the case with non-profit or community groups and particularly so with small organizations. In that situation, the media relations are done by you or a colleague. Focusing now on a direct relationship you may have with a media person (just like a media specialist would have), you may wonder how you can accomplish this.

Messages from the field

OMG, the media wants an interview!

Anne Atkins, Former Public Relations Official, Virginia Department of Veterans Affairs, Virginia Department of Motor Vehicles

Don't panic. Media interviews offer a great way to get your message out to thousands of people at no cost to you. But, to make the most of an interview, plan carefully.

- Identify a single message or point you want to make. Don't muddy your message with multiple topics.
- Tell the viewers or listeners what action you want them to take. For example, don't drink and drive.
- Make a list of all the questions a reporter might ask and have answers ready.
- Check the newspapers, web, radio and TV to see if there are other stories about your topic. Is there a unique point you can make about your story that distinguishes it from the others?

Many drunk driving campaigns emphasize the death toll resulting from drunk driving. However, the Checkpoint/Strikeforce campaign takes a different perspective by focusing on the consequences of being arrested and getting a DUI conviction. Like Checkpoint/Strikeforce, look for something that makes your message stand out from the rest.

One of the know–feel–do strategies is to prepare a press release. This is a brief announcement about an upcoming or recent event or service and provides information about this. It may trigger someone from the media to actually be present at the event, and it may also provide awareness to media personnel that this event or service is available. They, then, may follow up on this. More details on the specifics of this are provided elsewhere in this chapter.

Another approach is to call the media source directly. You may be contacted with one of several departments there, depending on the size of that media organization. Of course, if it's a small organization, just a call may put you directly in touch with the right person. You may ask for the news desk, the features department, the health division or other relevant group. At that point, you provide a brief introduction to your initiative and determine if this is the proper person with whom you should be talking. It's important to try to build the relationship quickly and also to be cognizant and respectful of their limited time to hear what you have to say. You'll want to get to the essence of your request fairly quickly, whether that is to cover an event, to be aware of a resource or service, or to take a stand on your health issue (e.g., through a feature story or editorial). If the media source is interested, you may be asked for more information, as well as to provide follow-up documentation and resource information. That's all good, as it is the beginning of a relationship that may result in what you want—coverage. It is very possible that the media person may not be interested in the issue, at least not at the present time; again, the emphasis should be on building the relationship and hoping there will be an opportunity to become engaged with them in the future.

A related approach is to call a specific individual. You may identify the appropriate person because you found their name associated with a specific title or department (e.g., on a website) and they seem like the most appropriate person to whom to reach out. Or, you may see that they authored an article on a related topic; for example if they covered sexual assault recently or in the past, and your issue is that one or something related to it, you might contact them directly. At that point, you may ask if they are the proper person and if not to direct you to the best person (there may be other specialists and individual assignments may have changed). If you have comments about the previous coverage, particularly positive ones or even gaps you noticed, you might briefly note these as a way of gaining their attention to what you have to say. Then, just as with the call to the general media office contact, pursue the conversation with a succinct version of your request.

With any of these approaches, you may find that you are not linked directly to a person, but to a voice mail system. You may decide to wait and call back, rather than leave a message, because you find that you are more effective with direct human interaction. However, it may be best for you to leave a brief message, highlighting the essence of your request and, hopefully, establishing some intrigue for a level of interest in your issue. As noted in Chapter 10, this is the perfect opportunity for the "elevator speech" that is quite brief and to the point.

Press releases and news announcements

Called a **press release**, a news release, a press announcement, a video news release and more, this is an opportunity to reach out to the various forms of media about something that you deem is newsworthy and appropriate for the attention of the news media (see Figure 9.1). This is a vehicle that can stand alone; it can also be part of a campaign (see Chapter 8) or can serve to support many of the other know–feel–do strategies highlighted in this book, such as workshops or speeches.

The Disaster Distress Helpline 1-800-985-5990 provides immediate crisis counseling to people affected by the Pulse Nightclub shooting in Orlando Florida

✗ samhsa.gov/newsroom/press-announcements/201606120500

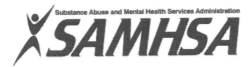

Substance Abuse and Mental Health Services Administration

Sunday, June 12, 2016

A disaster or tragedy is unexpected and often brings out strong emotions. The Disaster Distress Helpline 1-800-985-5990 can provide immediate counseling to anyone who needs help in dealing with the tragic event in Orlando Florida. The Helpline is a 24 hours-a-day, seven-days-a-week resource that responds to people who need crisis counseling after experiencing a natural or man-made disaster or tragedy.

Sponsored by the Substance Abuse and Mental Health Services Administration (SAMHSA), the Helpline immediately connects callers to trained and caring professionals from the closest crisis counseling center in the nationwide network of centers. The Helpline staff will provide confidential counseling, referrals and other needed support services.

"When disaster strikes, people react with increased anxiety, worry and anger. With community and family support, most of us bounce back. Some may need extra assistance to cope with unfolding events and uncertainties," said Acting SAMHSA Administrator Kana Enomoto. "People seeking emotional help in the aftermath of a disaster can now call 1-800-985-5990 or text TalkWithUs to 66746 and begin the process of recovery."

The Disaster Distress Helpline is a national hotline dedicated to providing disaster crisis counseling. The toll-free Helpline is confidential and multilingual and available for those who are experiencing psychological distress as a result of natural or man-made disasters, incidents of mass violence or any other tragedy affecting America's communities. The Helpline complements the U.S. Department of Health and Human Services, the Federal Emergency Management Agency and other disaster response capacities, and is available immediately anywhere within the United States.

The helpline can also be accessed at http://disasterdistress.samhsa.gov/ (link is external) and TTY for deaf and hearing impaired: 1-800-846-8517.

For more information, contact the SAMHSA Press Office at 240-276-2130.

The Substance Abuse and Mental Health Services Administration (SAMHSA) is the agency within the U.S. Department of Health and Human Services (DHHS) that leads public health efforts to advance the behavioral health of the nation. SAMHSA's mission is to reduce the impact of substance abuse and mental illness on America's communities.

Last Updated: 06/12/2016

1/1

Figure 9.1 Sample press release

Typically, the preparation and distribution of a press release is handled by an organization's public affairs unit or media specialist, if, as noted above, the organization has one. If your organization does not have this specialty office, then your responsibility is to do this in as professional a manner as possible, as you are serving as the de facto media relations unit for your organization.

Messages from the field

Don't settle for a good news release, write a great one

Anne Atkins, Former Public Relations Official, Virginia Department of Veterans Affairs; Virginia Department of Motor Vehicles

Write a great news release by picking an angle. For example, rather than writing that traffic fatalities are up by 5 percent, look at the statistics to find out why they're up or if they are up in a specific population. You may find that teen fatalities increased more than any other age group. Use that as your angle. Focus on teen fatalities in your headline and first paragraph, then fill in with information about overall fatalities.

Five tips for writing a news release:

- Start out strong. Use a compelling headline and put your most important information in the first three or four sentences. For example, if you are announcing a child safety seat check, answer the questions what, when, where and who in the first sentence or two.
- Explain why this news is important. In the child safety seat check example, explain that, according to the National Highway Transportation Safety Administration, 75 percent of children are riding in car safety seats that have been installed incorrectly. Boost the power of your release by adding that traffic crashes are the leading cause of death for children age 12 and under.
- Use quotes. In the child safety seat example, a quote from local law enforcement about the importance of child safety seats would be ideal.
- Keep it short. Double-space your copy and keep the release to one or two pages. The purpose of the release is to interest reporters in writing a longer story or providing additional coverage.
- At the end of your release, provide information about your organization, give your contact information and where reporters can find additional information about your topic.

The press release is designed to let the media know about something—an upcoming event, a new resource or service, an activity or something specific for which you or your organization would like some media coverage. The media may decide that they do want to send resources to cover the event, or that there is something newsworthy that warrants an interview or further attention. For something that may not be time-sensitive (such as the inauguration of a new service), the media may decide that they want to cover it as time permits.

When you write your press release or news announcement, it can be used in any of several ways. First, it may inform the media of the event or service. Second, the written announcement may be posted in its entirety in the media source, whether in a print publication or on a media website. Third, the announcement may be shortened and distributed. Finally, the message, in its entirety or shortened, may be shared more broadly with other media outlets, whether in the region, state or nation, depending on its perceived news-worthiness.

As you distribute a press release, a couple of points are important regarding how it may be received. First, you should know that a media outlet undoubtedly receives many, many press releases every day. Thus, as you prepare yours, make it stand out in some way. Second, there's a fairly typical format for preparing these news releases; you'll want to follow this. Otherwise, while you do want yours to stand out, you don't want to be perceived as not knowing how to prepare a news release properly. Third, even though your announcement may be viewed as newsworthy and the media may plan to have it covered, things do change. Decisions can be made at the last minute, based on what is most time-urgent and most newsworthy. Sometimes commitments that are made for coverage are changed, because something has bumped up in priority, or staffing changes have caused less availability to cover your event. That is often the case with the health and safety communications work, as much of it is proactive and, often, viewed as "optional" or "elective."

Your purpose with the press release is to inform the readership—quickly and succinctly—of your message (whether it is the media itself, or their audience, as described above). You might think of the press release as organized in the shape of a pyramid, with the most important information at the top, and the content then becomes increasingly more detailed as the press release proceeds (and gets lower on the pyramid). For example, the headline's purpose is to engage the reader with the essence, very briefly, of what is to come next. This is followed by additional detail, again in a summary format. Further detail follows this, perhaps with an illustrative quote from an expert or key official; it may also include a brief example as a type of testimonial about the value of the health effort or service, about the need for this and how this resource or approach can be helpful. Additional detail may follow, including paragraphs about background information, resource need, statistics, proposed initiatives and potential impact.

Sending a press release can be done by mail, but it is preferable to send it electronically (thus allowing for easy modifications if needed) or by fax. You want to be sure you have a date on the release, as well as easily found contact name, phone and email address. If you report statistics (which is usually helpful), you want to follow the standard of spelling out numbers less than ten and then using numerals for numbers or percentages that are larger than ten.

When writing the press release, be as active and current as possible. You want to demonstrate action. Typically, use the "who, what, when, where, why and how" approach, thus providing a succinct overview of the important elements of your effort.

Through the press release, your aim is to get some type of action from the media or other audience receiving it. Being clear about what you want them to know, feel or do is important here, just as it is with other health and safety communications efforts. Thus, you want to be clear with the content, be accurate and provide it within a context that is deemed appropriate and actionable. You want to be persuasive and hope the reader (whether media or otherwise) is responsive to your request.

Media advocacy

One way the media can be helpful with your health and safety communications efforts is with their own stands on various topics. The media can work with you and for you, as you seek to advance a policy or environmental shift around your issue or thematic area. In short, **media advocacy** is having a strategic engagement with the media for the purpose of advancing a social initiative or policy effort. Media advocacy is about engaging the mass media as a partner, to help you achieve your cause.

Some examples may be helpful in this regard. If you seek to obtain a smoking ban for a workplace, public area or other setting, the media can be helpful in promoting this. They may use their editorial influence to accomplish this by lending their opinion to the topic. One of the lead media personalities, such as an anchor on a radio or television station, may use his/her influence to weigh in on the topic. There may be an event that occurs and the media offers an opinion, suggesting the need for a more thorough review of policies and procedures, and ultimately, they would hope, an actual policy change. While this may sound like what you or your organization can do, that is precisely what is occurring, except that the media organization itself is taking a stand.

The media can also help advocate a cause by convening a topical discussion about the merits of a policy. Again with the smoking issue, the media may decide that it is timely to have a public debate on the issue, and thus they serve as a host or convener of an event where the pros and cons of the current smoking policy are debated. They may also decide to sponsor an event, such as having a speaker or speaker's series in the community (or, if the media has a national reach, more nationally). The media can basically use its prestige and influence to help achieve the goals that you and your organization ulti- mately have. Further, the media may accept your public service announcements, which may be print ads or audio or video, depending on the venue. They may also be helpful in preparing more professionally done PSAs, which may be beyond the capabilities of you or your organization.

Media advocacy is about policy change. It's not just about informing the public or another audience about a specific health issue or risk, or the availability of a resource. Media advocacy means getting them involved with efforts to modify the policy, with the belief that having a larger scale policy change will be more influential, in the long run, with behavior change.

There is a challenge with media advocacy—and that is if the media decision-makers have a viewpoint that is contrary to what you or your organization wants. If you seek a policy change on some issue—such as aggressive driving, water purity standards, nutri- tion labels or specific safety protocols—and they don't value that as a viable option, then this particular strategy won't work for you. Similarly, the media may have an exact opposite point of view, and their effort may not only not support yours, but may directly oppose your initiatives.

Part of the focus with media advocacy is to use your constituency and your coalitions to promote your message with the decision-makers in the media. You seek to have the media support your efforts, and you want your partners to use their influence with the media personnel also. The focus is on long-term change and not so much with the spe- cific, more immediate know-feel-do strategies with which so many health initiatives are based. With media advocacy, you seek to help set the agenda and framework, and your work (through your media relations activities) is to help the key personnel in the media to see your perspective. Your aim is to be persuasive and grounded, providing solid and current information, using the skills of testimonials, research, framing and pairing so they (the media) are convinced that this is important for them, too. While you will still want your health messages communicated, and while you wouldn't necessarily negate a media source supporting those messages, the ultimate aim with media advocacy is to promote healthy public policies and an overall shift within the environment.

In order to achieve this support, it is important that you work with your media rela- tions personnel in your organization, or directly yourself, to inform the media about the nature and scope of the issue. You need to be clear about the outcome you seek and the specific policies you believe would be helpful and advantageous for your cause. In this sense, you are helping the media to set the agenda. So a large part of the media advocacy process is to get great media attention, in general, provided to the issue. If your focus is healthy nutrition standards, you may work diligently to get the media to cover these issues. Through approaches such as linking and pairing, providing sound research information and promoting individuals who express their opinions with letters to the editor, you can demonstrate to the media officials that the topic is, indeed, newsworthy. As an alternative, if you remain silent, as do your colleagues, then limited attention may be provided to the issue, and then it appears to have limited importance relative to other issues. Thus, it is important to promote awareness of and interest in the topic, more generally.

Following this, you can help show the media how attention to these various issues is actually part of a larger area of concern. That is, you can demonstrate the importance of this specific issue, as part of a larger health or safety concern. With nutrition standards noted above, you may consider showing linkages with obesity, other diseases, learning capabilities and behavior. You can argue that attention to your specific issue would help to set a larger agenda that has a greater likelihood of making substantive structural changes with the area of concern. Involvement by the media at this stage helps demonstrate the need for policy change; the aim here is to persuade the media to take a leadership role in influencing this change. As long as the identified cause is perceived as fitting into the mission of the media source, this role for the media decision-makers can be a logical one. That's the case you want to make, so it appears quite logical and appropriate that they do become involved.

The final aspect with this is that the media personnel actually take a stand. Again, this may be through the sponsorship of an event, or, ultimately, with the endorsement of the health policy you have sought. Typically, this is found in the editorial pages; there may be other things they do as part of the media, including their own specific attention to it (it could be through a televised segment or an ad they take out in their own publication).

Following any involvement of the media, the actual work is not done. At this point, it is up to the policy makers to make their own decision. The media has become involved at a few levels—they have conducted the news activities, with publishing articles. They have decided to publish several op-ed pieces (perhaps yours). An **op-ed** is short for "opposite the editorial page" and is a newspaper article conveying the writer's opinion (see more detail later in this chapter). Further, the media may have orchestrated one event or more. Perhaps they sponsored your public service announcements. They may have taken a public stand, through advertising or editorials. Now it is up to the decision-makers, at the policy level, to make a decision. These may include local elected officials, such as a mayor, a council person, a legislator, or a member of a board of directors; they may be appointed individuals, such as town managers or administrators. They may also be governing bodies, whether elected or appointed. These are the individuals who make a policy decision—the precise outcome wanted from the efforts of media advocacy.

Your role continues, through your work with the media and your media relations activities (such as thanking them for their support, writing a letter to the editor for public attention and even preparing continued op-ed articles). You also continue your advocacy with the policy makers, themselves, through the involvement of you or your organization, or others, making testimony and providing information to them. That's not media advocacy, but it continues the work that you need to do to get the policy finally approved and implemented.

Letters to the editor and op-ed articles

Another aspect of media relations is writing an article that can, hopefully, get published in the newspaper. These include, primarily, letters to the editor. This is when you or someone in your organization (or several of you) write a letter to the newspaper or magazine (or other media source) and express an opinion. Here are some examples:

- You were upset with a certain event that happened locally and thought it should have been handled in a different way.
- You didn't like how the media outlet handled the issue; it may have not provided enough detail, it showed only one side of the issue, it appeared inaccurate or it provoked some other area of concern.
- You have noticed that the media source hasn't provided attention to a certain issue over an extended period of time, giving priority to other issues (that you deem less newsworthy).
- You have a point of view that is relevant, you believe, and should be shared.

These letters to the editor are not "out of the blue"; rather, they are associated with what is occurring in the media or in your surroundings, and you're providing some additional information or perspective that you believe warrants public attention. While it is called a "letter to the editor," its inclusion in the media outlet serves to inform the readership of the resource about your point of view. You are informing and attempting to influence, directly, media leaders (a type of media advocacy), but what you can expect is that this may get the attention of someone in the public. It could, ideally, be a policy maker (or his/her staff member) who affects policy change in your jurisdiction. More realistically, however, you may be trying to establish some public awareness and possibly some debate on the issue. Further, you will be advertising (at no financial cost to you) the organization or agency with which you are affiliated. This type of public awareness also serves as a type of media relation, as the reporter may learn about you or your organization through your public communication; for future articles or stories, they may decide that you are worthy of contacting for your viewpoint and perspective.

A good way to determine how to make your presentation in a letter to the editor is to review those that have been published in the resource with which you want to work. This gives you an idea of the types of arguments that have been made and accepted by the editorial staff. It helps guide you regarding the length, as well as some of the techniques that writers use to present their case.

Then, start writing. What is important in this process is that, if you have something to say, then do so. Start the process by writing down what it is that you want the audience to know, feel or do, as a result of reading your letter to the editor. You'll have a good sense of the length, but don't worry about that at the onset; just write what you believe is important for them to know. Once you have prepared it, then you can start editing your own work. Have someone else read it too, to be sure it communicates what you want to say. With a letter to the editor, timing is important. While you may wish to wait several weeks, to be sure your letter is "just right," this is not advisable as the timeliness will have passed and thus the letter may be viewed as outdated. You'll want to maximize the timing aspect, as well as having a product about which you are proud.

Very often, your letter will not be accepted. That's OK; just keep at it and prepare letters as you deem appropriate and timely. If you think strategically, you can identify periodic opportunities to share your insights and perspectives through your writing.

Related to this are pieces known as "op-ed" articles. This is simply an article that gets published on the page across from the page that has the editorials and letters to the editor. They undergo the same type of review processes that occur with letters to the editor. However, there are significantly fewer of these published and far fewer submitted.

What's different about these articles is that they are much longer than a letter to the editor. You should look in the publication to see the typical length of these; in a newspaper, this may be 12 column inches, presented as two 6" columns in a boxed location. These are much more in-depth and may provide you with the opportunity to make your case much more eloquently than is possible in a letter to the editor. The media sometimes has op-ed articles that were solicited by them; or these articles may be submitted by someone whose name is recognized by the paper's readership. Or, the op-ed piece may be unsolicited and may be from you or your organization.

It could be that you are invited to prepare an op-ed piece; that depends on the nature of the publication and their style. In any event, consider doing an op-ed piece, or having one ready to go that can be timed with something current (which could be a policy, a local event, a tragedy, a state or national initiative, or even a memorable date in history) through the linking and pairing functions noted elsewhere. It's a tremendous opportunity for exposure and you should maximize the opportunity to do this if you can.

Public service announcements

A **public service announcement** (PSA) is something that you want to have aired by the media, at no cost to you or your organization. Simply put, this is an advertisement, but without a budget. Why would a media source want to sponsor a public service announcement? After all, this does not generate income for them. One reason is that, historically, broadcast media were required to air a certain amount of public service announcements. The Federal Communications Commission requires that stations donate some of their airtime to serve the greater good of the public. Why? The radio and television airwaves are publicly owned, thus providing a rationale for some non-commercial use of these resources. The main reason now is that this is good community service for them. If they produce a reasonable amount (unspecified quantity) of public service announcements, this can be viewed to their benefit when they have their license reviewed, or if some ruling or policy affecting them is being considered. If they are viewed as a "good citizen," as evidenced by sponsoring PSAs, then the issue may be more likely to be viewed in their favor.

PSAs can occur with the radio, television and even in print media. Each of these may have different criteria and standards, and it's best to determine what the requirements are before you go to any effort to have these prepared.

When you think about the development of a PSA, you'll be thinking primarily of two main venues: radio and television. PSAs can appear in other locations too, such as a movie theater; you might even see a type of PSA hosted on a billboard, or as signage on a bus or at a bus shelter. While the concept is the same, the approach is what was described when doing these various types of print materials.

Focusing first on the radio, you can do a PSA in written form, or you may have it recorded and ready to play. PSAs are typically in a fixed time limit, and these are specified, so they can be inserted into the broadcast that has its own structure. You may have a 10 second, 15 second, 20 second, 30 second or one minute PSA. Obviously, if it is recorded, you can manage the time very precisely. If you provide a written script, you are specifying on the PSA what the anticipated length is, or how long it would take to read the script. Here, it is important to be honest with the actual time estimate.

For the written script, you'll be necessarily limited by the amount of time you have. Imagine a series of PSAs on a topic, something that would be typical to do when instituting a campaign. You prepare a series of PSAs, all around the same topic, and various lengths are offered. Ideally in the PSA, you want to be sure that the listener has a good sense of what you want him/her to know, feel or do. You want to be credible and clear, and you want to point them to a "next step." You'll also have the sponsor or host agency identified, as well as a follow-on phone number or website. All of that is encapsulated in a brief announcement.

With longer PSAs, you might have a quote, such as from an expert or trustworthy source that is appropriate for your audience. You may have a statistic or two; this is feasible in a short one, too, where you might start it by saying "Did you know that one in two Americans …?" With a campaign, you very likely will have a slogan that is used throughout each of the PSAs, as well as with other approaches you use (such as posters, fliers, fact sheets, billboards and more). Just as with the slogan "Friends Don't Let Friends Drive Drunk" for the impaired driving awareness campaign initiated decades ago, your PSA may have a slogan or tag line included within it.

Moving beyond the print version of the radio PSA, you might prepare an audio version and submit this as a .wav file or on a CD/DVD. This would be pre-recorded and available with the specified length. The advantage of this type of approach is that you could include sounds and voices of your choosing. You may wish to have background sounds (depending on your topic, it could be the ocean waves breaking on the shore, a train passing by, car horns, children playing, a car crash, a baby crying or anything else linked to your topic). These sounds may also include music, whether familiar or not to the listener, to capture the spirit or mood you seek. You may also record specific voices, whether it is a noted personality (such as a celebrity, elected official, sports legend, entertainer or high profile person), an expert (such as a doctor, nurse, traffic safety specialist, educator or other), or specific role (such as a parent or child). You may include one or more voices, depending on how you choose to choreograph the PSA. The PSA may include the sounds and/or voices, as well as any narration that prepares a complete, ready-to-go sound track for implementation at the radio station. This makes it easy for the station to implement and is included within the specified time identified on the PSA. It also adds diversity to the voices, so it is not the same broadcaster's voice reading a script. While it takes more labor to produce this type of product, it also lends itself to a greater potential impact due to its apparent professionalism.

Turning now to the television PSA, this becomes more challenging. However, it remains doable. Typically, your television station will want a relatively high quality PSA to air; this would not be done with the equipment or expertise that most health professionals have at their fingertips. What you do have are ideas, and you can develop a framework for what you want to have implemented as a television PSA.

As a starting point, think through this approach just as you would with other health and safety communications approaches. Think about the radio PSA, developed as an audio file for sharing with the station, but now do an overlay with visuals. As you think about the time for this (e.g., 30 seconds), think also about how you want that time spent with the PSA. You're thinking about the overall sequence of messages and images and sounds. You will probably end with a call to action, as well as specific next steps (such as a website or phone number). The rest of it will be up to you. Will you start with a dramatic beginning, or will you have a soft and slow build-up to your main point? Will there be a variety of fast-moving pictures (e.g., 20 pictures in 10 seconds)? Will you include pictures of scenes as well as of people? Will there be people talking? Consider the same situation with experts or "typical" adults or kids, as you did with the radio PSA. Will you use movie clips as part of the PSA? Will you use pictures? If so, how will these be displayed—will you have a montage of pictures, or will you have pictures that seem to move on the screen (e.g., using the Ken Burns effect, where the emphasis seems to zoom in or out of a picture, or pans the picture from one side to the next, thus giving the illusion of movement)? How will the sounds be incorporated within it? Some of these decisions will be determined by what you can afford or have available (e.g., if you only have pictures but want it to appear like it is moving, that would be different to taking new film footage of a scene). You may decide to incorporate words or graphics that overlay or frame the other images you have on the PSA. Many high quality PSAs are prepared without video footage.

With these considerations, you have made a big start to constructing the content and style of the television PSA. Whether you actually do it yourself will depend on your capabilities with design and editing, as well as the quality of the equipment you use. What would be helpful is to check with the potential source(s) you would like to have airing your work and see what they need in terms of production quality.

The other thing that this process does is to establish, at a basic level, a type of storyboard for your PSA. You can actually start with the storyboard, or use it to help frame your limited time on the air. That is, you would determine, in a sense "frame by frame" or "section by section," how you envision the PSA unfolding. Thus, you may want the first three seconds to be a black screen and then words appear that have a specific message or quote; at the same time, sound or music appears, gradually increasing in volume. You may ask for the multiple images (e.g., 20 images in 10 seconds), for the following 10 seconds, and then you specify what you want those images to be or feel like. These could use the Ken Burns effect, or you could suggest that they be presented one after the other, very rapidly. What you're doing with the storyboard is giving production guidelines to whoever will be preparing the final product.

While you may not be the expert in overall design, you may have some good and creative ideas based on your knowledge of your topic, your familiarity with your audience and its needs, and your available resources. The advice is to work hand-in-hand with the production team, so that your knowledge of these factors is blended with their knowledge of how to produce a high quality, and appropriately designed, PSA. This is more appropriate than simply letting the production folks do all the work, and also probably better than you doing all the production work yourself. You might also find that the television station (or a local community station, a high school or college station, or other resource) may donate their equipment and time to this cause; this can particularly be true if much of the work and background design considerations are prepared ahead of time, and for them, as identified above.

With these PSAs, the main theme is that your messages are getting aired on radio and/or television, with little or no funding. As you think about preparing these, you should be thinking about whatever radio and television stations are within your purview; if you're in a populated region, you may be looking at several, and if you're in a rural area and doing a local initiative, your reach may be much narrower. While ads could be taken out, and each of these can be professionally developed by a for-profit firm, the focus here is on how to accomplish the same end without substantive resources. The assumption, however, for many of these issues and many of the agencies or groups with which you will be working, is that funding is quite limited or non-existent, but the need for strong and effective communication remains high. With some savvy and creative networking, the aims can still be met.

Forward!

In summary, having a better understanding of the media is important for engaging them as a partner in the process of communicating your message. This starts with media relations, whether you initiate your contact with them, they reach out to you or you work through media relations specialists. This continues with media advocacy, where your aim is to have the media be an active advocate for your messages, and ultimately to help obtain policy shifts suitable for your purposes. There are op–ed approaches, letters to the editor and other ways of getting your word out. Finally, the use of public service announcements, whether produced by you or others, can be most helpful in communicating your messages more widely than might be expected through the more traditional approaches found with print know–feel–do strategies. Some of these approaches with the media are based on good skills, such as many of those outlined in this chapter. Others are obtained by hard work. And still others also require a sense of good opportunity or luck. Also, typical with an op–ed piece is that they are longer than the letters to the editor; while they have limits, they allow for greater detail and discussion within the context of the article. Blending these can be helpful in maximizing the chance that the media will be an effective and suitable partner for you and your health–oriented initiatives.

10 A public presence

Overview

Your health and safety communications efforts are often done in a quiet setting—your office, your home or as you travel. Much of your work will be conceptualizing and planning, thinking of ways to best reach your audience with your messages. Your creative work may just evolve passively given the luxury of time. Further, your work style may be such that you work better in groups, or it may be that you work better when you are alone. Much of your work will be "behind the scenes," drafting content for resources, writing PSAs and designing materials. In any event, the preparation of your health and safety communications efforts, to be done well, requires careful and thoughtful planning.

While some of your efforts will involve face-to-face interactions, many will not. Ultimately, you want all of your health and safety communications efforts to be public—your materials will be seen, the posters or billboards you designed will be viewed and your PSAs will be seen or heard. Further, you will have a public presence with your use of social media, whether through Facebook, Twitter or even your organization's website (see Chapter 12 on social media). There are even times when you will have a face-to-face presence with your communications efforts; an obvious one is with a workshop, addressed thoroughly in Chapter 11.

The focus of a **public presence**, as described in this chapter, emphasizes your active engagement. Specifically, it involves you making the case for your topic or issue in any of a variety of settings. This public presence may involve you directly in the "limelight," or it may be you working behind the scenes. Through this, it is important to be ready for having a presence of which you are proud; good planning and preparation can help in this regard. Further, some insights and tips about how to maximize the delivery and potential impact of your message will be helpful.

What are some of these opportunities? You might have the opportunity, or be asked, to make a presentation to a local government committee or governing body, such as a town council. You may also have the opportunity to make a case for your initiative with a smaller leadership group, such as the executive council of an organization, agency or campus. This may involve offering some brief remarks at a public event, such as when a keynote speaker is invited; or it may be that you are that keynote speaker! Consider also being interviewed for an article in a newsletter; it could also be for something in a newspaper or a magazine, whether at the local or national level. You may be called for an interview or an appearance on a talk show, or with the local or national news. And, some of these can be on the radio, on cable or on broadcast television.

The opportunities abound for having a public presence and for getting your message distributed more widely. Much of this is beyond what you expected; much of it may be

more than you actually want. In any event, it is important to be prepared for the opportunities and even to seek them out should you desire them.

Why go public?

One of the key questions surrounding having a public voice is why you might want to
do that. A related question is whether it will actually be you who is going public. Once
you address these basic questions, the focus shifts to identifying the best ways of being in
the public eye in the most appropriate ways, and doing so in the highest quality ways.
This section focuses on the initial questions, with the majority of the chapter emphasizing
specifics within the context of different settings and audiences.

So, why go public? Ultimately, consider what it is that you seek to accomplish with
your health and safety communications activities. Who is it that you want to reach and
what is it that you want them to know, feel or do? In short, going public broadens the
nature and scope of your message and thus affects its potential impact. When you think
about the basic communication efforts, you may have a brochure or a poster and you
hope that it reaches your audience. Blending multiple approaches within the context of
a campaign (where numerous know-feel-do strategies are offered over a focused period
of time), your opportunity for reaching your target audience is further enhanced beyond
those found with some basic know-feel-do strategies. With the public presence, these
opportunities expand even further. While the public presence may be part of a campaign,
they all-too-often are spontaneous, in addition to your regular planned efforts, and what
you might consider "beyond your wildest dreams."

What these various know-feel-do strategies all have in common is that they include
your direct involvement with an audience or a public, large and small. These are opportunities for you to get your message out in a personal way. You can inform, you can
inspire, you can cajole, you can motivate, you can educate, you can lead and you can
personally have a hand in making your voice heard. In fact, this is not just "your voice"
but that of your organization or agency. What this does is to put a personal face on the
issue as well as the organization and lets the opportunity appear for reaching people more
directly and personally.

Certainly, you may have hoped for these opportunities, but when they come, are you
really ready? Will you feel good about taking advantage of the opportunity when it arises,
and once it is completed?

All-too-often, these "public presence" elements are sought by health communicators, as they provide access and reach to audiences for you that are often difficult to
obtain. The down side is that these initiatives can cause a significant amount of stress. To
do them well, you want to prepare well, be organized and be proud of what you did.
Certainly you are taking on an extra burden, as you are doing something that may be way
beyond your traditional "scope of work" and are typically beyond your comfort zone.
You may also decide that it is not you who is best suited to become engaged in these,
whether because of the area of expertise required, or the venue (such as appearing on live
television). In any event, it is important to think about these opportunities and to view
them as just that—an opportunity. Through the tips and skills and perspectives offered
in this chapter, you might find that you actually look forward to participating with them
and to enjoying this as an opportunity to get your messages spread much more widely
and deeply.

A speech

You have been asked to give a speech. That can be one of the most overwhelming challenges of your life! All sorts of thoughts are likely to run through your head:

* What do I—me!!!—have to say?
* Why would they select me?
* Is there someone who can speak better than I can?
* How long will I have for the speech?
* Do I have enough to say?
* What if I go on too long?
* Will they ask questions at the end?
* To whom am I speaking?
* How do I keep their interest?
* How large a group is this?
* Who else has spoken to this audience and how did they do?
* How will I come across?
* What if they ask questions I don't know how to answer?
* How soon is it?

There's a lot to think about when planning to give a speech. Just as with other health and safety communications initiatives, your initial thoughts will be about the audience and who they are; then your attention goes to what, specifically, you want them to know, feel or do. From this general construct, you will want some more detailed information, all of which is helpful as you make preparations for the speech.

* What is the background of those anticipated to be in the audience? What are their expectations?
* What are the expectations from the sponsor about what they want from you? What specifically do they want you to address?
* How long is this scheduled to be? Will it be before or after a scheduled meal?
* How are the logistics of the setting—how large is it, how is it arranged, what flexibility is there in the setting?
* What arrangements are made for the use of visuals, should you wish to use them?
* How is the set-up? Will there be a podium? A microphone (fixed, lavalier, hand-held)? A stool and table? Other considerations?
* Will this be filmed? If so, does that cause any constraints on your presentation style, such as staying in a certain location and not moving around?

With this background in mind, you can now start preparing for the speech. Think about your outcomes and what you envision the audience hearing from your remarks. That is, focus on what you want the audience to take away from your talk.

Think also about how you envision this talk—is it designed to be informational, with primarily an educational flavor? Is it intended to be motivational or inspirational? Will it be persuasive, such as making a case for action? Are you seeking support for an initiative or cause?

Once you have some of these basics in mind, start constructing the outline of the speech. Think about the key points that you want to make and then think about specific ways that you can support and document your message. Think about how you might illustrate the message—this is because having a straight informational talk is not sufficient; that would assume that the audience will hear things only from a "logos" point of view. You will want to enhance the main points with illustrations, things that will help them understand what you are saying, as well as to be convinced that these are important points. These may be testimonials from individuals (such as those affected by whatever issue you are addressing) and these may also include evidence provided by experts or those whose opinions will be respected. You will want to find ways to make sure that the audience is "getting" your key points; you may decide to incorporate some light-hearted remarks, illustrations, data summaries or humor as well. The caution with any of these approaches is to make sure you are resonating with your audience; humor, in particular, can be tricky as it may not make sense to many in the audience, or it may offend others.

As you prepare this outline, be sure to keep it focused. There's a great tendency to try to put too much information into a limited amount of time. Be certain that your key points are identified and that you build the substance around those points.

So what are some ways to organize the talk? Lots of different approaches can be used. What you will want to do is to find a structure that works for you, and that you believe will work well for the audience. What you don't want is a rambling talk; you want to be clear with your message and with your approach. Here are a few ideas:

1   Identify the need, current know–feel–do strategies, considerations and know–feel–do strategies for action.
2   Suggest a specific number of steps (e.g., 3 or 4 or 5 or 7 or 10) for making a difference.
3   Offer main issues and consequences.
4   Specify primary controversies for this topic.
5   Incorporate storytelling with various examples.
6   Prepare an acronym around which the talk can be organized; with a talk on being a "leader," consider "listen, execute, advise, delegate, evaluate and rejuvenate" or any other words that best illustrate your key points.

These just serve as some ways of organizing your thinking. As you plan your talk, this initial outline may be replaced by something more appropriate for your audience. In any event, this process provides an overall framework for your talk, designed to get you started with your thinking and organizing of what you have to say.

As you start this process of organizing your remarks, you will undoubtedly be thinking about the overall "package" of your presentation. That includes the setting, such as whether you are on a stage and using a podium, or are in a more casual setting. You will be thinking about whether you will be making remarks before a meal, or after a meal; if the latter, you will probably want to make reference to the meal and it will be very important that you limit your time. You will want to consider whether you want or need to have visuals to accompany what you have to say. These are all factors that contribute to the tone of your speech; in a more formal setting, you may be reluctant to be particularly cute or folksy, and in a less formal setting, you don't want to be too stiff or pontificate.

Another classic framework for a talk is the following mantra, regarding how to structure the speech: "Tell them what you're going to tell them, then tell them and then tell them what you told them." In this, you're providing an overview of your outline and what you intend to accomplish during the speech; then, as you wrap up the speech, you summarize what you have covered and provide any concluding remarks.

Messages from the field

Incorporating examples for public health

Beth DeRicco, Ph.D., Drexel University and Caron Treatment Centers

In all of my public speaking I try to use real time examples, from my life, and then from the lives of my audience, that illustrate an environmental public health approach and the way in which health and safety communications have succeeded or not—think of the Crash Test Dummies and campaigns around tobacco cessation and seat belt use.

A final thought in preparation of the speech has to do with supporting materials. You may want to have some materials that support your overall message. These could be illustrative, such as an experiment or activity conducted for the audience, on stage. It could be some quick polling of the audience, whether by a show of hands or verbal comments. You may also want to have on hand copies of materials you reference, such as a book or a chart. These are helpful to bring to life your remarks; they also serve as a type of diversion from the words you are speaking.

Related strongly to these supporting materials is the use of slides. Found typically with PowerPoint or Keynote software packages and most recently Prezi, these can be helpful for illustrating key points and documentation throughout your remarks. They can provide visual displays of your points, such as tables or graphs with data, perhaps with point in time analyses or trend data. They can also offer visual illustrations of people, places or situations to which you refer. Slides offer the opportunity to incorporate quotes from key personnel, such as recipients of a health service, or experts reporting its value. The slides can serve as section breaks in the talk, particularly if you have organized the talk within several segments. Or, you may include some humor (such as a cartoon) or a video clip, to help break up the monotony of a series of wordy slides; again, you will want to make sure that these elements help make your point and you want to be careful, with humor, that it is not offensive to audience members. Often, these slides provide an outline of the speech, such as the framework for the talk as well as key points within the talk.

Some dangers lie with the use of these slides, however. One is that the slides may be far too detailed, with too much information included in them. Another is that a speaker may have a tendency to read from the slides; obviously, the audience can read, so if slides are used, cite the major points rather than read the slides. This means that you should know the content very well and just refer to the slides as you talk. A related issue is that slides are all-too-often word-heavy and are also organized with a series of bullet points. Further, with slides arranged in a sequential order, you may feel constrained to go through every one of them; this can be problematic if you find that the talk is running longer than you (or your planners) had anticipated. If that's the case, learn how to skip slides effortlessly and perhaps without alerting the audience that you are doing this (for example, in PowerPoint, type the number of the slide to which you want to go and then push "Enter").

As you prepare any materials such as slides, make sure that they bring value to your talk. Make sure that these are important to your message, or to the repository of information you are providing your audience. It could be that you incorporate numerous data slides so the members of the audience have access to these at a later time, for their own use; if so, it is helpful to state that point very clearly, so that you are not spending too much time on specific content slides.

At this point, you are fairly close to giving the talk. As you have now completed the overall planning and outline, and have identified the support materials, you are ready for some feedback. It's helpful along the way of preparing your remarks to share your outline with colleagues and perhaps with the sponsor. This can aid in determining whether the talk will resonate well for the audience, from their perspective; this is a type of pilot testing for you. What is important is that you gather honest feedback, because otherwise you may feel good about your talk, but it may not be effective or appropriate. Gather input and feedback and then make refinements as appropriate. This can also include a rehearsal where you actually deliver the speech to those around you. This process helps you gather input and make modifications as needed; it is also an opportunity for you to practice the speech, to be sure that your remarks stay on topic and are delivered within the specified amount of time.

Once you have finalized your talk, print out your content. This may include your written remarks as well as any documentation you are using, such as slides. Be careful about having a cumbersome set of print documents (that is, two separate documents, one with the slides and another with your speech content or notes). Try to condense your own materials as much as possible, as you don't want to be fumbling through pages as you are giving your talk. You would benefit from having all of your items blended into a single document. This may be a text version of your talk (or an outline and notes, if that is sufficient for you); then embed images or descriptors of the slides you will be using, at the location of the talk where you want to include them. Also be sure to include the slide number, in case you need to move ahead or back with the slides. This document can then serve as your working notes throughout the talk.

As you finalize the preparations for the talk, it is wise to consider various contingencies. You have been preparing your talk for delivery in a certain setting and have made various assumptions along the way, most or all of which should have been checked out. For example, you may have asked for a projection unit and screen; you may be expecting a podium and a laser pointer. It's vital that you verify these, but also plan for the situation when some of these may not have been accomplished, or where something is not working properly. You may arrive to find that someone forgot to get the screen; is an alternative projection location feasible, such as a blank wall? Or, can your talk be accomplished without the visuals? You may have a situation where you expected a clicker to advance the slides; perhaps you should bring your own, in case the provided one doesn't work or has low batteries. You may have prepared your slides on a flash drive; consider also emailing yourself a copy of it and preparing it on two portable devices in the event that one is corrupted. Check out the room and the equipment, and make any last minute adjustments as possible. And most important, have some back-up plans so you can still accomplish a quality talk if something is not quite right or malfunctions.

Now you're ready to give the speech; or, as some say, "it's show time!" You may be introduced, or you may be introducing yourself to the audience. The main issue at the onset of your speech is to connect with the audience. You will find the most appropriate way of doing that, whether it is by letting them know a little about yourself, telling a story, making a joke or offering an illustration (such as a recent news article). Whether or not you use a slide to get started, the important thing is that you resonate well with the audience.

Following the introduction, you will want to "tell them what you're going to tell them" and get started with your formal remarks. Then, you will proceed with your talk, monitoring your time and ensuring that you stay on track. Through this, keep an eye on the audience to assess their reactions (if you can see them; sometimes, this is not possible with bright lights on the speaker, thus not permitting you to see the audience). Stay on track with your remarks, and make adjustments with your content as you proceed, so that you end on time. To do this, make sure you have a clock, watch or timer very visible so you can gauge where you are throughout the talk. Then, with a few minutes remaining, you should start to wrap up your comments. This is the part where you "tell them what you told them"; you may review your overall objectives for the session and what you intended. Hopefully, your final remarks will encourage and motivate them to do what you sought as their next steps (what you want them to know, feel or do). You may close with some final, rehearsed words or a quote.

Throughout the talk, here are some specific suggestions:

- Monitor the speed with which you speak. Be sure that you don't speak too quickly or too slowly. Make sure your key points are made; you may wish to vary your speed to emphasize key points.
- Some of your messages are worth repeating. This may be done by stating something several times throughout the talk. Or, it may involve repeating a sentence right after itself.
- Insert questions to the audience periodically. These may be rhetorical questions, like "What do you think that means?" or "What would data like this suggest?" These help engage the audience.
- To the extent that you can (and this comes with more practice and comfort with public speaking), try not to read your notes. Further, if you are comfortable doing so, remove yourself from the podium and walk across the stage or into the audience.
- If you're using slides, try to use a remote clicker to facilitate moving through the slides. The laser pointer can also be useful for highlighting key points or data on certain slides. This also keeps you from being relegated to the podium, unless, of course, that is where you want to be!
- Watch the use of audio space holders, such as saying "uh" or "you know" over and over. To do so may result in participants counting the number of times you use those phrases. This may require some practice—so just pay attention to it. It may also mean that you have to slow down your pace and be more deliberate with your words.
- Attend to distracting behaviors. You may have a behavioral pattern, about which you are not aware, that distracts listeners from your key points. Just as saying "uh" over and over is distracting, you may click your pen or move your hands in a distracting manner. Consider videotaping yourself speaking to see if you notice any of these, so you can then attend to and modify them with your actual speech.
- If you use slides, the important thing is to know your content. Rehearsal is helpful with that. You shouldn't be waiting for the next slide to inform you what the content is on that upcoming slide; this should be printed out in advance with the slides and any relevant notes associated with them.
- Demonstrate that you know your topic. Since you do know your material, it is important that your speech demonstrates this. You should know the key points of what you want to say; what causes concern with listeners is when you are just reading your speech. There are undoubtedly parts that are key that require precision with the words; however it is best to use the prepared remarks as an overall guide for your talk.
- Feel comfortable looking at your notes periodically. There's nothing wrong with using your notes, to offer a quote, to illustrate key points or to remind yourself of what you want to say. Try not to belabor your use of the notes, even though you refer to them. If you have key statistics to share, have them on the slides so you don't appear unprepared.

- It is not vital to say everything that you planned to say and to tell every story that you had planned. What is important is that your overall message is heard, so watch the audience and watch your time. Remember that the audience only knows the "large picture" of what you want to cover and they don't know what you choose to leave out.
- Be careful with your use of acronyms, such as those found with organization titles, agency names, degrees or other uses. These can be helpful shorthand in talking, but be certain that your audience is conversant with their meaning.

Overall, there's a lot to think about when preparing and delivering a speech. These insights can be helpful in organizing your thinking, preparing your plan, thinking about contingencies and actually delivering the talk. The most important thing is to focus on the audience you are seeking to influence and attempt to monitor how that is going during the course of the talk. Sure, it may feel like a lot of pressure is on you as you are doing this talk; however, this can go smoothly with sufficient preparation and a lot of practice. Then, you can enjoy these opportunities more and more.

Messages from the field

Use of graphics, visual aids and technology

Kathryn Bedard, MA LCADC, Sojourner Consulting LLC

With your workshop or talk, tables and graphs can be an asset; however, if the graph or table is not straight to the point, and cannot stand alone, it will shut down an audience. Your data slides should be so clear that you can put up a slide and lecture about other details in the subject matter that enhance the graph without really delving into the graph itself.

When you develop your data slides, do not use gridlines, avoid too many variables of comparison, never put graphs on colored background and be simple. Anything with lots of details should be a full page handout. Your presentation should stimulate curiosity and result in the tendency of the audience to nod, and say something like "Hmmm ... interesting ... look at that!"

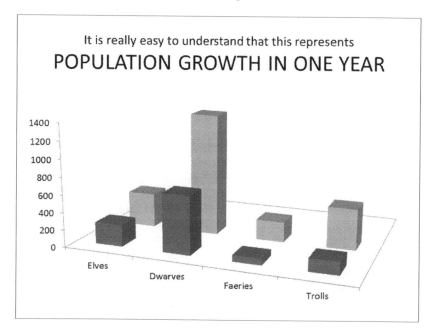

Software presentation slides can be a great asset to learning, if used correctly. A good slide will have some bulleted slides to enhance important points and some photo slides to bring impact. You can embed graphics, film clips, audio files—all kinds of bells and whistles. The goal with digitizing information is to abbreviate it, not put everything you know on the screen. The content of your lecture should be different from the content of the slides, or at bare minimum enhancing or elaborating the content of the slides in different words. The slides should never tell the story.

The most crucial part of using PowerPoint and similar programs is the structure of each slide and the size of the font. Structure means how many lines you can get on a slide. A good rule of thumb for how much information to bullet is the rule of sixes: confine it all to six lines. Yes—you only get six bullets, with six lines and six words per line—with a space between each line. Another rule of thumb in the sixes category is to try to have six slides or less. Go for high impact slides, bringing out emotional connection and response; the result will be a dynamic presentation, with the focus on you and what you say. You and your audience will find it to be liberating and refreshingly like human conversation. Aim for a "fireside chat" and facilitate discussion instead of preaching.

The type of font you use must be a common, easy to read font. If you choose some of the less used, or "informal" fonts, you run the risk of your slides being modified if you use someone else's equipment: if your computer is new, and you've chosen a font that you think is pretty, but the hotel where you are presenting has only Office 97, the computer will locate a font it thinks is close. The worst that might happen with the less formal fonts is that your presentation will appear as big red 'X's on each slide. Stick to the old standby fonts like Arial, Comic Sans, Lucida Console and Calibri.

Finally, with the beautiful templates easily accessible, anyone can create stunning presentations that look professionally designed, but you must always keep track of the fact that not all computers have the same graphics capability, so the colors you pick may project very differently elsewhere. To further complicate the use of color, the monitor you look at as you make your presentation has a lot more contrast to it than a projector.

Font Size Is Important

- Your audience is very far from the screen.
- You might think it enlarges on that huge screen behind you, but the opposite happens!
- Size and readability of fonts is very important:

Calibri	Angsana	Bradley Hand	Comic Sans
32 pt	32 pt	32 pt	32 pt
24 pt	24 pt	24 pt	24 pt
18 pt	18 pt	18 pt	18 pt
14 pt	14 pt	14 pt	14 pt
12 pt	12 pt	12 pt	12 pt

Never less than 24 point!

Avoid light colored fonts at all costs on white or pastel backgrounds. When you pick backgrounds for your slides, white with black fonts are a great choice for two reasons: 1. it is easy to read and looks the same everywhere, 2. it is easier to copy for handouts. Black font on white or soft gray, white font on black background creates a distinct and sharp image that your audience can easily see.

TED talk

Another approach found within the framework of having a "public presence" is with conducting a TED talk. While similar to a lecture, a TED talk has a very different style or flavor. In brief, a TED talk is brief, more conversational and storytelling in style and less technical. While TED talks have been around for several decades, these have taken off in recent years and have been adapted. Some organizations are using these as part of the training programs and these can also be used as work or class assignments.

In its origin, "TED" stood for "Technology, Entertainment and Design," and now covers many topics. TED talks and TEDx events provide the opportunity for individuals to learn different knowledge and ideas on countless topics. Further, the TED and TEDx experience provides an opportunity for individuals, such as you, to share your insights and knowledge with others.

What is important to realize as you consider delivering a TED talk is that this will be more than a talk for a given audience; it will be recorded and will have the opportunity to be made publicly available for individuals and groups worldwide to view. That can seem overwhelming, and indeed it is. However, if your aim with health and safety communication is to "get the word out," this is a perfect opportunity. While there is no guarantee that your talk will be posted, it is something to which you can aspire, based on the sponsoring organization's arrangements and the quality of the talk. The other thing to keep in mind is that the concept and nature of a TED talk may be adapted, so an event or conference in which you are participating may offer a "TED Talk-Like Event" that then may be filmed and made available. Whether through the formal TED or TEDx vehicle, or a locally prepared event, the link to your message—through a recorded "you"—can be disseminated through other communication vehicles, whether these are websites, print materials, public service announcements or other talks.

So, as you think about preparing to deliver a TED talk, remember that, while these talks have similarities to traditional lectures, they are very different in style and tone. The general rule is that they are 18 minutes or less. They are purposely shorter to provide a specific focus and to promote heightened attention by the audience. The main focus is on your engagement with the audience, so incorporate storytelling, examples and a visual presence. Further, make sure any slides are illustrative and of a general supportive nature. You want the focus to be on you and not on information or data in the slides. Finally, as you proceed in the talk, focus on the audience; don't look at the slides or visuals behind you. Emphasize the connection between you and the audience.

As you conduct a TED talk, you'll find that the time passes quickly. You do need to attend to the limited time that you have and maintain the focus on the audience and your connection with them. And, since this is being recorded, attend to both the in-person audience as well as the larger, ultimate audience you'll have when someone watches your talk at a later time.

Media interviews

Another consideration within the concept of public presence has to do with the media. While this book's Chapter 9 addresses media relations and media advocacy, attention to media interviews is included here because it focuses primarily on your presence and your messaging. It incorporates, just as with a speech, sound preparation and clarity of message delivery. Many aspects of this are different, but the essential components are the same. Here, it is about the presence you have with the audience, based on the intermediary factor called "the media."

An important starting point with media interviews is an understanding of what is meant by "the media," and the context within which the media operates. As highlighted in Chapter 9, when talking about "the media," think in terms of print media (such as newspapers, magazines, newsletters) and non-print approaches (such as radio and television). And with the radio and television segments, the focus is on the news or public affairs type of show. With changes in the digital arena, other areas often are, and can be, considered to be media approaches. For the purpose of this section, the focus is on the primary and more traditional media approaches.

So, why would you want to get involved with the media? In brief, this represents another opportunity for you to communicate your message and to do so in a much broader network than you might find with your more traditional approaches. This becomes an opportunity to be heard much more broadly, including by audiences that may be hard to reach. Further, having a presence in the media is typically done at no financial cost to you, except for the time and energy necessary to have a quality presence through this venue. Through your involvement with the media, you may gain support from various sources, that otherwise you would not be able to obtain. Further, your exposure may help bolster your efforts at the current time, as well as to set the stage for future support. By your presence in the media, you may become a "go to" person for this particular source, as well as with other media sources.

Similarly, why is it that you might not want to get involved with the media? One primary reason is that you are afraid that your presence in the media will undermine your overall efforts; you may feel that you do not have sufficient expertise within the topic area (let alone the quality of your presence that you may have encountered working with media specialists). You may not want to subject yourself or your organization to heightened scrutiny that may easily come through publicity with the media. Also, you may not have sufficient staffing or resources to handle inquiries that may come from exposure in the media.

To help understand the media, recall what is important to them, from an overall perspective. Media outlets, such as the print media, radio and television, are all businesses. From a simple perspective, they can be seen as having two audiences—one is the public that purchases or signs on to their services. The other includes those who pay for advertising, which in turn is reliant on the popularity of the paying or viewing public. Media's advertisers like a broad reach, so that their invested dollars (for a print or radio/television ad) reach as large an audience as possible. With factors such as ratings or sales volume, advertisers are increasingly willing to invest in the media source. And, individuals read the print publications, listen to the radio or view television shows because of topics, issues and approaches of interest to them. It would be reasonable to surmise that the public doesn't tune into a show because of the ads; rather, it views a show where you might be involved because of its news value, the commentary offered, the points of view included or some other factors of importance to them.

The same is true for print media; the reading public may be involved with a particular print publication because of its style, its overall emphasis or focus, its perspectives on key issues, its diversity or other factor. With any of these, the media source is all about ratings and profits. Certainly there may be a social cause for them and a larger societal contribution they wish to make. They may have a niche they seek to fill, whether as an entire publication or as a part of the publication. The thing for you to remember is that the media, whatever type it is, has its own agenda. That agenda may not necessarily be entirely lined up with yours; that agenda may be in direct conflict with yours, and it may also be something that provides you with an opportunity to get your message communicated to new audiences.

Working with the media does represent a tremendous opportunity for you to get your message shared. Yes, it is challenging, and it requires a fair amount of perseverance and focus to make sure that your message is, in fact, delivered. The media personnel may push you and challenge you; less often, but indeed present, are situations where media personnel nurture you gently.

First, consider the print media. One of the easiest approaches is with a newsletter. This may be a place where you are asked to write a column or a blog. It is helpful to know more about the audience of the newsletter, as well as the overall length anticipated for this written piece. Also helpful is to know about the context of the article, within the overall newsletter. Where does the article fit; is it a lead story, a regular feature within the newsletter or one of several points of view? The newsletter opportunity may also be one where you are interviewed, with someone else writing the article. In that sense, your perspective on a specific health issue, or what view you take with a particular controversy, will be helpful for the readers of the newsletter to understand. With an interview such as this, ask the writer questions such as how long the article will be and the context of any comments you may provide. Will you be quoted, paraphrased or simply have comments provided as background information? Very typical for this type of print approach is that the editor and writer are seeking to "tell a story" and to "get the word out" about various issues. Thus, generally, you could expect that they will want to serve you well and communicate that which you want to emphasize. For this, as with the other communication approaches, you will want to be very clear about your key message or messages. The length of these written pieces is typically quite short, so you will need to be focused with your language, wording and messages.

A second example is also with the print media. Newspapers and magazines are opportunities to have your messages distributed widely to their readership. With a newspaper, the timing is typically of the essence; for something to appear in the newspaper, there will be content that has a time urgency. For the magazine, this will be less urgent, as that print publication is typically produced much less frequently. You may be contacted by a reporter (or you may contact a reporter, as identified in the discussion on media relations in Chapter 9). Again, it is important to know the overall thrust of the article about which the individual is writing.

You should do whatever preparation you can, so you are well informed and prepared for the discussion. Very often, the reporter will inform you that s/he is working within the constraints of a publishing deadline; that may be part of the message when you are contacted for the interview (so if you call back too late, your comments may not be considered). However, just because you don't meet a reporter's deadline does not mean you should not call back; to do so may help establish a helpful relationship that can be nurtured for future such interviews. It may also generate interest in some follow-up writing to be undertaken by the reporter. One related advantage with the newspaper or magazine interview is that these can be done on the telephone; this makes much easier the logistics of getting an interview scheduled and can often be accomplished within a very limited period of time.

During the interview, take the necessary time to answer any questions thoroughly and thoughtfully. Knowing that the reporter won't be able to use everything you say, be particularly clear with your main points. Some of these would be worth repeating and emphasizing, to ensure that the reporter does hear your messages. You, and the reporter, may find it helpful to cite specifically data as well as real-life examples that help illustrate the points you are making. If you use data, be sure to offer to send specific references and documentation. This may be helpful for accurate reporting and may also be a nice way of establishing positive relations for your involvement in a future interview.

A final thought that may be useful with the interview—and can also serve as a deal-breaker—is for you to ask if you will be able to review the article and your quotes to be sure that they represent your views well and accurately. The resolution of this depends on how important it is for you, your prior experience with similar interviews, the timeline and the reporter's standards for this. The reporter may agree, provided that the timeline is honored. Or, the reporter may not agree to share the article prior to publication; at that point, you have to decide whether you will be interviewed or will not accept this opportunity.

The radio interview is the next level of media interview. With this, the interview can be done in several different ways. One way is that this can occur within a broadcast studio, such as at the radio station. You may be the featured guest, or you may be one of several individuals or panel members who are interviewed or involved in a discussion. Another way is that you can call in to the show as a guest. The advantage of being on site for the radio interview is that you can interact directly with the host of the show. This is helpful if you are a member of a panel, as you can have the attention of the radio show host, while those calling in will not have that same advantage.

Messages from the field

Staying on message

Kenji Matsumoto, Seattle-King County Public Health

As the media's job is to obtain information that is marketable, they will use many tricks to make you admit or disclose some issues that might be too sensitive to discuss in public. The media interview can be nerve racking and it is not your job to provide them with publishable materials; however, there are many ways to avoid such traps and use the opportunity to your own advantage.

If you are in the position to speak to the media, the most important thing is to stay on the message that you want to convey to public. Most of the time the media interviewer has a premeditated storyline that he or she wants to develop before the interview. At any point, if you feel uncomfortable, you can always defer to someone else—it is best to only discuss what you know.

It is good to draft the potential questions and their answers if you know about the interview in advance. Even at an unprepared interview, you always can ask what the media wants to discuss before the interview although the caveat is that the interviewer can change the topic. An interviewer can try to lead you to various directions to stir up the conversation or try to trick you to admit something that you are not familiar with. In order to stay on the message, you can use the phrases such as "That is an important point but today I want to talk about ..." or "I am not in the right position to discuss this but I can refer you to ..." to avoid such traps. Politicians are the best examples for this. They sometimes even give answers that are not what the questions asked. You can also then use this opportunity to convey your message to benefit your intention such as fundraising or advertisement of a resource or a company.

Another option with a radio interview is that it may be taped. You may be interviewed by a radio show host or a staff member who is gathering audio footage from an interview. Your interview may actually be very long, and the program director or editor may choose to air only a small clip of what you had to say (or nothing, too). Again, this is the type of situation where you benefit from being very clear with what your messages are and speaking in a grounded and thoughtful manner. Since this is the radio, it will be important that you articulate well, as all that the listener has to go on is your voice. You should speak clearly and do so with full sentences, knowing that, if this is taped, only a portion of what you have to say will be aired. If the intent is for the producer to have some quotes or segments from you, you are well advised to state various aspects of your key message numerous times; because there will be some selection of your content later, having the core messages articulated several times, and in different ways, allows for those making the editorial decision to select the one that is most appropriate. It's not a matter of repetition that the listener will hear over and over, although that in itself is not necessarily a bad thing. The importance of this repetition is that your message is heard by the listening audience. The same would be true of your website or other resource where the listener can go for additional information; make sure you highlight this multiple times, to maximize the opportunity of it being heard and included in the final radio work. Should this be a live show, you may wish to repeat several things, such as a key point, a website or other resource information, as some listeners may hear only a portion of the show, and you want to maximize their opportunity to hear your key message.

The final situation has to do with a television show. Again, the question of "live" versus "taped" is important; for a live television show, the emphasis is all upon the limited period of time, when everything that is covered is aired. For a taped show, there are shows that have the entire show taped, as if it was live; and there are those that, like a radio interview, will have segments extracted for later inclusion in the full-length television show. Knowing the set-up for these different settings is important for how often you may repeat yourself, and how you handle yourself.

Overall, with television, it is important to realize that a camera may always be "on you"; so be sure that you always have a television presence, and that you don't say or do anything that you wouldn't want aired. If a show goes to a commercial break, that is a time to get refreshed with your notes or key talking points.

Through a television interview on the air, again the most important things are to be clear in your own mind with your messages, stay focused on your key messages and not get distracted, and maintain your composure.

- Determine where to look. Some settings benefit from you looking directly into the camera, and others prefer that you look at the interviewer or host and ignore the camera. At some times, with multiple cameras, you may see the red light above the camera to know which one is live. Ask ahead of time where the producer or organizer believes is most effective for this setting. If it is directly into the camera, this can feel awkward talking into an inanimate object; that can become more comfortable with practice.
- Use your own words. If an interviewer or another person on the show uses a phrase that you wouldn't normally use, do not repeat that unless you, too, want to "own it"; that phrase, when it comes out of your mouth, becomes yours.
- Be wary of leading questions or conclusions attributed to you. Make your point clearly, and specify your main points over and over. If an interviewer or another guest tries to infer conclusions that are not yours, say so. It's important to not let these go unchecked or unchallenged. Make sure your point is clear.
- Maintain your integrity. Through the interview, say what you mean and mean what you say. Try not to be misled or to let viewers assume that you believe a point that is not, in fact, yours.
- Watch silence. If you are being interviewed, and you provide your response, an interviewer may use silence to get you to say more. If that happens, you can remain silent, unless you have something more to say. This is a strategy often used by interviewers to get you to say something less rehearsed and, perhaps, more newsworthy for the media.

- Aim to feel good at the end of the show. While you may think you need to please the interviewer or host, your primary obligation is to please yourself and to be proud of what you said and how you said it. If the host is annoyed at your non-response to his/her use of silence, that is really a statement about them and not about you.
- Use props and materials as needed. Sometimes it is helpful to have visuals that you can hold up to illustrate helpful resources. If you do this, make sure that these would be within the viewing area, such as at eye or shoulder height.
- Use gestures that can be seen. Also helpful is to use your hands, again at a level that can be seen with the camera, to further illustrate your points or to demonstrate your passion and commitment.
- Be sure to repeat yourself. With a taped show, this is most helpful to help ensure that your key points are picked up. For a live show, you can do this and acknowledge that you are repeating yourself, because of the importance of the key points.

The television interview can be particularly overwhelming. All-too-often, once it is over you will likely have regrets about what you said or did and what you could have done better. You might have experienced something that you never experienced before, such as having the sound not work well if you are provided an earpiece, if you are interviewed alone at a desk while the interviewer is in a distant location, or if others keep interrupting you. Know that you have done good planning and quality preparation and then do the best effort you can do. Then, learn from your experiences and prepare for another time on the air.

Messages from the field

The call

Thomas Krever, MPA, Chief Executive Officer, Hetrick-Martin Institute

Every non-profit person dreams of it; waits for it; yearns for it ... The call. The day when your phone rings and the voice on the line identifies themselves as a major news organization; a global news brand seen across the planet and their top show—PRIME TIME—wants you to be interviewed by their star anchorperson about an issue that you were "made to" speak about; that your organization and its mission have been working decades to address. A chance to tell the story of your work and spread the word on your knowledge, skills, organizational excellence ... And so on. IF you get that call—no, WHEN you get that call ... Don't do what I did ... DO NOT HANG UP!

'Cause that's what I did ... With an entire career in non-profit direct service and executive management, I've always begrudgingly settled for working in an environment where a communications strategy and infrastructure (staff, responsive database, marketing, etc.) has been a "frills" or "luxury." As a result, while you're doing the "good work," you're also generally relying on that work to "tell its own story," hoping that someone somewhere is going to pick it up and run with it.

Of course, you might ask, "Well, in the age of social media, isn't it so much easier to have your story told and heard by audiences on a global scale ...?" And I'd have to inevitably answer a resounding "YES!" But, the sobering reality is, that's what EVERY organization is doing these days ... It's just getting more and more difficult to have your story heard and more difficult still to have it "sink in" and "stick." So, here's what led up to "The Call" I received.

A board member won an auction to have lunch with this same "star reporter," and he invited me along to have access to this person—no pressure ... Just lunch. I showed up looking my best, press kit and brochure in-hand, ready to make my "pitch" (nothing overt or over the top).

After about 15 minutes or so of a lot of small talk, I was able to tell the story of how his own work internationally mirrored mine right here in the United States—right in his own "back yard!" He found it interesting and we began a deeper debate from the philosophical all the way through to the pragmatic. "What solutions would you propose?" "How would you address X, Y and Z?" When lunch ended, we bid each other well, promised to "stay in touch," and went our separate ways.

Soon after, I had made several attempts to reconnect, share more stories and engage in our work, I received no responses and eventually moved on to the next crisis of the day. I had finally given up hope; in fact, a year and a half sped by ...

Then my cell phone rang and a voice declared they "very much would like me to come down" to the studio for a live show airing in a few hours. I remember chuckling, thinking this was a "creative stunt" and disconnected. Shortly thereafter, a staff person told me there was a producer on the phone who remembered our meeting last year and very much wanted me on their show! And my inbox displayed several emails with red exclamation points next to that same name, querying *Could I be ready to go live on the air in a few hours with this person?* This was real ... VERY real. My staff person interrupted my combined panic and stupor, saying, "It's a producer and they are doing a story on the tragic incident that happened yesterday." The implications were national, indeed, global and the producer was seeking me out—the anchorperson wanted me on the show.

I picked up the phone, took a deep breath and forced the air out of my lungs and up into my throat and out my mouth ... "This is Thomas; I'd be honored to help you ..."

Clearly, this is the type of exposure that so many of us seek, yet most of us never get. But we might, and we should always be ready. Here are some brief suggestions to prepare:

1 Understand where, when and HOW your organization and personal mission intersect with others beyond your own constituents and affiliations.

2 Listen for the opportunities to understand, empathize and really connect with other people's missions. Ultimately, you WILL find a connection—usually on a deeper level—and it is from that place of connection that communication and collaboration can happen.

3 Remember, you are being asked to be on the air because you know something about the subject matter and as importantly, people want to hear your thoughts, understand more and join in on how to help.

4 News stories can happen at any time, so stay caught up on current events and know the basic facts.

5 You may not have too much time to prepare—so don't be afraid or embarrassed to ask for help and enlist others to do necessary background research, share your ideas and test your talking points.

6 KEEP BREATHING—I was really nervous as I stepped into the light of the studios and three people began quickly "wiring me up."

7 BE SUCCINCT when on the air. This is hard, as your impulse might be to "cram it all into your three minutes of fame" (not 15 minutes). Look for the "sound bite" and practice economy of words—it's usually fewer words than if you are in a regular conversation.

Testimony at community/state/national settings

Often, opportunities arise to make a presentation at the meeting of a town council, county board of supervisors, state agency, national hearing board or other similar setting. These can vary in length and style; they can be a great setting for garnering additional support for your health or safety initiative. You or your agency may be called upon to provide a report or an update; or you may be asked to have a presentation about a project or initiative. With these, you may be asked to do such things as offer programmatic descriptions, provide documentation of progress, summarize expenses and needs, and identify problems and challenges.

With this type of setting, what is helpful at the outset is to do three things. First, get as much information as you can about why you are being asked to appear before this group. Is it information gathering? Accountability? Inquiry? Justification? Try to assess the purpose in having you make a presentation. Second, learn what the parameters are surrounding the presentation. Is there a time limit? Would visuals or handouts be helpful or appropriate? How many people will be present? What is the setting like? Third, overprepare for the setting. While you may be informed that the purpose is one thing, other issues may emerge. It is helpful to have related information readily available, even if it is not part of your prepared materials or presentation.

Often with this type of setting, your time will be quite limited. You may, in fact, be offered three to five minutes, total, for a presentation. It is likely that you will be one of several individuals or groups making a presentation; sometimes these situations offer multiple presentations one right after the other. If this is the case, it is extremely vital that you know your material well and that you know that what you have to say will fit within the allocated time period. It's difficult to address your issue within such a limited period of time, such as three to five minutes. What you will need to do is be very well organized, and practice what you are doing to ensure that you are within the time parameters.

You may find that you are making a presentation from a podium, and you are facing a dais or platform where your audience sits (like a town council). Further, you may find that different lights appear to guide you with your time: green for continue, yellow for a certain time remaining (e.g., one minute) and red for your time being up. You will want to check with local personnel to determine what the specific colored lights actually mean in that setting. What you will need to do is to be sure that your presentation works well within that time period. Very often, you will find that the yellow light goes on when you think you have just begun—it's when you feel that you have barely started. Of course, when your time is up, you should end promptly; if the sponsors want you to continue, that is their prerogative, but you shouldn't expect or insist on that.

This type of presentation is quite challenging and nerve wracking; with the discussions throughout this resource about appropriate preparation and working well with the audience, a situation such as this makes it very difficult to build rapport and get them and you warmed up to one another. What is important through these is to be flexible and focus on your key messages in ways that the audience will truly hear and understand. While challenging, this situation does provide you with the opportunity to make your case and advance your cause.

Something else that can happen in settings such as these is interruptions—individuals to whom you are presenting may be interrupted while you are speaking. For example, you may be testifying before a congressional committee or to a town council, and an administrative aide comes up behind one of the elected officials and appears to be saying something to that person. How do you handle that? Should you stop and wait to resume? No. Should you make a point of repeating yourself once the individual is paying attention again? Not exactly. While it will be clear that this individual did not hear details of your points exactly, you can delicately blend them back into your remarks as a type of recap and summary of your main points. You want to be sure to not call attention to this interruption (although it will undoubtedly be noticed by many), nor to insult this individual; this type of situation with interruptions is not uncommon, and you should be prepared for this type of experience.

The important thing with settings such as these is to have your global points and to know them inside and out. Have supporting data, which may be illustrated by charts, quotes or expert opinion. You may or may not use visuals, whether these are with slides (e.g., PowerPoint), displays, handouts or other approaches. And you should be flexible, knowing that time will slip away from you easily and interruptions may occur. You should maintain the "big picture" in a setting such as this and strive to be as comfortable and knowledgeable with the main points you wish to make throughout the limited time you have. Your overall mission is to make your case in the most effective way; your planning and practice will be very helpful with accomplishing this outcome.

Panel member or debate at a public setting

Similar, yet different, from the other public speaking opportunities are those found with serving as a panel member or debate. Overall, this type of setting is one where you share the time with one or more other individuals, in a workshop or conference setting. This could, in fact, be on the television, with the various parameters and factors identified earlier. Also, in this sense, the debate is not meant to be one of the more formal competition styles of debate; it is meant to suggest a panel-type opportunity where different viewpoints are heard (e.g., pro and con regarding some issue).

In this setting, your preparation will be much the same as for the public testimony at the local, state or national setting. You need to be prepared with your key points, with documentation, with expert viewpoints and with situations that illustrate your point. You want to be engaging with the audience, striving to communicate clearly your points of view and why they should consider your perspectives. Further, there will often be some back and forth among panel members, whereby you have the opportunity to challenge, refute or reflect upon what others have said.

One of the key ways you can prepare for this type of setting goes way beyond the content preparation that you would normally do for any of these "public presence" situations. That is, it is vital that you determine what the "ground rules" are for this type of experience. Specifically, ask ahead of time, and ask at the time of the debate or panel, how the time will be allocated. Then, it will be incumbent upon the moderator to follow those standards. If the general agreement is that each person is allocated a specific amount of time (e.g., ten minutes), if the first person goes over time and the second person does the same, what time remains for the third person (e.g., you)?? Sometimes, a moderator will say "Well, we're out of time, so you need

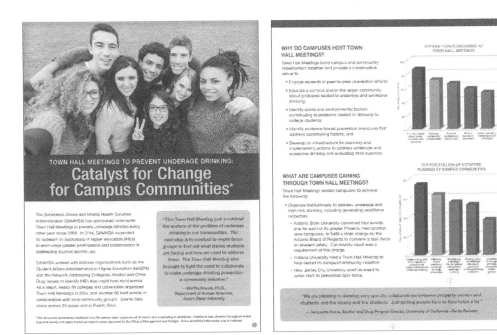

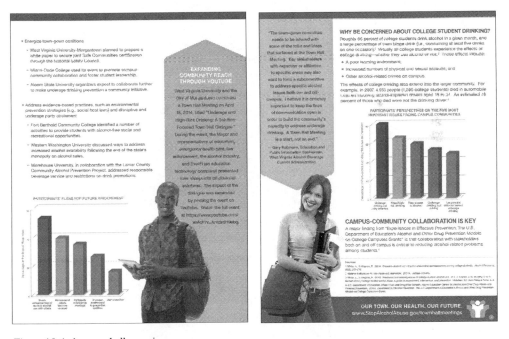

Figure 10.1 A town hall meeting

to cut your remarks in half." Your reaction, quite warranted, may be "baloney!"; however, you may not have much choice at that time. To avoid this dilemma, it is beneficial to do whatever you can at the outset to ensure that the time allocations are monitored; similarly, if you are the first person, honor your time allocations clearly, or even "offer up" extra time that you might not need. Of course, through all of this, the audience is watching how the moderator, you and the others are handling such balances of time.

With a debate situation, you may encounter someone who continually takes advantage of the setting and tends to monopolize the time. You can strive to have this balanced clearly at the onset (e.g., for every minute or two of time that one person spends, then the others are allocated that same amount of time). If this is promised at the beginning but not honored, you might want to challenge that during the course of the event. Again, remember that the audience is watching how this plays out.

The important thing with this type of setting is to have your work organized ahead of time and have your materials prepared in a way so that you, indeed, can be flexible and adaptable. However, be careful that you are not taken advantage of by others who monopolize the time or do not provide adequate opportunity to offer substantive responses. Again, as with other types of situations, you will find yourself more and more comfortable as you do more of these.

A flash lecture

You may have heard about a "flash mob," which is an event where people gather, rather spontaneously, for any of a variety of purposes. This could be for entertainment, to voice an opinion or to simply have a visible presence for passersby. Its presence is typically not advertised until the very last minute, made quite possible by the use of social media. For a **flash lecture**, this concept is applied to a brief lecture on a topic. For your purposes, think of a flash lecture as another opportunity to get the word out on your health topic.

How does this work? Briefly, the flash lecture is arranged by the program planners or sponsors and is typically in a location and time that benefits from a significant amount of foot traffic. Consider a public park, a campus quad, a town center, a bus or subway stop, or other similar location. The planners will ensure that appropriate approvals and permits are obtained, if needed. There will also be arrangements for amplification, so that your voice can be heard by those passing by. You will probably be in a setting where you are using a hand-held microphone and speaking to a growing or waning audience. You may or may not have a table nearby and probably not a podium; you may be on a riser. These are logistics prepared by the program sponsor.

Flash lectures will typically be brief in nature—probably 10 or 15 minutes. They may involve questions from the audience, or other audience interaction. The attendance will be fluid, with some people arriving after you start and some leaving before you end. Thus, you will want to organize your remarks in a type of fluid yet repetitive manner that doesn't require attendance at the entire lecture.

Since this is not advertised, who would attend a flash lecture? This will include those who are part of the social media outlets used by the program planners; they may also include your linkages as well as those of your organization. There may also be signs or placards prepared that are displayed just before the flash lecture. The advertising typically goes out shortly before the planned start time.

Attendance at these is challenging. You may have some persons showing up because they received a notice on social media, or saw a placard, and found the topic or speaker interesting. You may also have people who just happen to be walking by the area and decide to listen. People will be coming and going, and this can be disconcerting to you as a speaker, as you may conclude that they are not interested in what you have to say, which can be quite demotivating (it may simply be that they had an appointment).

It's also challenging to know when to start. Is it when a certain number of people arrive? Is it at a certain time? It's a fairly non-traditional approach with fewer organized parameters around it. However, it is something that creates an opportunity for you to reach some of your audience in a new way. Further, even the mere participation in a flash lecture can generate news coverage, a photo or other "buzz" that further communicates your message beyond the event itself.

An "elevator speech"

You may have heard about always having an "elevator speech" ready to go. What does this mean? Does it suggest that you will be doing speeches in the elevator, similar to speaking in a public place like the flash lecture? No, that is not the intent. The focus of the elevator speech is that you should always have a short "blurb" or synopsis of your message or initiative that could be delivered in the time of a "typical" elevator ride. Think about the elevator trip being about 30 seconds; you should have a pitch or summary of your work that can be delivered in that short period of time.

As you think about many of the other ways of having a public presence, you have much more time available. With a speech, it might be 30 minutes and with a flash lecture, it may be 15 minutes. If you're on a panel, you may have 10–15 minutes; if you're on a television show, it may involve 2–3 minutes of air time. If you're on the news, it may be only a few seconds, or a half minute or 1–2 minutes are aired.

With the elevator speech, there are two ways to think about this. First, this is a short interaction that encompasses, ideally, your key points or key messages. Second, this is designed as a stimulus or lead-in for further conversation or discussion with the recipient. Your intent with the elevator speech is to stimulate, motivate or suggest some specific action or new way of thinking. You may think about the use of intrigue as a strategy; you may quickly blend a statistic with a brief illustration; and you may offer a challenge to a widely-held point of view. Ideally, whatever you say, briefly, is designed to cause the person hearing this to ask further questions, to want to know where to get more information, to continue the discussion or, minimally, to ask for your contact information. All of this is good and is precisely the intent of having your elevator speech "ready to go."

To prepare this, think in terms of boiling down your key points into a summary message. With the various tools identified in this resource, think about something that would be memorable or intriguing, or would cause the audience (probably a single person or two) to follow up on the issue. You may find it helpful to have an acronym that spells out something of importance (e.g., LEADER could mean Listen, Execute, Advise, Delegate, Evaluate and Review).

Messages from the field

Gaining traction for an issue no one wanted to consider—the evolution of Erik's Cause

Judy Rogg MSW and Stephanie Small MA, LMFT, Co-Founders of Erik's Cause

Our journey began in 2010 after the blindsiding death of Judy's 12-year-old son, Erik, from what the detectives called "The Choking Game." HUH? WHAT? (See www.erikscause.org.) Very few people knew about this issue—and as we discovered, no one wanted to consider it. We began our uphill battle by creating a new solution—a skills based, non-graphic prevention program that educated but did not encourage this behavior. But we also needed credibility, to inform parents and educators, and then convince them of why to educate kids. In six years, we've gone from nothing to having our program known and sampled across numerous districts and formally adopted in one school district where it is both successful and generating data for study.

How did we get there? Here are some suggestions based on our grass-roots experience:

- Find others who have shared a similar tragic loss. Listen to what they've tried. Discern how you can move beyond the limitations of their failures.
- Dream big. Create a context for your message and who you want to reach (e.g., "stop this game and other risky behaviors," so we can reach "kids, parents, educators and communities").
- Understand your context. Let it be your "North Star."
- Develop objectives appropriate to your project but flexible enough to evolve over time. This is crucial when appealing to a wider audience and enlisting collaboration.
- Be creative. Think outside the box. Bounce ideas around with collaborators. We drew upon best practices being used to approach other risky behaviors since our issue has not had prior successful traction.
- Develop a succinct message that will catch attention: "If you only had 30 seconds to get the attention of a busy leader ..." Ours include:
  - Even smart strong kids can make dumb choices with deadly consequences.
  - Do you know everything your kids are really doing?
  - Do you think your kids would ever do something like this?
- Share it and don't be shy. Reach out to everyone, especially professionals. Some will laugh, others will listen. We sought out researchers, law enforcement, medical/mental health professionals, state/federal congressional representatives and all levels of educators. They all had varied experiences to contribute, some with content and some with furthering initiatives.
- Say "Yes" to all platforms offered to spread your message. You never know who will be in the audience.
- Be flexible. Listen to, evaluate and incorporate productive feedback. Also, know your boundaries. (e.g., we will not consider inclusion of any graphic material.)
- Talk to the media whenever possible. Media frequently wants to show the dramatic "shock" of this activity when there's an injury or death. We continue to educate them beyond the shock so they also report on our educational efforts.
- Keep current. We've stayed contemporary with the media. For example:
  - When the ice bucket challenge to support ALS went viral, the pass out "challenge" paralleled this, with an explosion of "how to play" videos including the word "challenge."
  - Track your efforts in writing and share it regularly with your supporters. This documents your progress as well as identifies where additional efforts might be needed. Further, it is a psychological aid when you feel like forward progress is at an impasse.
- Create an internet presence. This takes time. People reach out to us now from across the world.
- Display data in a visually compelling format. You might not think data exists, but it does, though it may take ingenuity to find it. Data speaks volumes.

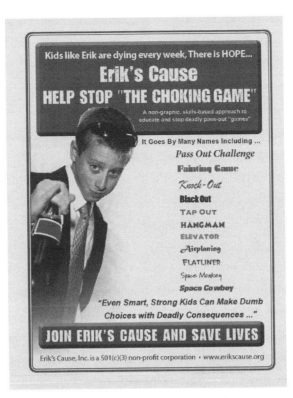

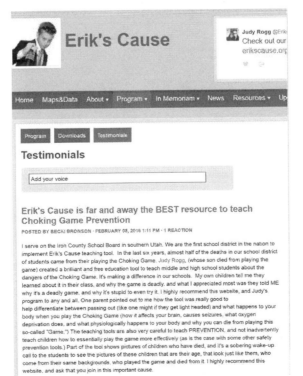

Emergency or crisis situations

Another situation that can present itself with health and safety issues revolves around an emergency or crisis. This could be an outbreak of a disease, a major health issue (e.g., water contamination), a weather-related situation (tornado, flood, storm), death (drunk driving, drug overdose, unexplained cause) or other situation. The emergency situation may directly affect you or your organization, because of its nature and the nature of what you do; because of this, you may be expected or required to have a voice or presence regarding the situation. This is included here because it is vital that you and your organization have a contingency plan, for handling situations relevant to your mission and topic specialization should they occur. For example, you may work in a public health agency and it is expected that you or your agency will speak out about a current or impending crisis situation, to provide information that is necessary to share and to highlight what you or your agency are doing to address the situation.

On the other hand, the emergency situation may be such that you don't have a direct relationship to the situation, but it could provide an opportunity for your voice or your perspective to be heard. For example, you may be in a setting, whether a city, town, campus, state or other environment where a crisis occurs (e.g., a horrific drugged driving automobile crash) and you may be part of a prevention organization focused around safe and sober driving. This tragic situation may be such that your organization views this as an opportunity to have its voice heard; this is not so much being "on the scene" with the tragic event, but responding to it within a timely way following the situation. You or your organization may want your voice heard, for example, about the prevention of such situations.

What is most important with these situations is that you are clear with your message and that you stay on message throughout this process. Particularly with a crisis situation, it is vital that you remain calm yet also engaged. There will undoubtedly be a lot of emotion associated with the crisis, whether it is panic or catastrophizing by the public or specific audiences. You will want to keep all of this in perspective, as you share as openly and honestly as possible what you know. You want to be clear, provide factual information and demonstrate your continual awareness of the feelings that may exist among your audience. You want to keep myths and rumors in check and should anticipate questions, issues and concerns so you can address them before they are asked of you.

Another issue that is often overlooked regarding emergency or crisis situations is the work that can and should be done before it happens. Think about how you will handle such a situation, should it occur. Depending on your role and your agency's responsibilities, consider the possibilities of the types of situations that might occur. Consider also who would be handling the public comments about the situation and what the overall message would be. Learn what processes should be followed to address the situation and to gain a clearer understanding of the details of the situation and ways of continuing to gather up-to-date and factual information. You may be tasked with the responsibility to share this with a broader public, but it is most helpful to have a plan already talked through and finalized prior to the actual existence of the crisis situation. Further, if and when the crisis situation does occur, you will have plenty to discuss and address, based on the idiosyncratic aspects associated with that specific event.

When you actually talk about crisis management in a preventive way and start to build the plans about how you will handle it, the obvious thing that happens is that you will build the key elements of a plan. The other thing that happens is that you can use this as an opportunity to talk through ways of avoiding a crisis and minimizing any negative impact this may have on you and your organization. While the external environment may be such that you cannot control the existence of a crisis, you may discuss ways that you can take proactive steps to reduce the severity or impact of a crisis, or reduce the frequency with which it happens. Just the process of talking through crisis and emergency situations can trigger new perspectives about how to prevent these or minimize the negative impact of them.

If and when a crisis does occur, you or someone in your organization should be designed to deal directly with the media. This may or may not involve the use of a press conference, or the preparation of a press release or a media advisory. This individual should be particularly skilled with handling the pressure and ongoing inquiries from the media. Again, it will be important for this person—perhaps you—to remain calm and also be informative. You will want to keep the media up-to-date on whatever new information you have. You should also be prepared to let the larger public know specific things that they should be doing to minimize personal risk or harm through the crisis situation.

Avoiding pitfalls

A helpful resource has been prepared by the U.S. Department of Health and Human Services and includes a section about avoiding pitfalls with crisis situations such as you may encounter. These pitfall examples, while prepared within the framework of a crisis situation, are also helpful for general planning purposes as approaches to avoid.

- Abstractions—use examples, stories and analogies to make your point. Don't assume there is a common understanding between you and your audience (even when you are using stories and analogies to make your point).

- Attitude/non-verbal messages—remain calm, attentive and polite. Adopt a relaxed, neutral physical stance. Don't let your feelings interfere with your ability to communicate positively. Never convey disgust, frustration, indifference or smugness. Never lose your temper. Don't allow your body language, your position in the room or your dress to affect your message.

- Blame—accept your share of responsibility for a problem. Don't try to shift blame or responsibility to others and don't magnify the fault to be found in others in order to deflect criticism or minimize your culpability.

- Costs—focus on the benefits to be derived, not on the costs entailed. If costs are an issue, voice respect for the need for responsible stewardship of public funds. Don't discuss issues in terms of their dollar value, or complain about a lack of funds.

- Guarantees—it is better to offer a likelihood, emphasizing progress and ongoing efforts. Don't make comments like, "There are no guarantees in life."

- Humor—avoid it. If used, direct it at yourself. Don't use it in relation to safety, or health or in describing risk.

- Jargon—define all technical terms and acronyms. Don't use language that may not be understood by even a portion of your audience.

- Negative words and phrases—use positive or neutral terms. Don't cite national problems, or make highly-charged analogies, e.g., "This is not Love Canal."

- "Off the record"—always assume everything you say and do is part of the public record. Don't make side comments or "confidential" remarks. (The rule is: never say anything that you are not willing to see printed on the front page of a newspaper.)

- Personal identity—speak for the organization. Use the pronoun "we." Don't give the impression that you, alone, are the authority on the issues being raised or the sole decision-maker. Never disagree with the organization you are representing, e.g., "personally, I don't agree," or "speaking for myself ..." or "if it were me ..."

- Promises—it is better to state your willingness to try. Promise only what you can deliver. Don't make promises you can't keep and never make a promise on behalf of someone else.

- Reliance on words alone—use visuals and handouts to emphasize key points. Don't rely entirely on the spoken word to explain your point.

- Speculation—stick to the facts of what has, is and will be done. Don't speculate on what could be done, or on what might happen, or on possible outcomes other than the intended one(s) or about worst case scenarios.

- Statistics—use them to illuminate larger points and to emphasize trends and achievements. Don't make them the focus of your remarks, or overuse them.

- Technical details and data—focus on empathy, efforts and results. Don't try to fully inform and educate audiences on the minutia of issues.[1]

Messages from the field

Staying calm amidst the crisis

Kevin Tunell, Communications Director/Emergency Public Information Officer, Yuma County, Arizona

One of the critical factors for anyone with primary communication responsibilities during a crisis or disaster—whether this is the Public Information Officer (PIO) or others in leadership positions—revolves around handling all the "white noise" during this time. The primary aim is to get good information to the public and to do so in a way that provides the public with a sense of calm and trust. Significant challenges to that effort during a crisis are rumors, half-truths, inaccuracies, speculations, lies, fear, anxiety, anger and other emotions.

Like no time in history before now has the white noise challenge been so daunting. The immediacy of the media, social media, news feeds, 24 hour news and the allure of rumor to sell, can spread (mis)information today in seconds when it used to take days or more. And what is spread can create and perpetuate panic, feelings of despair, anger and even riots before a lead communicator is tasked with restoring calm in the community. Dealing with media requests, executive emergency staff meetings, social media monitoring, news feed monitoring and all associated responsibilities are enough to make the best PIO confused if not overwhelmed. Thus, it is critical to keep the basic needs of the public in the forefront of thinking during these crisis situations.

During emergencies of any magnitude, chaos in varying degrees will exist. Therefore the communicator (whether a PIO or other leader) must be able to mine the needed information and make sound decisions quickly when disseminating that information.

What leads to the best results in this type of chaotic situation is to try and think like the people with whom you are trying to communicate. The general public has three basic needs during and after an emergency situation:

1 How do I protect myself?
2 How do I protect my family (including pets)?
3 How do I protect my property?

This is the nucleus of human nature and it mimics most forms of nature, much like the animal kingdom. It is important for information leaders to consider these three questions as the ingredients to reestablishing a sense of calm into the community, while also providing an organized message to the audience:

1 What happened?
2 How does it affect me?
3 What are you doing to make it go away?

It is vital that the lead communicators transmit usable information, and do so clearly, throughout the crisis or disaster situation. Further, realize that the situation can evolve and can be further compounded by chaos that continues to occur from multiple directions. The communicator should attempt to filter through the "white noise" and develop a sound framework which delivers the answers to the three basic questions the citizens need; by doing so, the community should be well on the way to a healthy status.

Messages from the field

Get up, dress up, show up and raise up

Sandy Spavone, Family, Career and Community Leaders of America

When I took on the role of the Executive Director of National Organizations for Youth Safety (NOYS) in 2003, I inherited two boxes of papers and a very old, small laptop. My first duties were to see where we were and present a plan of where I thought we could and should go. What I found was we had one official member and a year's worth of funds. To deny waking up in a panic at first would not be truthful. However, I knew NOYS had great potential and I had amazing support from trusted friends in the field. Working from home and running NOYS out of my home was also new. Determined to make NOYS work, I got up early just like I had a place to get to, got dressed up and showed up at every relevant meeting to which I could get an invite. Those allies who had been with NOYS before it became a non-profit were my strength and counsel. They listened, provided ideas and secured me a seat at meetings where I could share the potential of NOYS. Although I was the only paid employee, I wasn't alone, as I did have cheerleaders and guides. Within that first year together we converted participating organizations into active members and grew in funding with our first corporate donation. Seven years later, NOYS had over 50 non-profit and corporate members, office space and four staff members … as well as an annual budget of over 1 million dollars. Our motto was "If we were doing anything about youth, do it with youth and not to youth." This message resonated with leaders in the health and safety community. Through many long days and nights and the support of so many, we built NOYS into a vibrant well-known coalition that received quote placements in magazines including *Seventeen* and *Teen Vogue* as well as on the front page of *USA Today*. Was it easy—no. Was it worth it —yes.

In 2013 I left NOYS to go back to FCCLA as their executive director. In these past three years we have updated our Student Body program, held a rally with thousands of FCCLA youth on Capitol Hill advocating for family and consumer sciences and are releasing two updated programs addressing financial literacy and teen traffic safety. If you are in the world of working with teens and in the health and safety arena, know if you continue to get up, dress up, show up and don't try to do it alone—you will make an impact larger than you ever dreamed possible. Our youth need us to make a difference and include them in our work. It's up to us to raise them up! There will be failures and doors will not open when you wish they would—but you will succeed and your work will save lives and prevent injuries.

Forward!

In summary, the idea of a public presence is an important one for you. This is offered in contrast to much of the alone, behind the scenes work that you will do with your communications efforts. The "public presence" does not necessarily mean being in front of an audience or a camera; numerous approaches have been identified as contributing to this.

What is important is that many of the same concepts and principles highlighted through the various segments of this book are also found in the different approaches highlighted here. You need to have good planning undergirding your effort, and you need to be clear with your ultimate message of what you want the audience to know, feel and do. Whether the reach is large (e.g., through a nationwide television show) or small (e.g., with a flash lecture), the messages to you are the same. It is important that you are focused and provide a clear direction for the audience. You can draw upon the various general know-feel-do strategies (planning, message development, pilot testing, ethical factors) and specific tools (e.g., social marketing, positioning, creative epidemiology). No single magic approach is appropriate; you are the creator of the approach you want to implement, and your unique combination of elements and your personal style help you with organizing and orchestrating an effective effort.

Note

1 U.S. Department of Health and Human Services (USDHHS) (2002). *Communicating in a Crisis: Risk Communication Guidelines for Public Officials.* SMA02-3641.

11 Workshops

Overview

A workshop is an important vehicle for communicating about health and safety issues. It is a unique opportunity to convey messages to an audience compared to other communication approaches. A public service announcement, an interview in the newspaper or a poster each tries to engage or get the attention of the target audience. By contrast, a workshop has a relatively "captive" audience, participating in an event with some structure. Nonetheless, the opportunity for effective communication is central to the workshop and poses its own unique opportunities and challenges. This chapter explains how the health and safety communications model detailed in Chapter 1 can be used to ensure an effective workshop, from planning and implementation to review and refinement.

In short, a **workshop** is a time-limited opportunity to prepare the participants with a specified set of knowledge, attitudes and/or skills. Participants come to a workshop with an expectation that they will learn something specific—and they know what that is. Generally, workshops are limited in size, have a specific focus and incorporate a variety of know-feel-do strategies. Workshops may be fully voluntary and they may also involve participants who are required, encouraged or even coerced to attend. Workshops can be long or short; some, in fact, may be held over multiple days.

Some examples of a workshop:

- a one-hour session on how to manage your time more effectively;
- a refresher training on skills with CPR;
- a three-hour session that prepares you to make a skilled intervention with an individual with a drug abuse problem;
- an all-day training for teachers on how to teach middle school youth about good nutrition and healthy eating habits;
- an evening parenting, grandparenting or sibling class for expectant parents and their families;
- a train-the-trainers session that prepares potential workshop leaders with the knowledge and skills to conduct topic-specific workshops with others.

From a practical perspective, most workshops can be viewed as a type of training. The aim is for participants to learn as much as they can about a specific content area and within the defined amount of time. The person conducting the training is, ideally, knowledgeable on the topic area and skilled with working with a group of people. That's where this chapter comes in—enhancing the skills of you as the practitioner!

Content and process

Workshops encompass both content and process. Both are important, as one without the other results in a training or event that is not very engaging, or one that does not achieve the desired outcomes. Obviously, it is vital that the content be present—that individuals learn something as a direct result of participating in the workshop. Otherwise, you have a "feel good" session with little to show for it. For learning to occur, the process should be of good quality as well as appropriate for the audience. While the content may be excellent, individuals don't learn well if the delivery is poor. Similarly, if the learning environment is not conducive to receptivity, then quality learning does not happen.

You have probably experienced some particularly high quality workshops or courses, as well as some that are not done as well. When you think about what makes a workshop or course high quality, what comes to mind? Undoubtedly, you think of things like the following:

- The workshop leader knew the content.
- The participants were respected by the workshop facilitator.
- The environment was conducive to learning.
- A variety of approaches were used.
- Participants' questions were addressed.
- Attendees were able to identify how to apply what was emphasized.
- The time was used effectively.
- Examples were provided.

On the other hand, you know of some elements that are to be avoided. Although many more could be identified, here are some:

- The workshop leader was disorganized.
- It started late—or—it ended late.
- There was too much time between breaks.
- The speaker was not engaging and often just read paragraphs at a time.
- Many of the slides were too detailed and had too much information on them.
- The room was too hot/cold.
- Participants felt like they already knew all the information; it was so basic.

In order to have an effective workshop, you should balance both the process and the content. Each is vital for an effective workshop. While some of the process is not directly under your control (perhaps the seating in the room and sometimes the room temperature), much of it can be addressed successfully. The important thing is to have balance between each of these elements.

Regarding content, "As a result of an individual participating in your workshop, what do you want them to know, feel or do?" Once you are clear on this, you can create your workshop design, content, flow and supporting resources. Further, you will be able to establish objectives for the workshop and then design an appropriate evaluation to assess the extent to which these aims are achieved.

For process, the focus is on how you do the workshop. This has everything to do with how you run the workshop and the extent to which you engage the audience, to the temperature of the room and the promptness of starting and finishing. The process is all about how the participants feel and the extent to which a comfortable and appropriate learning environment is present. If the room is too hot, for example, participants don't learn well. Thus, the workshop facilitator should take appropriate action to address this, whether through adjusting the temperature, relocating the session, having more breaks or another strategy; the leader should not ignore something that clearly gets in the way of learning.

Preparing for the workshop

When planning the workshop, it is most helpful to begin with some of the basic parameters and draw upon the health and safety communications model used throughout this book. Basically, there is no one best way of doing a workshop. For example, some topics lend themselves more readily to a "hands-on" approach with practice sessions; others may be more emotional or affective in nature. Some topics or issues may necessitate a more intensive approach and other topics may be more academic or scholarly in nature. Within this overall context, the foundations begin to be laid. In preparing for the workshop, you will find that it is much like a piece of art. It's quite organic, blending the expectations of the planners, the nature of the audience, the time allocated, the setting, your skills, the content to be covered and the unforeseen.

A key consideration with the workshop has to do with several other factors. What are the expectations of the planners or organizers of the workshop, particularly if that is not you? Learn as much as you can about what they expect as a result of the workshop. Try to understand why the workshop is being done and what its desired outcomes are. See what you can find out about the audience; for example, who is expected to come, who is recruited, what they are expecting and whether they are required to attend.

Other parameters include the length of the workshop—whether it is envisioned as a half-day training, or is limited to a one-hour time period. Find out whether this will be offered during a time that includes lunch and, if so, whether this is a "working lunch." How many people are expected and what is the room like?

Messages from the field

Handling time parameters

David S. Anderson, George Mason University

I recall a workshop that I was asked to prepare for staff members of elected representatives in the U.S. Congress. I thought a minimum of 90 minutes would be appropriate, particularly since lunch was being served as a motivation to encourage attendance. The planner insisted that the maximum would be 60 minutes. I tried to encourage a compromise of 75 minutes and the time of 60 minutes was all that would be allowed. The reason was that attendees knew they could get an hour away from the office for lunch (and the training), but more than that would be a deal-breaker in terms of their participation.

How do all of these parts fit together? That's the creative and artistic part of the workshop. Once you know the parameters, you can start designing the content. For example, if you know that you will be doing a workshop with 10 people, the result may be a different design than if you are preparing for a workshop with 40 people on the same topic. Or, if you know that your aim is one of increasing awareness or knowledge on a specific topic, your approach will likely be more content-based; alternatively, if you seek to enhance a participant's skill level on a specific area, you will probably have more hands-on know-feel-do strategies with some practice sessions. For example, with the issue of how to install a child safety seat safely and properly in a car, you may have vide-otapes of correct and incorrect know-feel-do strategies; you may also include a child safety seat and a car seat mockup or car where participants can actually practice installing this. If you have a specific content to be accomplished, you will do it in different ways if your time constraints are 45 minutes versus 90 minutes.

In a similar way, if the workshop is being prepared for individuals who volunteer to participate, and are true volunteers for the session, the approach will be different than if the workshop is developed as a mandated approach for participants. The workshop leader may or may not say "I know that you all are required to be here"; in either event, this awareness of the mandatory nature of the workshop must be included in the planning and design of the workshop so that the workshop content and approaches are, because of this factor, more engaging and directly applicable than it otherwise might have been. The leader will, in this case of "mandated" participants, have to work harder to maintain their interest in the workshop.

A common error is to try to cram too much into a limited period of time. Thus, all the planning goes together so that the time limitations and the workshop objectives are handled together and consistently. To try to accomplish a large amount of content is reasonable; however, sufficient time must be available for this to occur. If the time allocated is limited, then the objectives and activities must be similarly limited and focused.

Through the planning process, an overall guiding principle is that there is parallelism between the workshop objectives, the various parameters (such as audience, size and length) and the content used to accomplish the objectives. Throughout the workshop, the leader must pay attention to these, particularly since unexpected interruptions or challenges will appear.

Selecting and preparing the space

One of the first things to do with having an effective workshop is to have the space prepared in a way that is suitable to your style, the size of the group and the nature of the workshop itself. Your aim is to make the space as conducive as possible to what you are seeking to accomplish with the workshop. As indicated earlier, if you seek to have more hands-on activities, you will want to be able to move around. If you envision having workshop participants role play in a fishbowl type setting, you will want to have the setting so that those doing the role play can be engaged with one another, yet visible to all workshop participants. If you envision having small group breakout sessions, you will want the space or moveable furnishings that allow for this to be accomplished.

There are often occasions where you are assigned a space for the workshop; if you are provided a room for your workshop, you will want to check it out as early as possible to determine the extent to which it meets your needs and also to identify ways of making adaptations to the space so that it maximizes the workshop experience for your participants. Similarly, if you are in a room with fixed seating, that format necessarily limits your ability to have participants arrange themselves in small discussion groups.

Most of the discussion, however, is about how to arrange the space or to specify the room configuration, as it is typical that you will have a choice. The space arrangements will need to be in line with your workshop plans.

- What set-up will best promote the type of learning environment you seek to promote? What set-up will make your audience most comfortable?

- How many people will participate? If you have a small group, you may want to arrange the room in a circle or open square, so that each participant can see every other participant. You can even do this with a medium sized group of 30 or so participants. If you have a large group, this type of set-up would be cumbersome; you would be better served with a different arrangement (rows and tables).
- What audiovisual arrangements are needed? Will there be a specialist to help? Will you need a screen, projection unit or sound equipment? Consider having redundancy, by bringing your own equipment to be sure you have what you need.
- Is there someone available for technical assistance, whether with the audiovisual equipment or with other room arrangements?
- Do you or one of the presenters need a podium for notes or materials?
- Do you need flip charts or newsprint for posting?
- What materials are needed—note cards, tape, markers?
- Will you need a microphone?
- Will you have a remote clicker for slides? Does it have a laser pointer?
- Do you want a head table?
- Where will you and other leaders be situated? Will you be at a head table? Will you be standing? Will you be moving around?
- Do you need a table or place for additional materials, such as a resource display or materials for distribution?
- Do you want tables for the participants?
- If you have conference-type rectangular tables, what is the arrangement? Square? Open square? U-shape? Two-layers?
- Will you have extra chairs on the outskirts?
- Watch the lighting for any items projected on the screen; make sure that the screen can be seen from all places in the workshop setting.
- Learn what you need to know about the space—directions to the site, local directions to the building, parking arrangements, signage, access to the room.
- Identify the location of resources, such as restrooms, drink or snack machines.
- Will food be served? Where? When will it be set up?

Many of the answers to these questions and issues will be based on other factors associated with the workshop, including the workshop goals, the number of attendees, the topic and your style, among other factors.

- With a workshop of ten people, you probably would not have a podium.
- With a group of 50 participants, it is unlikely it would be arranged in a circle.
- With a topic of increasing skills, such as with CPR, having fixed seating would not be appropriate.
- For a workshop having a dozen people, you may want to all be seated in chairs around a table so you can see all workshop participants easily.
- With a workshop having teams or small discussion groups, you may want to arrange for seating at round tables for participants to work together.

Again, there is no one approach or single best way of conducting the workshop; it all depends on the variety of factors associated with the workshop topic, place, participants and you.

Messages from the field

Creating positive learning environments

John Kriger, M.A., Kriger Consulting, Inc.

Many facilitators don't fully utilize the tools of influence available to them to create engaging and enlightening presentations. The more you set the stage for your participants before they arrive, transitioning them into the training environment and fully engaging them, the more impact you will produce and the greater the potential for satisfaction.

Orient participants early. Provide an opportunity for participants to mentally transition themselves into the training space. Provide transition time to allow participants to adjust from the activities required to get into room or setting. Facilitate their physical, emotional and psychological transformation from commuters to participants. By providing a smooth transition from the external world into the physical setting, participants will be far better prepared and adjusted for the learning process.

Minimize distractions in the learning environment. Make sure it is comfortable and free from overt or more subtle distractions. Learning does not just happen in our heads. It is impacted by our ability to maintain focused attention to tasks and the information being provided. Make sure your environment does not distract from your information.

Contain clutter. Keep the front of the room clear of distracting materials, pictures or training aids. When you maintain the front of the room in a neat and uncluttered manner it allows participants to focus on the material and not be distracted by debris in their field of vision.

Make it predictable. At the very beginning of your training let them know where things are: restrooms, vending machines, where lunch will be held, secretarial support, phones, copy machines and anything else they might need. Go over the expectations of the day. Let them know when breaks will be held, what time lunch is and if there is even the smallest chance that the session will deviate from the scheduled time for ending.

Attend to sounds. Make sure what you want participants to hear can be heard. Make sure sounds you don't want are eliminated. I remember being in one training and the presenter kept bringing his hands together and clicking his rings, which was very distracting. At the break I went up and mentioned it to him; he was totally unaware that he was doing it, let alone that it was distracting, and thanked me for the feedback. When confronted with an external sound don't try to compete with it. If someone's cell phone goes off, there's noise from another room or there are other temporary distractions, wait until the distraction passes and then continue. If participants' attention is diverted they are not learning anyway.

Maximize safety. In order to participate fully and avoid distractions, participants need to know they are in a safe, secure and predictable environment. Let them know that you want them to raise concerns if they have them; if there are unresolved concerns, they are not listening. Your brain cannot function optimally when it needs to attend to multiple agendas. Encourage them to bring up concerns to be addressed, so you can move on.

Workshop approaches

The workshop itself comes down to the content that is included in it and how it is delivered. Two main recommendations are found here. First, incorporate approaches that best help you achieve your desired outcomes or results. Second, have a variety of know–feel–do strategies. Workshops are based on the variety of factors such as your preferred instructional style, the nature of the audience and its experience, your setting, the time available and your desired outcomes.

Imagine a workshop that is entirely a lecture—that would probably not be the most engaging for the audience. Add to that some background informational slides; including these now provides two different modes of delivery. If you now incorporate some visuals within those slides, and some video clips, you have further adapted the range of workshop delivery processes. Beyond that, you could include some queries of the participants, like asking a question and getting a show of hands. You might have a workshop where attendees report similar experiences to what is being highlighted in the content, or offer perspectives about how they might implement the strategy being noted. Engage in processes that maximize the participants' learning during the workshop setting.

The other consideration with having multiple approaches is the acknowledgment that people learn in different ways. While you have particular content to highlight, the participants will be engaged in different ways. It's helpful to be clear, in your own mind, about the key point(s) within a segment and then proceed to develop that point in different ways. For example, you may make the point, provide further detail about what the point means, offer any research or documentation that supports the point, provide one or more illustrations of it and engage the audience in discussion or an activity to ensure that they understand the point. This broad-based approach helps individuals learn. Further, it acknowledges that people learn in different ways; some are primarily visual learners, others learn through reading and others learn by practice. The contextual point here is that many workshops will be conducted with adults; these adults will be of all ages, backgrounds, education level and cultural context. Helpful for you being effective with the workshop is to acknowledge the implications from the field of study of adult learning theory.

What follows are brief descriptions for each of a variety of approaches that can be considered for the workshop. As you plan your workshop, think of a parallel scenario with cooking: when you look at your spice cabinet, you won't use all the spices in a recipe, but you might consider ways of enhancing the food that you are preparing. Similarly, look at these various know-feel-do strategies as those from which you can choose, as you prepare the workshop. Some of these require more advance preparation and others can be incorporated much more easily. You might blend or adapt some of these; other know-feel-do strategies certainly exist and you might even create some of your own!

- Lecture—the lecture provides prepared remarks or insights on the topic. The workshop presenter has specific content that is highlighted. This is basically the content narrative that incorporates the knowledge, practical applications and suggested directions for the workshop participants. Typically, this is complemented by other approaches to "bring it to life."
- Guided discussion—this is a modified lecture, whereby the group leader develops the content in ways that involve the audience. The leader may ask a question and get some initial reactions or feedback. The leader may have an overall flow of the content and then engage the participants with specific activities, questions or other interaction elements.
- Large group discussion—this is often done throughout the workshop and provides the opportunity for participants to go into more depth on a specific topic. The guided discussion previously noted is more focused and allows for give and take with the workshop facilitator through a process and issues identified by the leader. The large group discussion is often more free-wheeling and around a general topic or issue.
- Small group discussion—when the workshop leader seeks the opportunity for more in-depth discussion among group participants, this approach can be implemented.

The topic or "assignment" may be the same as would be done with a large group discussion, but the workshop leader may want to have the opportunity for more individuals to speak and be engaged in the dialog; thus smaller groups of four to six people may each address the same, or different, issues. This also provides the opportunity for each small group to provide a summary or brief report of the main findings or highlights of its discussions. With a relatively small number of workshop participants, small group discussions will probably not be needed. This approach gives individuals, particularly those who are hesitant to speak up in a larger group, the opportunity to be involved and have their voice heard.

- Audiovisual materials—these complement the lecture or guided discussion. Typically, these are found with PowerPoint slides that organize the key points. These slides may have specific content, bulleted points, quotes, visual illustrations and applicable know-feel-do strategies. Audiovisual materials may also include sound or visual clips, such as public service announcements, segments from a film or newscast, pre-recorded interviews and more.

- Sample materials—it may be helpful to bring samples of whatever is being illustrated or demonstrated. For example, if the aim is to illustrate how nutritional labeling occurs on food packaging, you might bring in some food containers or boxes to illustrate this.

- Handouts—materials are helpful for participants to have as a reference or guide following the workshop. While some of these may be used in the workshop, others may simply be referenced over the course of the workshop. Sometimes, handouts are incorporated into a workbook that includes content, resources, worksheets and other materials. These can also be made available for later access, on a website or on a flash drive distributed to workshop participants. There is no need to just have handouts; items should be helpful and relevant for the attendees. Further, to the extent possible, it is also wise to not print materials that may have no relevance for a particular person; think of ways to be as environmentally friendly and budget-conscious as possible.

- Worksheets—just as with the handouts, worksheets can complement the achievement of the goals. Sometimes approaches require a printed document. If an exercise is fairly brief and can be done without a printed worksheet, the instructions and content may be prepared and displayed visually. However, there are times when it is most helpful and expedient to have a printed worksheet that individuals, or groups of individuals, complete on site.

- Audience response systems—often known as "clickers" or "decision software," this equipment allows for polling the audience on key questions or issues; further, their use helps keep the audience engaged. The technology allows for stand-alone software and hardware and increasingly through the use of cell phones. This approach allows for querying the audience's knowledge, attitudes or perceptions, gathering pre-workshop and post-workshop responses and sharing results with participants as a foundation for discussion. The important thing is to be comfortable with the fact that you may obtain responses about which you may be concerned (e.g., if you find that a large number of respondents engage in some inappropriate behavior); you must be prepared for dealing with whatever findings emerge.

- Testimonials—this approach involves personal statements from individuals, helpful for illustrating specific points in the workshop. It may involve their reflections or insights about a specific incident or strategy, their perspectives, their recommendations and other views. This can be done in person individually or with a panel, through pre-taped comments or in writing to be read or shown to the participants.

- Reflection pages—there may be times in the flow of the workshop when you want participants to do some thinking, planning or reflection. This may be done to give them the opportunity to think about how they are reacting to the content of the workshop, ways in which they might apply the content, or concerns about implementing this when they return to their work, community or home setting. These worksheets may be shared or may simply be used to aid the participants with self-reflection.

- Sentence completion—this can be done with the group as a whole, or within the context of completing a workshop. They may be done privately (e.g., writing it down) or shared with others (e.g., in a dyad, a small group or the large group). Participants may be asked to complete the sentence stem such as: "Right now, I'm feeling …" or "What I've learned most during this workshop is …"

- Dyads or triads—there may be times when it is helpful to have small groups of participants discuss a topic, or work on an issue together. Not only does this help break up a standard approach, but it is also helpful in promoting interaction among participants, as well as keeping them engaged. Often helpful with this is to have some or all small groups report on their results; it will be important to manage the time, however, so that sufficient time is available for reporting.

- Small workgroups—this provides the opportunity for individuals to have a more intimate discussion than can be achieved with the larger group. The workgroup size will be based on the nature of the assignment and what most effectively helps accomplish the goals of the activity. This may include three or four individuals, but can also involve eight to ten individuals. This will also be determined by the nature of the set-up of the workshop space; if you have a room constrained with round tables, your workgroups can include those sitting at each table; if you have flexible workshop space and the opportunity to regroup in a different format, you can arrange this in a different way. The designation for specific workgroups may be random (e.g., by counting off or a pre-assigned group number or color), by professional role, by a demographic (e.g., age, gender) or by an issue of interest (such as one developed on site).

- Case studies—this involves a summary or example that describes a real-life situation. These can offer summaries of a situation that ended up poorly, that had good conclusions or that could have been better. These can be helpful for stimulating discussion about how a situation was handled, what was done well or poorly and how to handle similar situations in the future. These can be prepared in narrative form as part of attendees' print materials, read to the group or distributed as a handout. With smaller breakout groups, different case studies can be provided to the groups.

- Brainstorming—creativity underlies the brainstorming activity, whereby "rules" or "standards" are identified. With classic brainstorming, typical guidelines include "be creative," "no idea is stupid or silly," "no criticism" and "please do piggyback on others' ideas." The concept is to generate as many ideas as possible and to discuss and critique them later. This can be done in a regular workshop format, with eyes closed, or having participants reconfigured so that no one faces anyone else (e.g., with backs together in a circle formation, facing outward).

- Skill practice—with workshops focusing on the enhancement of skills, it is appropriate to actually practice the new skill. This can be technical (such as how to install a child safety seat correctly or how to do CPR) or interaction (such as doing a television interview). This approach has participants actually perform the activity (appropriate equipment or props are required for some of these and can be helpful for others). This can be done in smaller groups, or as part of the entire workshop group (depending on the number of participants in the workshop and available time).

- Role play—similar to skill practice, the individual is involved in an interaction that seeks to enhance the skills. The role play situation asks an individual to respond to a situation or type of individual (such as an angry person) and demonstrate appropriate interaction skills. The aim is to have the opportunity to actually experience the situation and to handle it as appropriately as possible. This may be done in the larger group, to illustrate key points for being effective with the skills being addressed. The workshop participant is then provided feedback from the workshop facilitator, and often from the other participants, about what was done well and what could be done better. A variation on this approach is to have workshop participants "tag themselves in" during the role play situation if they would like to attempt a different approach for addressing the situation.
- Fishbowl—this is an approach used when the number of workshop participants does not allow the time for everyone to be involved; it incorporates other approaches, but only involves a few of the workshop participants directly. This could involve a role play with two or more people, a small group discussion, skills development or other approach with the individual(s) doing their activity, yet being surrounded by other workshop participants (thus, like being in a fishbowl).
- Computer simulation—it may be helpful to offer a simulation, where workshop participants engage in a process using online resources, and see what results emerge. Similar to the audience response systems where participant feedback is gathered, this may be a situation that illustrates how to obtain various findings based on the information provided.

Messages from the field

Practical tips

Thomas E. Legere, Ph.D., https://thestudyofthesoul.com

Public speaking—whether delivering a workshop or giving a speech—is an art. There's not a set format or style and there's no one best way. I offer the following tips based on my experience of doing large and small, and long and short, workshops and talks over many decades.

- Never show up with just a "canned" presentation. Otherwise, a great message may fall on deaf ears. Ask yourself, "Who, specifically, is my audience? What is the average level of education? Is this primarily an academic group or is the audience made up of clinicians or practitioners? Is the audience likely to be sympathetic to your message or is the group likely to be skeptical?" Keep asking yourself how you might "tweak" your message and words to be a more effective communicator. For example, with health care professionals, it is fine to use terms such as "neurotransmitters" and "neurons"; with non-professionals, use more everyday, less technical words like "brain chemicals" and "brain cells."
- Clarify your purpose. Be clear with whether your purpose is primarily didactic or motivational. Do you wish to cram in as much information as possible or do you wish to highlight several points and steer the participants as to how they can follow up on future reading on their own? Is community building important with this group or is it a disparate group only interested in professional information?

- Begin by giving an overview on what will be covered. Ideally, this should be projected on a screen or at least written down in an outline form. Be specific. Show how and why the material is being presented in this order and format. Lay out the general time that will be allotted to each section. After each major section, recap how the previous section has led to the current and future material.
- Be truthful and current with information. If a point that you wish to make is in dispute, acknowledge this. Only say something that represents "Best Practice" and "Best Thinking." Otherwise, you run the risk of sending people forth with erroneous information that may discredit their message in the future. For example, if you are speaking about the impact of "ecstasy" on the brain, state that when scientists talk about ecstasy causing "holes in the brain," this fact is not literally true; rather, clarify that there appear to be "pockets" in the brain where electrical activity is not apparent. Also acknowledge that information is always changing in the health field. Although "old" sources may still be valid, audiences deserve to know when research was conducted. Keep up to date on the latest audiovisual material available. Even DVDs or film clips where individuals appear to be from another decade can cause mental "flak" for an audience. If a matter is still in dispute, try to present both points of view fairly. It may be tempting (and is fairly easily done) to present a point different from one's own in an unfavorable light. This is unethical and unhelpful to the audience.
- Enhance your presentation with the point of view of an expert. This will lift your presentation from the realm of anecdote and personal opinion and give your delivery more credibility. However, keep in mind that, as a rule, the use of authority is the weakest approach. Always try to stick with human experience as the best touchstone.
- The worst thing to do in giving a speech or leading a workshop is to come across as giving a speech. The best communicators are relaxed, self-deferential, not married to the podium, not confined by power points, comfortable with some eye contact with the audience and open to feedback and even challenge by the audience. Remember, it is not about you or your opinions. It is about the subject matter and how this might serve the needs of those in the care and assistance of those in the audience. Of course, every presentation should be substantial and worth the time of all present. One of the best compliments I ever received was, "I feel like you work very, very hard to make it all seem very, very easy and relaxed."
- Every workshop should contain at least some process, otherwise it is just a long lecture. The trick is determining the right ratio. Usually, audiences like to feel like they are "getting their money's worth." Consequently, it is best to lay out your case, with plenty of notes and resources, and then introduce the process; this process can include, besides group interaction (dyads, triads, etc.), the use of music, DVDs, clips from YouTube and almost anything to ensure a multi-model learning experience. One of the greatest compliments that you can receive at the end of an all-day workshop is, "I felt like the time flew by."

Messages from the field

An alcohol educator online

Foundation for Advancing Alcohol Responsibility

In an effort to demonstrate how alcohol affects individuals differently, an online program using the latest science available helps demonstrate an individual's blood alcohol concentrations (BAC) after the "virtual consumption" of alcoholic beverages. Differences in BAC are cited based on gender, weight, height, age, amount consumed, type of beverage and elapsed time. The Virtual Bar app also shows how the individual might actually feel at different BAC levels, as well as specific consequences associated with various BAC levels. This program also illustrates comparisons with other individuals (different genders and weights) with the same amount of alcohol. This app also allows users to select different food options to better understand the potential impact of food consumption on their BAC; the app also provides a sense of how long it takes for the BAC to return to 0.00.

In addition to the online Virtual Bar a corresponding mobile app was created to allow for micro-moments, with real time relevance, to happen anytime and anywhere. The target audience for the mobile Virtual Bar is young adults of legal drinking age and provides the same experience and BAC information as the web-based program. The Virtual Bar may be downloaded for free from the iTunes or Google Play stores.

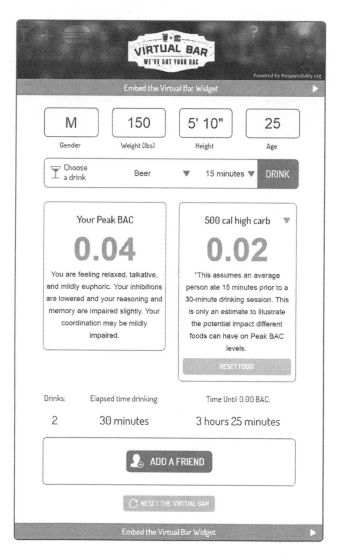

In summary, these know–feel–do strategies are not intended as the entire repertoire of options for what can be included in a workshop; however, they do represent the wide array of approaches that are typically used. As noted with several of these, different strategies can be blended together. Further, as you grow more comfortable with workshop preparation and delivery, you will find your own adjustments and enhancements and determine your own areas of expertise and comfort.

Starting the workshop

Most helpful for an effective workshop is having a strong start. This helps set the tone for the entire workshop, whether it is for one hour, a day or several days. You will want to be organized and clear with the workshop framework and how you envision it flowing. If you want to stay on time, and to have breaks at various intervals, please be clear with that. If you want individuals with questions to interrupt you, please be clear with that also.

You will want to share with participants the overall outline for the workshop—your workshop objectives as well as how you anticipate the time will be allocated. This helps provide participants with a framework about the overall workshop experience. This outline with objectives and timeline is also helpful for you to reference throughout the workshop, particularly if it is a longer workshop. You may say, halfway through the workshop, "here is where we started, here is where we are now and here is where we are heading." This shows the overall context during the workshop; it provides a "bird's eye view" of the workshop experience and can be helpful for participants as they think about applying the content in their home setting.

Another helpful process is having participants introduce themselves. The way this is done really depends on how long the workshop is and how many people are present. With a large workshop, or with a relatively brief workshop, this won't be feasible; for the large workshop, this would take too long and for a brief workshop it just isn't worth doing. A way of doing this for either of these situations is to ask some questions briefly, such as "By a show of hands, for how many of you is this the first time attending a workshop on this topic?" or "What is one thing you expect to gain from this workshop?"

The overall reason for doing introductions is to establish a type of comfort level among workshop participants. Thus, if this is a workshop that will last for several hours, it can be helpful to have all participants do a very brief introduction, such as their name, institution/ organization, role and one learning outcome they'd like to see addressed during the workshop.

A challenge is to have the amount of time used for introductions appropriate for the amount of time available for the workshop overall. Thus, it would be inappropriate to spend one-half hour for introductions with a two hour workshop. Another concern is that, sometimes, introductions go on too long and many people just want to get on with the workshop itself. This is a problem when some participants go way beyond what you expect as the workshop leader; you may ask for a brief introduction, but then someone gives a lengthy introduction. Model good leadership by establishing your parameters and then make sure that participants follow those instructions. If one of the first participants to provide an introduction goes on too long, you can address this by commenting that future introductions should be briefer. Overall, establish the tone that you find most helpful for enhancing the workshop's learning outcomes.

Another thing that is part of the opening, noted above and sometimes as part of the introductions, is to have clarity about what participants expect and the planned workshop objectives and activities. Sometimes, participants may read the advertising of the workshop to mean one thing, when you intend for it to mean another. Other times, individuals come with their own agenda, and that is not what you anticipated covering, nor are prepared to cover. Thus, some brief input from participants about their expectations and then sharing the extent to which various items will and will not be covered would be appropriate. If the workshop is at a conference, and an individual has some choices, this "back and forth" framework can be helpful so that the participants can decide to leave if they find that the workshop won't meet their needs or wasn't what they expected.

It is very important that the objectives stated for the workshop, whether through the advertising or with the initial outline presented at the workshop, actually are those that will be covered. It is up to you, the workshop facilitator, to maintain the integrity of the workshop with appropriate time management, already discussed, to be sure that every opportunity to address these objectives is met.

As part of setting the tone at the start of the workshop, you should demonstrate good energy for leading the workshop. This can be with enthusiasm regarding the workshop process and preparing to embark on this with the participants. The other part is exuding confidence with the workshop content and process. This may be a challenge, particularly if the topic is new for you, or the audience is one with which you have not worked before. It is also a challenge when this is one of your first workshops! Demonstrating this commitment and energy can also be difficult when you are doing a workshop that you have done many times. Your participants should feel like you are treating them as special, as if they are your only audience (even if you have done the workshop 20 times previously).

Several other things can be considered for the start of the workshop. These include both logistical issues as well as the overall way that you envision the workshop proceeding. These all help set the tone.

- Acquaint participants with the location of restrooms, drinks and snacks, and whether and when breaks will occur.
- Discuss any materials and resources, and how you will use them. This includes whether you will be using handouts, worksheets, a workbook and whether you will have materials available online or electronically following the workshop.
- Talk about how you'd like electronics used, such as computers, tablets and cell phones.
- Describe the overall plan for the workshop, including the need or desire to stay on schedule (or not), and the plan to end on time.
- If you intend to gather data from participants before the start of the workshop, such as with a pre-test or assessment, incorporate this at this time.
- Discuss how you want to handle questions or comments from participants. If you want interruptions or queries, make that point clearly.
- Depending on the nature of the workshop, it may be helpful to announce that the workshop has limitations, often due to the length of the session as well as the setting in which it is held. You may describe what the workshop will cover, as well as ways that participants can gain additional information or resources on the topic.

Once the workshop gets going, it will be helpful to maintain the tone that you'd like to have, so that the attainment of the workshop's goals and objectives can be maximized. You want to be respectful of the participants' engagement with the workshop and you also want them to be respectful of your expertise and time, as well as the time of the other participants.

Keep the participants engaged

Throughout the workshop content, strive to keep the participants engaged. This can be challenging for lengthy workshops. However, even in a relatively brief workshop, such as one that is one hour long, do everything you can to keep the participants focused on the content of the session.

What are some ways of doing this? One strategy is to be clear about what you seek to accomplish with reminders or references to the outcomes throughout the workshop. Keep your eyes on the "end product," which is what you want the participants to know, feel or do as a result of participating in the workshop. Continue to monitor the time to be sure that, in a general sense, you are remaining "on track" for meeting your end goals.

As you proceed through the workshop, watch the audience. If you see that many of them have glazed-over eyes, or are doing something else such as checking their messages or working on their computer, then incorporate some strategy to get them engaged. Watch for verbal as well as non-verbal cues. Observe how participants respond to your comments, your queries, your questions and the overall flow of the workshop. You may find that participants are following your presentation or guided discussion through their evident head nods or smiles; similarly, you may find no reaction to what you have covered, with no eye contact or droopy eyes. That's where asking questions of participants overall can be helpful.

Another way of maintaining participants' engagement with the workshop is to walk around. To remain behind a podium or table can be quite limiting and structured. What is helpful is to move around so that there is continuous action within the workshop room. If audiovisuals are used, then the use of a remote clicker can be most helpful for moving the slides forward and for highlighting specific content areas with the laser pointer; this can be done from anywhere in the room. This movement can also serve as a relatively inoffensive way of attending to those who may appear less engaged. Similarly, if you move around the room, the attention of all participants is not focused on only one setting or location.

Similarly, if the workshop involves activities with participants working individually or in small groups, walking around the room is helpful for determining whether or not they are "on track." If small group discussions are used to discuss a specific point, walking around and listening can help determine whether or not participants are working on the activity. Further, if the assignment is in several parts (e.g., to identify specific parts of the problem and then discuss how to proceed), listening in on the discussion can be helpful to determine if they are balancing their time so they can do both parts of the discussion. If they are not proceeding with the discussion, you can work with the group to problem-solve and try to move them forward so they complete the assignment.

Another way of keeping people engaged is to ask questions of the audience—this could be a query that links to your content, such as "how many people do you think die each year due to cigarette smoking?"; it may also be a generic question such as "does this discussion we have just had make sense?" or a more focused question like "do you see any inconsistencies between this recent content and the earlier discussion we had?" Having questions like these provides the opportunity to get audience reactions along the way; they also provide you with the opportunity to ask a specific individual, or group of individuals (such as those sitting in the back of the room) about their responses.

You might also use periodic assessments to keep the workshop participants engaged. One way of doing this is pausing the workshop delivery and asking participants about their workshop experience. While this is less necessary with a shorter workshop, it becomes more helpful when the workshop spans a half-day, full-day or multiple days. For example, when proceeding with the workshop, take a few moments and ask the participants how they are doing, whether they have any questions and whether the content and process is making sense to them. You can also ask them a question, such as to complete a sentence stem; this might ask how they would describe the content and/or the process thus far in the workshop. In short, this is a type of "pulse check" where you ask the participants about their reactions to the workshop at that point in its delivery. This can be an opportunity for you, as the workshop leader, to make revisions if needed. For example, if it is apparent that participants are not clear with a message or key point in the workshop, you can go over this again, or perhaps ask other workshop members to provide their description or interpretation of this content. Another thing you can ask is whether the flow or speed of the workshop is appropriate—whether the workshop is moving too fast, too slow or at just the right pace; based on the feedback, you can make modifications.

You might envision this process of checking on the status of participants as a type of "bookends" approach, with some additional "dividers" in the middle. This means sharing the overall outline and schedule with participants at the beginning, reminding the audience of "where they are" throughout the workshop and then reviewing the flow and content at the end of the workshop. This is a way of reviewing "where we are and where we are heading" for the workshop as a whole.

If, when conducting the workshop, you find that you need to spend more time on an issue, then you may need to do some readjustment with the scheduling of other content items. You need to take caution, in your planning phase, that your workshop flow is not so tightly regulated that you have no time for flexibility or adapting the content. If you need to spend more time on a specific topic, then balance that adjustment with less time or a different approach on another topic. If you have some part of a workshop take longer than expected, you know you have to adjust the overall flow by modifying the time from another part of the workshop. For example, if you have situations where you plan to have each workshop participant role play a series of activities, you may find that you have to modify this so that only some participants role play this; this could thus be accomplished by modeling the situation for the entire group.

One of the most challenging times for keeping participants engaged is right after a meal. If your workshop starts after lunch, or if it continues after the meal period, attend to the natural mechanism of an individual becoming tired after having eaten. Thus, in your planning, make sure that your post-lunch workshop content involves more activity than would otherwise be the case. It would not be wise to have a detailed or lengthy lecture right after lunch; rather, consider having an activity, watching a video, engaging in a discussion or having some other approach that involves the participants' engagement.

Manage the time

Parallel to the considerations about keeping participants engaged in the workshop is the emphasis about managing the time. Highlighted in the previous section was the importance of engaging the participants throughout the workshop. Maintain attention to the objectives that you seek to achieve as a result of the workshop. Thus, if you need to adjust the time spent on a particular activity or topic, or to modify how you are addressing an issue, this can be done. However, as the leader of the workshop, keep an eye on the overall picture of these objectives and how much time is being spent on various activities.

From an overall perspective, manage the time throughout the workshop. This means three concrete things: (1) start on time; (2) end on time; and (3) balance the time during the workshop. Honor the time of the workshop participants. Thus, make sure that the workshop both starts and ends on time. If a start time of 9:00 is advertised, then the workshop should start as close to 9:00 as possible. Adjustments would be appropriate because of weather or traffic conditions; however, the general rule is to start when you say you will start. If you have a group gathering for the workshop, and you plan to start at 9:00, it would be appropriate to pass the word that the workshop will be starting shortly and to do this just before the planned start time. Similarly, you should manage your time so that the workshop ends on time. Individuals are well known to be watching the time, as they may have other responsibilities or commitments. You should start winding down the workshop well before the advertised ending time. Thus, if the workshop is scheduled to end at 3:00, you would be well-served to start talking about the final workshop content during the last hour of the workshop, leaving time for any necessary questions, reminders and evaluation.

During the workshop, it is also helpful to manage the time by being conscious of the time constraints. For example, you might highlight that during the first hour of the workshop, various items will be accomplished and what would then be done during the second hour of the workshop. You can have your participants also help manage the time as you comment periodically about the current activity, how it fits and where you are in the overall flow of the workshop; this can help them take ownership of the overall process and content, so that all stays on track.

There are times in the workshop when you and the participants are highly engaged in a discussion. You may observe that a group discussion is going particularly well, but also note that it needs to end so that you stay on time with the rest of the workshop. Since you have the "big picture" in mind, you know that if you spend a lot more time on this discussion, then this comes at the cost of reduced time on another topic or issue. You may want to continue the discussion; or you may note that you will come back to that discussion if time permits. What can be helpful is to engage the participants in decision-making about how to spend the time. This is always a type of decision for you as the workshop leader, as you can decide whether to move ahead (by ending the discussion) or offering this as a choice for participants. When you offer the participants the opportunity to help shape the schedule, let them know what they will be gaining (e.g., more discussion time) and what they will be losing (e.g., less time on another topic). The advantage is that the participants can "own," to a greater extent, the workshop; they may also very much appreciate the extended time on a specific topic. The disadvantage is that time may not be spent on another topic or issue. This may be acceptable for an issue that is not particularly central to the workshop; however, if the content of what is to be eliminated or reduced was a highly salient point, or one which was advertised as a key part of the workshop, this can be a concern because individuals may feel that their needs were not met. Any negotiation about a schedule adjustment should take this into account. Maintain your perspective about what is most important through the course of conducting the workshop.

Ideally, your leadership with running the workshop is such that you are continuously monitoring the content and flow of the workshop. You are aware of the overall time allocation that you have, what your desired outcomes are and what tools or know-feel-do strategies you will use to achieve these outcomes. You are monitoring the participants' engagement and you have enough flexibility in the schedule to allow for modest changes here and there.

Thus, if you are given a situation that is unexpected (e.g., a longer discussion on one issue, or the need to provide greater explanation on a specific topic), then you have the flexibility to make those changes. In an ideal world, your mastery of the content as well as the process will be such that you won't need to have an "either–or" situation with the workshop content.

Related to the issue of managing the time is the importance of managing the attention of the workshop participants. Breaks are necessary during the workshop, as it is unreasonable to expect participants to maintain their attention non-stop. A typical rule of thumb is to have a break at least every 90 minutes. What you will want to do is look at the overall schedule of the workshop and break it up so that there are breaks at appropriate times; you can then plan your activities with the breaks as part of the schedule. With these breaks, stress how long they will be. You may have different kinds of breaks—a longer break would be appropriate mid-morning or mid-afternoon, for bathroom and/or refreshments. Similarly, you may want to have a brief stretch break sometime between longer breaks; or you may modify the activity within the workshop so that participants are moving around, or regrouping into smaller groups for discussion; this can serve as a type of modified break.

Manage the participants

When conducting the workshop, the focus is on having a quality experience for the participants. To do so, attending to the various elements described above will be most helpful. It's wise to have good organization, vary the approaches used, manage the time and engage the participants. When all of this is done well, the opportunity for participants to have the best possible learning experience is heightened. The overall aim is to maintain a quality learning climate for all participants. Of course, this is done with the knowledge that individuals learn in different ways, with some being more engaged with one type of approach (such as lecture, story-telling, discussion or reflection) and others being more engaged with another type of approach.

There are factors, however, that can get in the way of a quality learning environment for all. As noted earlier, the idea of engaging participants is most helpful. There will be participants for whom engagement is low. They may seem disinterested, bored, distracted or otherwise uninvolved. You may use some approaches such as moving around the workshop setting, standing in various places, or posing a specific question of an individual or a group of individuals surrounding the unengaged person. You may also ask a person, ideally in a more private setting such as a break period, how things are going with the workshop. If you feel comfortable doing so, you might cite that you observed that they seem disengaged or bored and ask if there is anything that you can do to make the workshop experience more engaging for them. Try not to embarrass or threaten an individual, but seek to get them more engaged with the process. There may be factors that affect their participation, whether it is not being well rested, having concerns with a family member or other things that have nothing to do with the workshop. Make an appropriate effort to engage participants and to do what you can do to maximize the learning experience for them, to the extent that this is possible.

There's another type of situation, which is the opposite extreme. You may encounter individuals who like to talk. This could happen during an introductory segment (such as when you ask all participants to introduce themselves briefly). Of course, this would not be done with a workshop of 200, but it may be done with a group of 20 or 30. You may intend for individuals to be very brief, such as their name, title and one outcome expected from the workshop; typically, this would be ten seconds per person. The first thing to do is to be sure that your instructions are clear; you may even model it yourself.

Then if someone, particularly someone at the beginning of these introductions, elaborates significantly, remind participants of what you wanted. If you let this go unaddressed, then this implicitly provides permission to others in the workshop to do the same. That can throw a big challenge to your time management, if all others are following the lead of, and permission for, a longer introduction.

There are other situations that also require your management. For example, there may be someone who is antagonistic with you; s/he may challenge what you say, your documentation or your illustrations. Similarly, there may be someone who offers comments that are contradictory to what you have said. You may encounter participants who are disruptive, such as having side conversations while you are making remarks or when others are talking. You may have individuals who are doing other things, such as reading the newspaper, checking their email or other work. Some of these may be more disruptive than others. Fortunately, the overall reaction of workshop participants is positive and engaging and these more challenging situations, while present, are manageable.

Generally, how you handle these situations speaks to the overall tone of the workshop environment. You can establish some "ground rules" at the start of the workshop, such as not interrupting others, demonstrating good listening, being an active participant and not checking email messages or surfing the web. How you address situations when individuals do not follow the standards is most helpful. To not follow up implies that the behavior is acceptable. One possibility is to remind participants (without identifying anyone in particular) of what was identified and/or agreed to at the beginning of the workshop. Another strategy is to relocate yourself, as the workshop leader, right next to or behind an individual who is participating in the specified inappropriate behavior.

Another way of handling disruptive people is much like the recommendation for the quiet individuals—talk with them individually and ask for their engagement with maintaining an overall positive tone of the workshop. This can be done in a cordial and professional way, seeking their involvement for a good experience for all workshop attendees.

The main theme with this segment is that you are the person who is orchestrating the workshop. While the workshop is designed for the participants present, the main message is that you are in charge of maintaining this for the group as a whole. Your overall responsibility is for the entire group of attendees—individually and as a collective whole. The aim is to have a good experience and you can do that by being an effective manager of the overall group environment. That means trying to draw out some of the more quiet people, who only need a little encouragement to be able to share their views. It also means trying to maintain a good sense of order with individuals who, left unchallenged, could disrupt and actually ruin the learning experience for others. Thus, your role is one of maintaining a good learning setting.

Manage yourself

In addition to managing the group, you also need to manage yourself. To have a quality workshop, you need to feel good about it as it is proceeding. That means that you have to keep your spirits high and your energy up.

Perhaps the best way of managing yourself is to be well prepared. That means having your thoughts clearly identified, in your mind, about what you want to accomplish over the course of the workshop. It also means having the smaller details outlined for yourself. Have a checklist with the various things that you want to cover, at the various times of the workshop, to help keep you on track; this may include notes about stories or examples to share with the participants. While you can think of these things when you are alone and not challenged with the time constraints of the workshop, it is often difficult, even for an experienced workshop facilitator, to remember everything.

Another helpful way to manage yourself is to arrive in plenty of time for the workshop. It's helpful to be present significantly ahead of time to be sure the room is set up the way you want it; you may need to rearrange it, or get help doing that, if it isn't the way you would like it. Similarly, if you need equipment, make sure that you have the extra time to be sure it is working properly.

What is helpful over the course of the workshop is to have a perspective about how things are going. In a sense, this is like watching and listening to yourself, as well as watching the audience, as you are presenting or facilitating the workshop. It can be a challenge to do this, particularly if your experience conducting workshops is limited.

Through the process of conducting the workshop, try to maintain good energy. As noted, being well prepared can help you do this. Managing the time, so that you have plenty of time to accomplish what you want to accomplish, is also helpful. If you get frustrated or annoyed, that will affect your delivery, your facilitation and the overall tone of the workshop for attendees.

If you are faced with challenging situations, such as a quiet group, a disruptive person or being off schedule, maintain your overall leadership of the group. Remember that your aim is to provide a quality workshop experience for the group as a whole. So there may be times that you would like to have participants involved in decision-making about how to proceed; if you spent too much time on a specific topic, there may be a choice about how the remaining time is spent and the group can discuss this. The role of facilitation is to manage the overall experience and to try to remain balanced throughout this process for the group participants. Try not to take personally negative situations or challenges; remember that you are dealing with people and that there are different circumstances that constitute the group experience.

To help further with this, remain hydrated and nourished throughout the workshop. Stay refreshed with breaks for you as well as for the group. As you have the break, consider taking a few moments to review where you are and where you are heading with the overall workshop objectives.

Through the process of the workshop, try to be as real as possible. If you become frustrated with the lack of time, or feel challenged with how much (or how little) attention is being spent on a particular topic, you may want to raise that concern with the group so all can discuss this. Similarly, if you are pleased with the insights of group members, share that. As you become impressed with the ways small group discussions are going, or issues the groups have identified, share those positive reactions.

Overall, the best way to manage yourself is to be well prepared. This means having a clear outline and timeline about what you are seeking to accomplish. It also means knowing your material and being prepared to address various questions that may arise regarding the content. It is wise to maintain a positive, upbeat approach throughout the workshop; this permeates the tone of the respondents and helps them have a good workshop experience.

Planning for the unexpected

Workshops do not always proceed smoothly. Even when you have done all the preparation, and when participants are well engaged, something can go wrong that is just beyond your control. This can happen to all workshop presenters, regardless of their level of experience.

There are situations such as bad weather, resulting in delays starting the workshop, as well as the need to end the workshop earlier than anticipated. There are fire alarms and external noise, such as construction or airplanes. Some of these can be addressed; others simply need to be acknowledged and then decisions made about how to proceed. Sometimes the workshop can be modified, or issues can be addressed in different formats after the workshop (e.g., through a follow-on webinar, written description or other format). Other times, the workshop just needs to be modified and not rescheduled. Whatever the situation that occurs, you should make the best judgment possible and engage the participants in this also. Your demonstration of this human quality carries a significant amount of influence for their engagement with you as the leader.

As noted earlier, there are situations when an individual is disruptive, non-engaged, quiet or otherwise not an active participant. These are dealt with through various know-feel-do strategies that you may use as the workshop leader, including smaller group discussions, repositioning yourself in the room and private discussions with these individuals. Your role and response help model the appropriate tone for the workshop learning environment.

A challenging situation in a workshop is when there are questions for which you may not know the answer. The best way of addressing this is to be honest; you may cite your limited understanding, or that it has not been an area that you have examined or about which you are knowledgeable. You may also note that this is an area that is controversial or for which research is limited. It is helpful to be honest and straightforward with your response.

Most participants understand about that these types of situations are beyond your control. Most participants are also willing to make adjustments; while they may be disappointed, they will likely problem-solve with you for an appropriate and satisfactory resolution.

Working with others

One of the challenges—and opportunities —of workshop design and implementation is when you work with one or more other workshop leaders. This type of situation with having a co-facilitator (or more) can work very well, and it can also pose some logistical challenges. If you are new with facilitating a workshop, it would be very appropriate and helpful to do this with another person or two; let the other person handle the overall workshop, and then you can implement a portion of the workshop as a segment of the overall experience for participants. This will be helpful as you become more comfortable with presenting and leading an entire workshop. It provides you with the opportunity to present in front of a group, to handle challenging situations and to guide a discussion to a successful conclusion.

How can having a co-facilitator be helpful? First, it is beneficial because having one or more other presenters allows for dividing up the responsibility for handling the materials as well as the process. Second, it means that you don't have to be "on your feet" or "on stage" for the entire time; having someone else present gives you the opportunity to reflect upon the segment that you have coming up. Third, with a co-facilitator, you don't have to remember everything and balance everything there is to know with the content and the process. If you are presenting your segment of the workshop, the co-facilitator can check on logistics of the room, see if the refreshments are ready or even talk with an individual if needed. Also, the co-facilitator may notice things that you don't, since you are focusing on your presentation. Particularly as a new workshop leader, you will be intent on your content and may not notice some of the nuances with individual responses. The co-facilitator may notice that some participants may not understand what you said, due to any of a variety of reasons (lack of clarity, novelty of the concept, conflicts with existing approaches, applicability for personal circumstances or other factors). The co-facilitator may also, when listening to your presentation, want to offer some clarifying remarks, or may encourage you to elaborate on a specific point or two. In short, having a co-facilitator can be helpful in maintaining the desired balance and tone of the workshop.

Now, where is having a co-facilitator not as helpful? One of the challenges is with having clearly defined roles. With a co-facilitator, you will want to divide up the responsibilities about "who is doing what" for the workshop. It is best to have a clear outline of what is to be done, by whom and how long is to be spent on each segment. Even when this planning is done, there are times when the co-facilitator will cover material that you had agreed would be done by you; the challenge is how to handle that. What is important for the workshop itself is that the attendees have a good experience; they may not actually know who was supposed to take which part of the workshop. Through the process of co-facilitating, it is important to maintain a quality tone and to demonstrate good teamwork and a collegial spirit with your co-facilitator. If there are issues or concerns you have with how things are being handled during the workshop, it is best to address these in a private setting, whether that is during a break or following the workshop.

Through the course of presenting the workshop, it is best to have the person who is the primary facilitator for a particular segment to actually be the person in charge of that segment. That means that the co-facilitator, for that segment, does not interrupt or try to manage the entire workshop. There are occasions, however, when a point is not clear, or questions may exist among attendees; with that being the case, the co-facilitator may interrupt at an appropriate time and suggest that a topic be clarified, or that some questions may be worthy of being addressed. All of this should be negotiated with a co-facilitator prior to the workshop. Further, debriefing "how it went" is helpful following the workshop, particularly if you plan to co-facilitate with the individual at a later date.

One of the disadvantages of having a co-facilitator links with how some last-minute things get handled. If you are conducting the workshop alone, then you can make these adjustments alone, with or without the involvement of the workshop participants. You may be thinking about how much time to spend on a specific topic, or whether to transition to another issue or not based on how the discussion is going (whether it is going well, or is not going well). If you have a discussion or part of the workshop that is going longer (or shorter) than planned, it is wise to talk with your co-facilitator—even in front of the workshop attendees—about how to proceed and what should be adjusted with the workshop.

Evaluation

As highlighted with Chapter 6 on evaluation, take every opportunity to gather information that helps support your efforts with health and safety communications. With a workshop, even a very short workshop, it is helpful and appropriate to have some evaluative activity. The data gathered from your evaluation efforts helps with improving the content and the process of your efforts. The results from these assessment activities can be very helpful in assessing what you would like to change for the future. They can also be used to demonstrate to others, such as a funder or sponsor, how things changed with the participants over the course of the workshop itself. Even a short workshop can demonstrate remarkable changes over the workshop time period and these can be attributed to participation in the workshop experience.

In addition to what the evaluation findings tell you about the impact of the workshop, they can also be helpful in identifying needs among this audience for future similar or not-so-similar workshops. Further, the process of completing the evaluation can be helpful for workshop participants, as they typically like to express themselves and report what they liked and did not like with the workshop.

Messages from the field

Using clickers for data assessment

Audience response systems ("clickers") can be used during a workshop, both at the beginning and the end. At the beginning, ask questions focusing on issues such as knowledge, attitudes and confidence sought for accomplishment during the workshop. At the end of the workshop, ask the same questions. For each question at the beginning, record the score (such as the average or mean score); at the end of the workshop with the same questions, re-solicit responses from attendees, gather the mean scores and compare them overall. Respondents like to see where they have made change over the period of time of the workshop, further demonstrating, overall, that the workshop was worthwhile. The challenge is whether demonstrable results are achieved; that is, the workshop leader must be prepared to have no change reported.

Similarly, at the end of the workshop, questions can be asked about various process factors, such as whether various objectives were addressed, the quality of the workshop, the materials, the presentation style and other factors. The summary of results can be displayed for all attendees to see, or not shown. Again, the challenge is whether the workshop leader wants to show attendees these results; this may be of concern if some aspects of the workshop did not go particularly well. However, the other factor is that this process helps model transparency and desire to improve.

When preparing the evaluation, it is vital that parallelism exists between what you seek to accomplish during the workshop, what you do and what you measure. While this sounds logical, some workshop leaders often try to measure things that are not covered, or don't seek to find measures of issues or topics that were deemed important. If you want participants to gain knowledge on some specific items, make sure that you cover the topics with enough specificity and clarity to maximize participants' understanding of the topic. Then, build measures that assess whether or not, or the extent to which, this was achieved.

In order to be sure that it was your workshop that made the difference with the desired outcomes, having data from before the workshop as well as at the conclusion of the workshop will be helpful. You may have participants do the "pre-workshop assessment" prior to arrival at the workshop, or once they arrive on site. The "post-workshop assessment" can be done at the conclusion of the workshop, as one of the last activities; alternatively, the post-workshop assessment can be done as a follow-on activity after the workshop. If you are interested in knowing how participants changed over the course of the workshop, gather some pre-workshop data; this can include issues such as their knowledge, attitudes, self-assessment of skills, confidence or other factor that may be addressed during the workshop. You may also want to ask about their expectations with the workshop and what they hope to get from it. At the end of the workshop, ask the same questions and subsequently prepare comparisons between the pre-workshop and post-workshop findings. With the post-workshop assessment, you can also ask additional questions, such as how well the workshop met their expectations, what they learned, what specific plans or actionable items they have based on the workshop, which parts of the workshop were most helpful, what concerns or remaining questions exist, issues about logistics or resources and recommendations for improvement.

The importance of having both types of questions is that the former (using the pre- and post-assessments) are focused on the learning outcomes that would be achieved from the workshop and the latter emphasize the process. Both are important. Unfortunately, all-too-often the workshop evaluations include only the process type of questions.

An additional insight with evaluation is that the pre-event assessment can be used as a type of needs assessment. If this is gathered before the workshop, the results can be helpful for the workshop leaders in planning the details of the session, providing greater attention to areas where gaps or needs exist. If the information is gathered on site, this can be helpful if it is collated by a co-presenter or aide, or if it is done with immediate feedback (such as can be obtained with the use of audience response systems). With this information, adjustments to the workshop content or approach can be made on site.

A few additional things help with data collection and evaluation. First, be sure that the data collection is done, at least at some level. Second, the data collection process should be time-appropriate and as efficient as possible. For a very brief workshop, make the questions as well as the administration of the assessment as brief and quick as possible. Third, use the data collected to improve the workshop delivery for the future. There may be areas that you, as the workshop leader, thought were very clear; however, the results may demonstrate greater confusion after the workshop. There may be areas that show remarkable change over the workshop; it is helpful to understand why this is the case, so that similar processes can be incorporated in the future. Finally, quantitative data gathered at the end can be shared with the audience to demonstrate the results achieved over the course of the workshop, as well as to model the importance and use of evaluation data; this is particularly true when using audience response systems. Evaluation is designed to help you improve the process as well as the outcome, so you want to maximize its use as well as its impact for your own professional enhancement.

Forward!

This chapter provides many details and considerations associated with running a workshop. Key points range from developing the overall design and content, and preparing the logistics associated with the workshop, to actually implementing the session and evaluating the results for improvement with future workshops. A workshop is not as simple as showing up and talking extemporaneously with a group of people. A well-executed workshop requires a significant amount of planning and understanding about the audience to be served. Indeed, the same content for a workshop that is conducted with different types of audiences may require different know-feel-do strategies for implementation. Attention to balancing content and process is important for effective workshop delivery. Further, experience with conducting workshops will be most helpful with enhancements of confidence and skill. Through the process of planning and conducting workshops, as well as having a range of challenges and hard-to-manage situations, you will gain more and more confidence with how to address the situation for attendees. You will gain experience through opportunities to do workshops, even if it is a small part of a workshop. Those can be very helpful as you learn about human interaction, group dynamics and effective communication within a workshop setting.

12   Social media

Overview

When you think about social media in health and safety communications, the focus is upon you remaining current and, to the extent possible, on the cutting edge with efforts to promote your messages. To accomplish this, you must remain vigilant and creative with your know-feel-do strategies and approaches. Just as it is important that you remain up-to-date with the latest research and best approaches for addressing your topical issue, it is also important that you remain up-to-date with what approaches might best reach a variety of audiences.

Attending to emerging approaches is, indeed, a challenge. This means being aware of and interested in current ways of reaching your audience. It's not about the changing needs and issues facing your audience; rather, it is about the changing ways in which people gather information, and the evolving ways in which they make decisions about their behavior. It's not about being cute or fashionable; rather, it is about being relevant and appropriate for your audience, and thus being more likely to reach them and achieve the results you seek.

This chapter addresses the broad issues of why it is important to focus on emerging approaches and some ways of doing this. More specifics are addressed with some of the current know-feel-do strategies, such as Facebook, Twitter, Instagram and YouTube. The caution with any chapter such as this is that some of the specific content can immediately be out of date. To have written about social media five years ago looked different than it does today, and will look different five years from now. So while some of the specific know-feel-do strategies and approaches are timely and appropriate as you read this, others will have been updated, modified, enhanced or replaced. That is precisely why this chapter is located at the end of this book. The approaches continue to evolve, and some become more popular and others less useful. As highlighted with campaigns (the focus of Chapter 7) which have evolved from print to online approaches, social media strategies are in flux. Also, social media approaches can be incorporated with and complement so many other approaches, whether campaigns, workshops, or other. In short, it is because these approaches are continuing to evolve.

Why attend to social media?

The context of emerging technologies is important for your work. You want to remain relevant and appropriate for your audience. You want to connect with them, and you want them to connect with you. Whether it is a print approach or one that is more interpersonally based, you have a greater likelihood of having the desired impact if you are current with your content as well as with the processes of delivery.

Imagine for a moment that you are doing a workshop. Consider further that this is the same topic about which you have been doing a workshop for years and years (decades, perhaps). You may use certain approaches because, for your topic, the content just hasn't changed. So you use the overhead projector with transparency slides (you may even have a couple of them in color!). You then have some illustrations with your slide projector. You may even have a short film clip to show—that may be on a film projector, or, if more modern, on a Betamax tape. How well would this workshop be received? Probably not too well. If you were to update the same materials with current technology, including PowerPoint, Keynote or Prezi, and embed some YouTube or other video clips, you would be received much more favorably today. In this example, the content hasn't changed, but the available technology—and appropriate use of that technology—has changed. In the future, you may likely look back and see some of the current approaches, now viewed as standard or even cutting edge, as antiquated and needing to be updated.

Messages from the field

Social media is social

Patrick Wade, University of Illinois Police Department
David Closson, M.S., Illinois Higher Education Center

The simplest definition of social media is described as forms of electronic communication through which users create online communities to share information, ideas, personal messages and other content.[1] It is that phrase "create online communities" that we would like to focus on.

Picture yourself at a physical social event—a dinner party or other get-together—and you try to start up a conversation with another party-goer, only to be ignored. Imagine if you ask that person how they are doing or what they do for a living, and your counterpart walks away without saying a word. You would not be likely to develop a very good first impression of that person, or you would be confused at the very least.

The same goes for social media. Users expect all agencies and institutions to be proactive in engaging with others. If they ask a question, they expect an answer. More often than not, it is very simple—a user asks a simple question about contact information or a service, and the agency responds. This dialogue creates an open and engaging online community.

Here's an example: "Unofficial St. Patrick's Day" is an enforcement nightmare for police local to the University of Illinois at Urbana-Champaign. The student "holiday" typically occurs on the first Friday in March every year, and is the students' replacement for the official St. Patrick's Day, as the actual holiday usually falls during spring break. The day is mayhem—binge drinking and all of its associated activities are taken to the extreme, and Unofficial St. Patrick's Day has gained notoriety as one of the largest and chaotic college parties in the country.

One of the ways police in Champaign County combat illegal, unsafe or unhealthy behavior is by saturating social media with safety- and health-related messages. In between, they engage users who talk about binge drinking or use Unofficial St. Patrick's Day hashtags.

The voice of the messages is important. In traditional communications like press releases or news articles, the flippant tone the departments use on Unofficial St. Patrick's Day might be seen as making light of a serious health and safety issue, but it is important to remember that social media are independent venues. This tone is common on Twitter or other social media, and it is a language that resonates with the most active social media users.

It worked. The vast majority of the response was positive, including when a popular local TV news personality mentioned the department's "good work" in a tweet—further amplifying the department's messages.

Lesson learned: promote dialog and conversation around your content through engaging with your audience.

Similarly, it is important that you are attentive to current approaches for reaching your audience with the whole range of health and safety communications. If you rely on channels or vehicles that are no longer popular or appropriate to communicate, your message will likely go unheard. For example, you may rely on newspaper advertisements because those have worked for years; however, your audience may have shifted its ways of learning, and they may no longer be reading newspapers, at least in the print form. Thus, it is vital that your approaches change too.

There's another reason that it's important to incorporate emerging technologies. The book *Future Shock*, written by Alvin Toffler in 1970, described the rapid pace with which society was changing; and this was said nearly one-half century ago.[2] Technology, cultural shifts, social upheaval and change throughout the society were, in his view, overwhelming for individuals. These widespread and fast changes resulted in significant uncertainty and malaise among individuals and groups. Knowledge kept expanding, new technologies appeared and ways of addressing problems and issues were constantly modified. Since that was in 1970, what would he write today? And what would he write tomorrow?

It is within this context that the important tool of "positioning" is reintroduced. With more and more messages—a "clutter" of advertising and marketing with all sorts of messages—the challenge is how you can get YOUR message seen and heard. An overwhelming number of messages are present and seek to gather the attention of your audience. You need to find ways to have your messages stand out. So with current approaches enhanced by emerging know-feel-do strategies, you have a better chance of your message being seen and heard by your audience.

As you work with preparing your approach, the challenge is to do as much as you can, as best you can, to stay abreast of current know-feel-do strategies and approaches, and also be watching for potential adoption of some emerging ones. This helps keep you relevant and connected. It may mean, but doesn't have to mean, that you (or your organization) get a reputation as a technological "can do" or cutting edge "guru"; that may occur, and can be an asset for you. The important thing is that you remain relevant and appropriate for your target audience.

Messages from the field

The virtual printing press and direct access

Patrick Wade, University of Illinois Police Department

Communications and marketing professionals today are fortunate to be working in an age where they do not have to rely on the traditional media to pass information to their audiences. Social media is a virtual printing press. When used properly, it can be a very powerful tool—especially in times of crisis.

To communicate with the general public, health and safety institutions historically have been subject to the whims of the people who own the printing press or radio frequency—very expensive enterprises with extreme limitations. To get access, a message would not only need to be deemed newsworthy by an editor or producer, but the final product would be abridged, filtered or otherwise distorted to fit the physical or editorial constraints of the newspaper space or the time slot.

Today, social media continue to grow more powerful, and they are a tool which give you direct access to the audiences communications professionals wish to reach. According to Twitter, the social media platform had 310 million active users throughout the world in 2016[3] – nearly the population of the U.S. Meanwhile, Facebook says it has surpassed 1 billion active users.[4]

Based on those numbers, a good social media presence is like having an email address or phone number for one in every seven people in the world—and even better, if you do it well, it is an active process. Communications officers can deliver content right to their audience's phones and laptops, instead of relying on the passive process of hoping they find a newspaper article or TV spot. No longer must communications officers rely on traditional media to spread their message. They can do it themselves with just a few clicks.

But big numbers present a problem, too. All of those users have their own voice, and without careful audience selection, communications professionals run the risk of having theirs drowned out or ignored by the others. Strategies like hashtags and geofencing, as well as deliberate community engagement, can help mold your audience so it fits your organization's needs. Just like traditional media, social media have their own limitations, and social media publishers must be aware of these things if they wish to be most effective in managing their message.

Just like a real printing press, the virtual printing press of social media requires constant attention and effort. Particularly for those which deal with real-time crises or emergencies, an agency would not want to find itself in a position where social media is part of its communications plan—only to find all their followers have long ago left them or stopped paying attention when the agency needs them the most.

This type of community building must take place regularly and its form must be one useful or compelling to the public. Virtual communities notice when an agency only posts content from which it has something to gain—calls for donations, media releases, safety tips, or other types of common posts—are easily ignored by an agency's online community when that agency has not spent the proper amount of time building rapport and credibility with their online audience. But if that agency invests time in developing a voice, a reputation, and a relationship with its online community, those community members are more likely to pay attention to the messages when they have a more direct purpose.

How to stay up-to-date

The context of emerging technologies is that these will always be emerging. The only thing that is stable through this process is change. Thus, be aware that change will occur, and that you strive to be as up-to-date as possible. This does not mean that you have to incorporate every new approach, or be the cutting edge person or agency. It just means that you need to be relevant and appropriate for your audience.

One of the ways of doing this is to watch what is happening around you. This is true particularly with respect to your audience, as you monitor ways in which they communicate, learn, interact, and ultimately modify their behavior. Some audiences may not be engaged with emerging technologies; that is, if you rely on some cutting edge approach for an audience that doesn't use that, then your message will not be received, just as with an audience that has moved beyond a certain approach. For example, think about a group of elderly adults who are not using Smartphones or iPads, and who may even be challenged with searching for information on the internet; how will you communicate with them most effectively?

Another way of staying up-to-date is to ask your audience about the ways in which they learn. You may find that they use a specific website, or Smartphone app. These technological resources continuously emerge and evolve, so a good way is to learn about these resources directly from them. As you watch your audience, you may observe them engaged with some application or process; that's a great opportunity to ask them about it, and then to assess the usefulness and appropriateness independently. For example, they may find a particular app very helpful; however, you may learn that it has questionable underpinnings (e.g., based on the aims of its developers or funding source) or that it is not grounded with good science or research. As highlighted in Chapter 3 on aims and goals, you have an opportunity to educate and inform, and hopefully modify, your audience about their own sources of information.

In a similar vein, ask colleagues what they use to engage their audiences. You may learn that they use clickers or Twitter, or that they incorporate blogs or webinars. You may then determine that some of these approaches (or none of them) would be appropriate for you as you work with your audiences.

Further, as you engage with various know–feel–do strategies, identify ways in which you might be able to incorporate some cutting edge, emerging approaches. For example, if you are doing a workshop and would like to poll the audience, consider the use of an audience response system (i.e., clickers). Similarly, if you are conducting a webinar and would like to do a similar assessment of your audience, determine if the technology you use has the capability to do this polling activity during, before and/or after the planned event.

Another strategy goes back to the original discussion in this guide about monitoring what approaches are used by the commercial business sector, as it does its own marketing and advertising. As you see different approaches used in the business sector, continue to ask yourself whether and how these may be adapted by your health promotion effort. Undoubtedly, your budget is significantly smaller than that found in the private sector; but some of the approaches and technologies may be appropriate and adaptable.

The overall context of the "how" is to remain vigilant, and to have an open and creative mindset. Continually ask yourself whether and how a certain approach or tool might be appropriate for reaching your audience, at this point in time. Whether it is with phraseology, signage, technology, imagery or other approaches, think about whether and how this could be adapted for your effort.

Here are some ways that messages are being communicated, found in the commercial marketplace, that were not present just a few short years ago:

- Wraparound, cling-on signs on busses or trains, as with artwork; from the inside the imagery is not seen, but from the outside the inside cannot be seen.
- Movable displays on the sides of a flatbed truck that drives through town.
- Billboards that change their imagery on their visual screen every 20–30 seconds.
- Television screens in public locations, whether in the hallway of a shopping mall, in a waiting room or at a gas pump.
- LED lit signs with changing messages or images, at the entrance to arenas, schools, churches, recreation centers, shopping malls or other settings.
- Scrolling words across a horizontal sign or at the bottom of a television or computer screen.
- Small signs on shopping carts at grocery stores.
- Advertisements on the back of receipts provided for purchases at stores.
- Lighting on the side of buildings or walkways with ads or imagery or messages.

These are offered as examples of messages communicated in ways that now seem commonplace, but were not common at all in recent years. Some of these may have been found in certain urban, high density settings many years ago, but with the expansion of technology and more widespread and cost-effective approaches are now finding their way into more rural or suburban areas.

These are basic examples of the know–feel–do strategies often used for communicating messages. While these examples highlight primarily commercial approaches, they, and others, could be adapted for your health and safety communications efforts. The important thing here is for you to be alert for opportunities may exist for your efforts, whether they are currently used for commercial products, or whether they may just be available as a general opportunity to reach your audience.

A final thought in this process of attending to emerging technologies is that you should remain true to yourself. It's important that you remain ethical throughout the process of engaging in new approaches. You may, indeed, be trying new approaches, and also pushing the limits of your capability (be sure to ask for assistance and guidance!). If some part of this technology or outreach effort doesn't feel right for you, explore it more fully before you commit to the process. Make sure that using the approach is consistent with your overall design, even though it may be a bit uncomfortable, at least at the beginning. You should be as conversant and relevant as possible for your audience, and incorporate know–feel–do strategies and use tools that help to accomplish this. You can only do this if you, yourself, are committed to trying something new and assessing the extent to which it works favorably for you.

Messages from the field

Social media tips and tricks

Amanda Harvey, M.S., CHES, Eastern Illinois University
David Closson, M.S., Eastern Illinois University

At the Eastern Illinois University Health Education Resource Center, we give our graduate assistants the opportunity to manage our social media accounts. This allows them to practice their health messaging skills and brings students' perspectives to our messages. During their orientation we teach them the ins and outs of social media. We also invite them to bring their own voices into the messaging as that will help the messages resonate with our students on campus. Our training follows the tips & tricks highlighted in the infographic. This graphic serves as a reminder to the students on how to best use social media. The graphic is available for others to use as a resource at www.eiu.edu/ihec/Social%20Media%20Tips.pdf. Our main lesson is to connect, interact and engage with the students through our social media accounts.

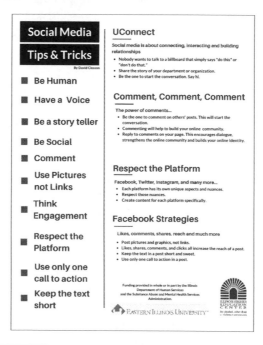

Social media basics

Social media is a relatively new, yet growing, phenomenon that is used primarily to promote interaction among individuals. Through the use of technology, social media includes Twitter, Facebook, blogs, photos, Instagram and much, much more. Through social media, individuals exchange ideas, make comments, create new information and test out new and old content. Social media involves extensive use of the internet, and involves specific sites as well as applications found with personal computers as well as mobile devices. Social media appears to have its underpinnings in the social interaction among individuals, including current friends and acquaintances and extending to those linked to these individuals as well as total strangers.

Social media, in contrast to more traditional approaches, is built on the themes of high usage, prompt engagement, widespread reach, currency and immediacy. Social media is based primarily on the interaction of individuals on a social level, through the vehicle of technology. For the purposes of this chapter, however, attention is provided to a consideration of various ways in which social media approaches can be incorporated into your health initiative. Specifically, attention is placed on ways in which many of the currently existing social media approaches can be included. Undoubtedly, this will not be all-inclusive, and, as noted earlier, will not be able to keep up-to-date with the plethora of changing approaches. What it does do, however, is suggest new ways of thinking about how to stay current and, ideally, expand your reach and ultimately your impact.

A critical foundational point with social media approaches is that they do not replace face-to-face approaches or other, more traditional, approaches with your communication on health and safety issues. In fact, it is helpful to look at social media not as technological tools, but relationship tools. While they encompass technology, it is helpful to think of these numerous approaches as tools or know-feel-do strategies that help you enhance your relationships with various constituencies. Again, consider the context of social media, such as Facebook; the question is how you, as a health or safety professional, can engage this type of approach with your programmatic or strategic initiative. You may use it to learn more about your target population or the issue; you may also use this resource as a way of helping to get your message out there.

Another foundational point with social media know-feel-do strategies is that it may take a while for you to learn how to use these tools, and how to use them in an effective and appropriate way. Consider email, for example. In the earliest days of its existence, and for late adopters of email today, some behaviors or know-feel-do strategies are just not appropriate; the concept of "email etiquette" was something to be considered when using this strategy. Related to this, you will establish your own "rules" in your interaction with others. For example, just because an email is sent at 2 a.m. doesn't mean that you necessarily have to respond to it within the next few minutes or hours; or, just because an email is sent it doesn't demand a response. You need to determine your standards, and those of your organization, to determine the guidelines for these approaches. Similar guidelines would be appropriate for you and your organization's involvement with text messages, tweets or Facebook posts; these may include what frequency, timing, circumstances, tone or messaging is appropriate.

Similarly, you may find some social networking activities to be inappropriate or unethical. Alternatively, what may have been too avant-garde or inappropriate several years ago may have now become an acceptable norm among the users of the technology. As stressed throughout this guide, it's important that you find your own balance and do what is appropriate, and what feels appropriate, for you and the audience you are attempting to reach and engage. If you find it inappropriate to promote professional consulting or speaking engagements on Facebook or LinkedIn, then don't do it yourself. Similarly, don't endorse someone else's behavior that you find unacceptable.

With any of these tools, the important thing is that they work for you; you are not subservient to them. These can be a part of your overall repertoire of know-feel-do strategies and approaches; they are not intended to define you, unless that is what you choose to have happen. They are designed to complement your efforts.

Further, with these approaches, it is easy to have them take over a large part of your entire operation. Said another way, social media could be something that monopolizes your time, with continuous responses to emails, sending out tweets all day, monitoring and making Facebook posts, blogging and addressing others' blogs, posting on YouTube and much more. If that is the intent of your organization or agency, and it may very well be the case based on your size and function, that is fine. However, for smaller, more focused health promoting efforts, which is probably the case for the majority of individuals communicating about the range of health and safety issues, it is important to keep the approaches incorporated with social media in context. Use social media and engage it to meet your needs, and to achieve the output or results that you want to have. Strive to not let these know-feel-do strategies define you, command your time and attention, redirect your focus and divert you from your overall purposes.

The context of this is that it is important for you to focus on your output, with relatively less attention on your throughput. Emphasize those strategies and approaches that help you achieve your desired outcomes. Otherwise, your attention will be focused on the throughput with limited results (output or impact) to show for all of your effort.

Acknowledge that, within this context of emerging approaches, there are hundreds of tools available for your use. These will continue to evolve and change. Your aim is to keep up with them, as much as you can, and to use what is reasonable and appropriate. You need to set time limits that help you stay on task—your task—with attention to the output that you seek with your audience and the specific issue. You need to set parameters or guidelines, and train yourself to attend to these. Further, just as with the importance of having evaluation to assess your programmatic impact overall, consider evaluation and monitoring of how you spend your time, and whether you are staying on track within your own established guidelines.

A digital presence

With social media and the range of technologies, the focus is on your impact, as well as upon the relationships you have and are seeking to establish. Your aim is to have a positive or favorable set of results with your audience, however you have defined these results. The role of social media and emerging technologies is one of establishing a digital presence. In fact, you and your organization may already have a digital presence, whether or not you have done anything to help formulate or establish this. Looking ahead, your preferred digital presence is not a new definition of you or your organization; it is simply taking it and putting it together in a different way—digitally.

A basic starting point for you and your organization is a quality and functional home website. This was viewed as more optional a decade or so ago; now, if your organization doesn't have a website, it is typically viewed as not being current. Further, as people seek information and resources to address a health or safety issue, they often turn first to an internet search to gain an awareness of what the issues are as well as to learn who is dealing with them. If you don't have a reliable, updated home webpage, then your organization's presence just won't be seen. This is now fairly standardized, and computer programs exist so someone with basic computer skills can create this online presence without having to know HTML code or hire a website specialist. However, for more advanced functions on the website, specialization can be helpful. An attractive and sound website is viewed as a basic and essential attribute; your organizational website is the foundation of a quality digital presence.

Beyond your website, the context is that change is omnipresent, and more and faster change is undoubtedly coming. With technology so widespread, it is only likely that your digital presence will grow and evolve. The question is whether your digital presence is what you want it to be, and whether it is such that the maximum desired impact is achieved. If you haven't worked to establish a digital presence, then you stand the likelihood of being obsolete for the increasing numbers of people who rely upon the digital world to gather their information, validate their approaches, identify new know-feel-do strategies and seek to achieve their own impact. Said differently, you will benefit from assessing whether you (and your organization) are part of this process or whether you are left out of this.

To achieve this presence, you and your organization need to become digital leaders. You can be transformed or reformulated in this way, reaching different markets and audiences. Again, this doesn't mean that you and your organization's mission or priorities change; it means that how it is presented and communicated will change. Digital leaders are not born, they are made. Thus, you can take your existing mission and aims and become more engaged from a digital point of view. With the change that will undoubtedly occur around you, you can assess the ways in which you choose to embrace this; you can determine the way in which you harness it, and where you will have a presence.

As a digital leader, a starting place is to think about your reputation. How are you, and how will you, be viewed? Are you "out there" with whoever your audience is? Whether you want it or not, you do have a digital reputation, a digital image, a digital stamp, a digital footprint or a digital shadow. Increasingly, your digital reputation is your reputation. And, as you have this presence, what is it? Is it what you seek? If not, what can you do to adjust it so it is more in line with your espoused and desired views? From a more proactive perspective, ask yourself what you want your digital view to be. How do you want you or your organization viewed? If you were writing your résumé, your life accomplishments or your obituary, how would it read? What can you do, now and in the near future, to make it read the way you want it to read? Or, said at both an organizational and a personal level, what legacy do you seek for yourself, and how do you want to be remembered? Then, what is it that you can do to help achieve this desired outcome?

As you envision this digital reputation, and seek to shape it, consider what you want it to look like in the very near future. Also consider what you envision this reputation to be, one and five years from now. This reputation, in conjunction with your mission statement, can serve as your moral and digital compass. Within this, consider what others think of you, your organization and your overall "brand." How do others envision your relevance and appropriateness for their lives? In order to have an impact on others, you must be relevant and current; plus, you must be perceived as relevant and current. This is all part of what the digital presence is; knowing it can aid in your reshaping it into something most helpful for you.

This concept of a digital presence is something relatively new. It expands how an individual's and organization's reputations have been determined historically, and is different from what has previously been the case regarding reputation. In essence, new rules about reputation exist. These new rules do not replace the face-to-face interactions, and the relationships that you build; these expand and augment the traditional ways of building your reputation. These "new rules" are necessary because of the rapidly expanding nature of information and knowledge, and the context of busy lives, high stress, uncertainty on so many things and competing messages. Time and distance become issues, and thus the use of digital media can be helpful in addressing this while maintaining your traditional know-feel-do strategies and your standard approaches.

How does your reputation work through a digital presence? You can communicate broadly, and immediately, through Facebook and Twitter. You can engage, through "Socialnomics," a whole range of digital approaches.[5] You can inspire others, surprise current and new audiences, challenge people and delight individuals. These tools can aid you expand upon and even modify your relationships. These digital tools help establish your digital legacy.

Are there some risks with this? Absolutely. Erik Qualman, the author of *Socialnomics*, describes the process of engaging a digital presence as being "flawsome." He cites the importance of being present and being immediate, even if mistakes (or "flaws") are made. This is different from refining and modifying and making sure that everything is "just perfect" prior to its release. While this is not meant as permission to be sloppy or inappropriate, it does reprioritize some of the planning and refinement activities that are traditionally done.

There are some other considerations with establishing a digital presence. One is to have a social media policy. If your effort, and that of your organization, is relatively small, your social media policy will be commensurate with your ability to manage this process effectively. However, if you have a larger organization and want a presence beyond what you have traditionally had, you will want to engage in a policy regarding your organization. This isn't necessarily about what is and is not appropriate for employees or organization members to be doing with their personal blogging, Facebook, Twitter, YouTube or other social networking (although this may be appropriate to have); the focus is on what your organization's policy is regarding these digital approaches, who will be involved with them, their frequency, their content and the timeliness. You may have a general social media policy, or you may have policies for specific media issues as they emerge for your organization. The issue of having a policy is helpful to have in advance of a situation so that you and your organization have a sense of what to do, in both a reactive and proactive way. The reactive approach is relevant if there is a situation or crisis that involves you or your organization; from a proactive perspective, these become opportunities for you to have a larger presence, and in a sense to be doing some branding of your name and image.

The other conceptual piece within having a digital presence revolves around the importance of helping others with their own digital presence. With the perspectives that you are a leader on health and/or safety issues, and that digital approaches will continue to grow and evolve, it is important to acknowledge your responsibility for others to be digital leaders. Everyone has a reputation, and your reputation becomes established, in part, based on your digital presence. Your role expands beyond your own digital presence, and is one of helping others establish themselves as digital leaders with a positive, desirable reputation. This can be viewed as a type of digital citizenship, so that others are learning how to use, most appropriately, digital approaches. As noted at the start of this chapter, email had challenges at its onset with what was and what was not appropriate;

similar situations exist with current digital approaches, and will undoubtedly continue to evolve with the increasing plethora of digital know–feel do strategies to be established for years to come.

In establishing a digital presence and being a digital leader, it will be helpful for you to continue to monitor what others are doing, and how they engage these digital approaches. These would be individuals and organizations with a mission similar to yours; it will also be those who have very different goals, such as those in the private sector with commercial products on the market. This does not mean that you will necessarily adopt these approaches; what it does mean is that you remain aware of various know–feel–do strategies, and that you consider whether they are appropriate and desirable, and even feasible, for your efforts.

To determine how you are being perceived, several know–feel–do strategies can be used. First, to assess your influence, you may use a resource such as Klout; this provides a level of influence on a scale of 1 to 100. You may then mention those sources that have a high Klout score in your various digital approaches, such as with a tweet or on Facebook. These sources can be found with the individual list of followers. Another strategy is to use a search engine optimizer. This helps your website become listed higher on the summary of results when someone conducts a search. Through the use of "spiders," the listings are continuously being rebuilt based on various factors determined by the search engine (e.g., Google).

In review, thinking about your digital presence benefits from several questions:

- First, what is your overall mission? How is it that you want to be seen?
- Second, in what ways do you differ from others, who seek to do similar things?
- Third, what would happen if you were no longer present tomorrow? What impact would you still be making, and how is that relevant today?

With this, your effort to address health and safety issues goes beyond the standard approaches, and the digital know–feel–do strategies complement and enhance your aim.

Messages from the field

Competitive marketplace of ideas

Patrick Wade, University of Illinois Police Department

The ability of the masses to self-publish is a double-edged sword. On one hand, communicators now have the ability to reach a global audience at the click of a button and at no cost. On the other hand, so does everyone else—for free, with fewer limitations and in real-time.

Think of social media as a crowded city street, maybe during a concert or festival with no entry fee. The street is full of vendors trying to sell their items and all kinds of customers with different interests. Everyone is talking, so it's very loud—especially with everyone's attention momentarily drawn to the rock concert. The vendors begin to speak over the guitars and the drums to hock their goods or ideas, and they insist that what they are selling is the best. The customers express their own opinions to each other about whether the wares are good or bad. Some of those people have more listeners than others. Some of them are yelling louder—maybe even fighting with each other. Some of them are not willing to listen at all.

For one person to speak to the whole crowd would be a very difficult and frustrating endeavor—there is too much chaos and competition in this ever-growing marketplace of ideas.

So there are two options: be the loudest voice to reach the people nearest to you, or select and recruit your audience carefully and speak directly to them.

Being the loudest voice, in the case of social media, means producing quality content native to those platforms. Shares, likes or retweets amplify your message so it reaches more people, but for this to happen, your message must be relevant, compelling or otherwise entertaining to your followers in the first place.

Take this June 2015 post by the University of Illinois Police Department of a squirrel which had entered the department and run amok in an office. The video itself is 13 seconds long, and it was shot on a cellphone. Pay attention to voice and content—the department takes advantage of typical language used in the policing business to enhance the entertainment value of the post.

 University of Illinois Police
June 15, 2015 · ✪

The University of Illinois Police Department is a very secure building. Only authorized personnel are granted access.

That being said, we had a security breach today when a detective walked out a back door and a squirrel walked in "like he owned the place," according to the witness. The squirrel evaded us for some time before he was detected rifling through computer equipment and sensitive documents. He escaped through a door that had been left open specifically for him and ran off without being caught.

We're still investigating as to whether said squirrel obtained any sensitive information that he intends to take back to his squirrel associates. We are releasing this video footage with hope that the squirrel can be identified. If anyone recognizes this squirrel or has any information as to his whereabouts, you are encouraged to contact the University of Illinois Police Department.

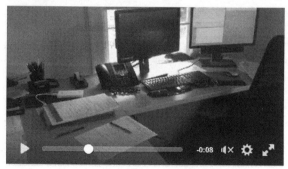

-0:08 ◄× ⚙ ⤢

26K Views

Facebook's algorithms further propel posts which include content native to the platform (in this case, a video uploaded directly to Facebook rather than, say, a link to a YouTube video) and posts with which Facebook users interact more often (likes and comments, for example). These factors helped the post stand out from others in the loud, crowded social media environment.

The hardest part of creating an engaging post is recognizing the opportunity—social media might not be the first thing on your mind when a squirrel breaks into your office. This loud post itself might not necessarily be furthering the mission of the police department directly, but now more people are listening when the department has something more pertinent to say.

The lesson here is to always be ready, thinking about what kind of content can engage your community. If you think it is something you might share with your friends in person, then it might also be appropriate for social media.

Facebook

The question of where to start with specific social media approaches can be daunting. One of the most common know-feel-do strategies, and perhaps the simplest to understand, is with Facebook. Established as a social networking site, this has evolved into more of a blend of personal and professional networking. Individuals use it for updates, and organizations and associations as well as the commercial sectors often find places on Facebook. While advertising does occur, your role with Facebook can be without any financial cost, other than the time and effort to make posts. It is also worth noting that some companies review Facebook or other social media accounts prior to hiring an individual. Within Facebook, individuals or organizations can create profiles and include photos, images, graphics, noteworthy events and resources. You can incorporate the website of your organization or special projects, as well as video content.

For your organization, you may have a presence through various know–feel–do strategies. Once you set up the site, you can invite others to "like" the page. On the page itself, you can have individuals who share a link related to the topic. Individuals may join groups of interest, so they can have specific linkages to others with a shared interest who also belong to that group.

How can the organization utilize Facebook to its benefit? It can post notices and pictures about what they are doing; for those who are friends with the organization, this can be a quick reminder or an advertisement about something that is occurring. Individuals may then "like" the notice, as well as make comments; this can promote conversation among participants. With various friends, an individual can see who else is a friend with whom they, individually, might want to become a friend. Your organization can post a public awareness ad, including information about an upcoming event, a map to a location for an event and ways of accessing tickets or other information. The organization can, itself, be a member of other like-minded or supportive groups, and it can provide links to other helpful resources and their events and activities; by supporting others' events and notices, a positive networking reaction can evolve. The organization may have a section on Instagram, linked to the topic. You can post smaller events, too, to simply have a presence; for example, you may have a photo of someone using your resources or information, or someone else claiming a gift card for a contest you are offering. You may have someone post a link to some other website, such as myths and truths. Further, having individuals "like" an announcement, a photo, a blog or other content, as well as incorporating specific comments, can provide you with feedback about your current activities and efforts, as well as provide input for future planned efforts.

Messages from the field

Four global tips for using Facebook

Steven Clarke, Ph.D., Applied Prevention Strategies

A Facebook page can be a great tool for reaching and engaging your target population. Here are some recommendations offered within four global areas.

Developing a strategy. The first step is to determine the goals and objectives for your Facebook page. In particular, whom do you want to reach, and what do you want to share? For you, think about what other types of information will engage your target audience and encourage interaction on your page. Most social media experts recommend that only about 20 percent of your posts be directly related to the cause or idea that you are promoting. You don't want to be "selling" all the time! You want to engage your target audience on other related issues that are important to your target audience.

The next step is to determine the "who, what and when" of posting. You will need to answer a few questions, for example: Who will post? At what time of day and week will you post? How often will you post? What will you post, and how will you find that content? Will you have contests or giveaways? There are many things to consider, and sorting through the options may seem challenging and may take some time. The important thing is to develop an initial plan that you can execute, and then get started, adjusting over time as you see how your audience interacts. Set a posting frequency and then stick with it for a period of time and track likes and comments to monitor your success. An Excel worksheet works well for setting up a schedule, plugging in links and creating posts that could then be scheduled for posting at a later time. It may also be helpful to find tools and applications that can be used to schedule posts.

Setting up your page. Once you select the page type and name, you need to set up your page by creating a profile and cover image, and creating a description in the page. To write a page description you will need to think about the goals for your page. Once your page is set up, it is important to populate the page with some initial content for your fans. Posting 20 to 30 posts over a 7–10 day period will provide content for new users to browse when they find and like your page.

Executing your strategy. The key to developing a great strategy is to monitor your page analytics. This information tells you when people are interacting with your page, which posts get the post likes and comments, and perhaps most importantly, which content is being shared. By keeping an eye on this information, you can begin to understand what your fans are interested in and the best way to engage your fans. The most important thing is to have patience, experiment, but above all, persevere!

Growing your fans. One you have your page created and are ready to launch, you will need a strategy for growing your fan base. This can be accomplished in a number of ways, including, direct mailing or emailing your target audience, use of traditional media (i.e., posters and flyers), and Facebook advertising.

Since your friends are notified of changes to your profile through their own news feed, having a presence on Facebook can be very helpful. You can change your profile picture periodically, to continually update your followers that you have something new to share, or simply that you are "present" and to remind them of your message and focus. While users can control what type of information they see from their friends, you can have a presence with their Facebook activities. With the linkage of Facebook with other services, such as Instagram, the use of photos can be very popular and useful in furthering your message. Individuals may also "follow" others, as they can subscribe to others' public postings without actually being a friend.

Twitter

Twitter is another social media and social networking tool that can be helpful in promoting interest in and support of your health initiative. Limited to 140 characters, this approach has, by definition, focus. It's not overwhelming, nor is it cumbersome. What can be challenging is the management of the various Twitter accounts or feeds that you may have.

The power of Twitter is that it forces you to be short and to the point. You might look at this as a type of essay or blog, but very direct. This approach really gets to the heart of your message. Twitter gives you the opportunity to have opinions on various topics, and to have these all separated. It's not a coherent whole, nor is it intended to be. It's more about having a presence, and being noticed by others. It's about creating awareness and, to a large extent, a "following." As noted at the start of this chapter, the essence of these emerging approaches is one of having a digital presence; with Twitter, this presence is such that others are reminded of you and what you (and your organization) stand for. These are like reminders about your key message, whether that's about healthy living, safe behaviors, prevention approaches, fire safety, driving courtesy, exercise, balance, stress management, financial wellness or ethical behaviors. When you "tweet," and if you do so often, what you stand for will be apparent among those who follow you.

With Twitter, you have the opportunity to both learn about what is happening around you, as well as to have others learn about you and your organization. You can watch what others tweet about, related to your area of interest. However, most important is the presence that you actually have—make tweets, whether it's an original tweet or it is retweeted from someone else's tweet.

Your activity with Twitter is accomplished through three main vehicles. First, you have a user name, written as @username; ideally this is prepared as closely as possible to your name or your organization's name (e.g. @FDATobacco, @healthfinder, or @USDAFoodSafety); this helps create a public awareness about you or your organization. Second, there is something known as a hashtag (#); these are helpful for organizing or categorizing messages and are prepared with no spaces (e.g. #Safety, #Safetyfirst, #Health, #Diet, #Stressed, or #healthandsafety). Clicking on a hashtag shows you all the recent tweets that include that hashtag. When you add a hashtag within a tweet you prepare, you expand the linkages to other organizations and initiatives, thus demonstrating your connectedness and potential value to those who follow up. You can create your own hashtag, provided it is unique and serves a strategic purpose of relating to your topic or issue, and promoting the development of community or discussion around your initiative. The third main Twitter approach is retweeting someone else's tweet; this makes their tweet a new update of yours. The appropriate etiquette is to make sure that their name (@username) is included with this. However, if you are involved with social movements, and attempting to garner greater national attention, someone may say "steal this tweet"; this means they want you to remove their @username so that you are making a tweet as if it is your own initially.

Once you get more established on Twitter, consider setting up tweets to go out at a specific time. In that way, you can have a presence without you actually being present or "live" for sending out a tweet. The resource HootSuite is a social media management system, prepared with a dashboard look; this can help manage the process for you. This also blends various other social networking approaches, such as Facebook, LinkedIn and WordPress.

As an active user of Twitter, you can do all sorts of things. You can respond to others, link to relevant news feeds or announcements of other organizations; there may be a new study about which you want to comment; and there may be an event that is upcoming that you want to recommend, or an event which you are attending or recently attended. You may comment on what others have posted, whether a generic announcement or specific personal item. You may include a photo or link in your tweet.

With some of the more detailed services found with Twitter, you can obtain a summary of your followers, mentions and retweets; you can also gather reports and summaries that can be helpful for your planning and outreach efforts.

Messages from the field

Seven Twitter tips for health and safety communications

Ed Cabellon, Ed.D., Bridgewater State University

After you have been on Twitter for a few weeks, here are points of information that will be helpful for you to remember.

1 Be "active" on Twitter. It's important that you stay "active" on Twitter once you sign up for an account. Don't let too much time pass between tweets! My assumption is that if you haven't tweeted in a month, you probably weren't using your account anymore. Twitter is about building community and being active in the ongoing conversations. While it is fine to "lurk," don't expect anyone to follow if you don't tweet every once in a while.

2 "Unprotect" your Twitter stream. Many new Twitter users check that little box under their account settings to "protect their tweets," but I'm not sure why. The power of Twitter lies in its openness and the ability to search tweets for keywords, hashtags, etc. Unprotect your tweets and give yourself the opportunity to have a full Twitter experience.

3 Use your real name as your Twitter handle. While this may be about user preference, part of using Twitter is building your own professional digital identity … and what is better than your own name? If your name is already taken on Twitter, try and use another combination of your initials, your name, an underscore, and/or numbers to create your new Twitter handle. This goes a long way in creating your brand, and once you establish that, use that to brand your Facebook and LinkedIn URLs for consistency.

4 Fill out your Twitter profile completely. I am surprised to see how many Twitter accounts still aren't completely filled out. Many are still missing part or all of the four main pieces of information. Adding your full name, current location, a website and bio goes a long way in proving to people you are who you say you are. Some quick tips about this: 1. If you don't have a website, use your LinkedIn or Facebook profile. 2. When you fill out your bio, make sure you use the key terms from your chosen profession (e.g. "Health and Safety," "Health Care," "Communications") so you show up in Twitter profile searches that have those keywords in them!

5 Use Twitter lists to build connections. What is useful to know about creating Twitter lists is that you don't have to follow everyone in them. Lists are powerful for two reasons. First, creating lists shares common interests in one place. Second, when you click the ones you are listed in, you get a sense as to how people perceive you on Twitter. Be sure to thank everyone who took the time to add you to one of their lists. UPDATE: Twitter Lists are harder to find in the latest version of Twitter.com. To access them, go to your profile and look about midway down on the left side for the "lists" tab. A nice feature of lists is that you can list whomever you want without having to follow.

6 Participate in *all types* of Twitter chats. Once you have actively engaged in any of the different weekly Twitter chats out there, you have the foundation for participating in other ones! Introduce yourself and don't be shy to give your opinions on things people tweet about. Ask questions and challenge their thought processes with your experience and perspective. Finally, offer to help when given the opportunity. It goes a long way in building your "Whuffie" (online reputation).

7 Follow *and* unfollow as necessary. The longer you use Twitter, the more you may need to "unfollow" people, places and brands. Sometimes, it has to do with something they said or what they haven't said. Other times, it's just because you feel the need to for a variety of random reasons. Engage with other Twitter users whose tweets you find interesting and don't be afraid to disconnect from them when the need arises!

Twitter can be an engaging online network, filled with information and connections ready for you at a moment's notice. Take your time to explore and understand its value in your professional area and you might discover a whole new world of professional development you never knew existed.

Social media dashboards

With various social media approaches, it can be helpful to have a "master" dashboard to monitor various aspects of your accounts. TweetDeck is available as a dashboard that includes the various aspects of your Twitter account. HootSuite is a vehicle that allows you to merge together various accounts you may have; in that way, you can monitor the various "feeds" and updates you have from the various sources, using a single approach. While this represents the status of a dashboard approach today, this fact can change dramatically over a short period of time.

With TweetDeck, you will find several columns that can be established. Consider having the primary newsfeed, notifications (e.g., someone new who is following you), selected topics set up with the hashtag (#) and a list. Twitter lists can be helpful for following certain people, such as a listing of those who are involved with health efforts in your region. You can have several accounts, including a default account as well as those where it makes sense for you to initiate your tweets. You can also send out a tweet from multiple accounts, if that's helpful based on the different followings that you may have.

With your dashboard, this always stays the same. You can search for and then follow a hashtag. You may find it in a tweet, and then decide that this is worthwhile for you to follow. For sending a tweet from the dashboard, it's easy to create a new tweet, as you write it (remember 140 characters). You can add an image and you can also schedule it for a later time for tweeting.

The same basic standards exist with HootSuite. However, the focus is on the various social media sites that you use. The specifics about retweeting and how to manage the columns will be different. The main point with this is that you can establish your own look based on what you want to follow, and how you want to keep up-to-date with the various content areas. Of course, you can change these over time.

Prezi

When making presentations, you may move quickly to an approach that has been used for years: PowerPoint. When working with a Mac, you may use Keynote. These programs continue to be enhanced, allowing for images to be moved in and out, embedding sound or video, and much more. These enhancements are incorporated to bring to life the content that you're providing.

Prezi is another type of presentation software, that allows for more of a storytelling approach. As you do a talk or workshop or presentation, it will be important that you are really connecting with your audience—this is about building a good relationship, and that the audience is understanding your focus and main messages. With Prezi, you will find very clearly that fewer words are better. In fact, for any type of presentation, major errors are when a presenter has too many words on a page, or an image that is quite cumbersome, confusing or overwhelming. Further, a major error is made when the presenter reads what is on the screen; a good presenter uses the support materials for just that purpose—to support the key points. While you can do this within the constructs of PowerPoint or Keynote, you may find software such as Prezi easier to use.

When using this software, you can start from scratch or import an existing presentation, such as one from PowerPoint. Basically, you start with a central point and then work your way out. You can replace images, include hyperlinks, add slides and edit the path. Then, one of the best features of this software is that you can zoom in on an image and point there. What this allows you to do is to guide the viewer deeper and deeper, and toward a final conclusion. In essence, you are leading the viewer toward the points you want to make. With the use of its top menu with frames and arrows, you can insert items, add video, diagrams or images, embed voiceovers or sounds, and much more. You can share your presentation in various ways, whether live at a presentation or workshop, during a webinar, on Facebook or even on your website.

Finally, here is a consideration for you with this software, as well as other related software. If you create something, share it among other know-feel-do strategies you use! Specifically, if you create something for one venue, adapt it for or incorporate it within another venue. This can be a relatively low-effort (low-cost) value-added approach. You may have an image, like an infographic, that you have developed as a poster. Then use that infographic as a background for a presentation or media event, including it as a fixed image PDF. Or, make the infographic come alive through the zoom-in features found with a resource such as Prezi.

With Prezi, you are digging deep and, simultaneously, being brief. Your challenge with using this tool is to make your message memorable, and make it glitzy. You need to be cautious, however, with not making it too overwhelming, so that the viewer gets dizzy. Movement within the presentation can be a good thing, but be careful about overwhelming others with too much "flying in" and "zooming" functions.

Webinars

A webinar is a workshop or presentation that is done remotely, using the internet. It is short for "web-based seminar" or "web conference" or "online workshop." In brief, it is scheduled, sometimes with limited registration and sometimes with open access. These may also be recorded so they can be accessed at a later time or played back on a schedule.

Webinars can be offered with various functions typically found in a face-to-face workshop. Consider having the PowerPoint slides, embedded video and voice narrative (the workshop leader). The webinar may have questions from the participants, whether done with voice/video chat functions or through the use of text messages. They can include the use of a pointer, highlighting of word or phrases, and even polling of the audience (see the use of clickers in Chapter 11). This may also include a video function, through use of a webcam, where the presenter is seen in addition to being heard.

When doing a webinar, there will typically be two main roles. One is handling the logistics, such as getting the webinar established, managing the software, monitoring the text questions or discussions that occur, noting when someone "raises their hand" and making sure the technology works well (such as muting a person's voice). The other is managing the presentation and its contents—that is done by the presenter, who is doing the talking and moving through the webinar content and slides. There are occasions, however, when both of those functions are handled by the same person—you may be the person making the presentation, but you are also handling the logistics. This type of multitasking is challenging, and requires some familiarity with the software's functions and comfort with managing these various processes simultaneously.

Some tips are helpful with conducting a webinar. First, presenting to an audience without seeing this audience is quite challenging. It feels awkward to make a presentation without getting any verbal or non-verbal feedback. When addressing the topic, make sure that your presentation style is such that you are not just reading a script; you want to feel engaged, as you try to keep the audience engaged with you. Second, make sure you practice the logistical arrangements, including the use of the following, if you choose to use them: the pointer, the audience polling, highlighting, text messaging, moving slides forward and back, incorporation of video, use of webcam, answering questions and other features of the software program you use. Third, manage your time well; it is easy for time to slip away, just as with a live interview or face-to-face workshop. You want to make sure that you know where you are based on the scheduled time, and how you are covering the content in a thorough yet understandable manner. Finally, if the webinar is recorded for later broadcast, you may find that some segments may need to be re-recorded; this may be the case because of some technical problem, or because of some content that would be better presented with a revised approach. That can often be accommodated, except that any audience polling or live questioning cannot be recreated, if those are the parts that need revision.

The webinar is a helpful tool, as it allows for a presence beyond a specific time and place, without the costs associated with travel or space. It does require equipment and quality software so it can be accomplished with high quality and appropriate engagement of the audience. It is not the same as face-to-face approaches; however, it does have its value. This approach can accomplish a more widespread distribution of your message. You can also create a digital repository or library of content areas where targeted audiences (and others, if it is open access) can gain perspectives, knowledge and skills for better addressing their health and safety issues. The main challenge is on your end, to be able to implement a webinar so it accomplishes quality results.

LinkedIn

With so much of health and safety communications being about relationships, the social networking service called LinkedIn serves the purpose of professional networking. Its role is primarily promoting professional identity, networking and sharing knowledge. This is a place where individuals can get expert opinion, as well as market their initiatives; it is a setting where you can discover new potential partners and those with shared interest.

With LinkedIn having over 450 million members as of 2016, it represents a powerful opportunity within the theme of nurturing quality relationships. LinkedIn can provide a way that you can offer positive accolades for others' work, thereby promoting their own good will toward your work. This allows you to incorporate basic information in your profile, including a photo, a descriptive headline or tag line, contact information, job experience and education. You can link content, images, video files, audio files, presentations, publications and much more. You may include links to other creative or start-up projects, using sites such as Kickstarter as well as Behance.

You can also incorporate various organizations with which you have affiliation, your volunteering activities, projects or courses, honors and awards, and other activities. These become helpful for others to know about your capabilities and services. With the broadest profile, while still accurate, you can increase the times that you are viewed by others. You can follow others, seek endorsements and recommendations, provide recommendations, endorse your connections and manage the endorsements you receive. Very important is your customization of your URL so it is easy for people to find you. Again, this is a way of maximizing your presence through digital, online approaches so that you, and your messages, can be accessed easily, thus enhancing your influence.

Video use

Video can be a valuable tool for a variety of purposes. This section provides brief comments about some know-feel-do strategies to maximize the quality of the videos that you prepare for any of a variety of settings. You may use video as part of your training activities, you may include video as a part of an interview and you may decide to use video to enhance your communication efforts; this can be done through Skype, Blackboard's Collaborate Feature, Apple's FaceTime, Google's Hangouts or other software.

As you think about preparing for a "presence" using a live video interview, it's important that you be present and visible as much as you can, and in ways that mimic, to the extent possible, how you would be in person. Thus, make sure that you dress as you would if you were having an in-person meeting or face-to-face interview. You will also want to pay attention to the lighting. Part of this is having an appropriate camera angle, and that you arrange lighting in front of your face. The shot should be a medium shot—so that the viewer can see your facial expressions. You want to be able to be seen for what is happening with you, how you are reacting and how you are engaged. You don't want an extreme facial close-up, but one that gives a good perspective of your head that includes some room above your head. Ideally, the visual image is one from your mid-chest to above your head. You want the viewer to be able to see your hands move, thus demonstrating engagement and interaction with them.

The angle of the camera is also critical. You want to be looking head-on into the camera, so that the picture seen by others is one that they would see—eye-level—if you were face-to-face with them. You don't want an awkward angle, nor do you want to be looking down at the camera. If you're using a laptop, consider raising it so that the camera is actually level with your eyes.

As you record, be careful not to make unnecessary noises, such as tapping your finger, as this is amplified by the sound device. Also, make eye contact with the camera; this is awkward, just as doing a webinar can be awkward, as you cannot see the audience's responses. Look into the camera and wherever the lens is located. Try not to look at the computer screen, or where the images of others are, but look into the camera as often as possible. You might consider having a sticky note or two on your computer, with arrows pointing to the camera, saying "look here." You will be multitasking, but this is important to demonstrate your confidence with the viewers and with the process, and to enhance the connection you have with them. Finally, as you interact with others and find that you encounter some technical difficulties such as hearing others clearly, feel comfortable asking them to repeat themselves.

Attention to lighting is very important, to maximize your engagement with others. You will want to have some level of direct lighting, as well as some indirect lighting. Realize that overhead lighting is not appropriate, as it may promote more bags under your eyes. Indirect lighting can be helpful with providing you a bit of a glow, and make you look better. You will also want to be sure that the environment surrounding you has some character; you won't want to have a messy office or desk or bookcase, nor will you want to film with a cinderblock or plain wall behind you. You also don't want a window right behind you; you want to have the camera and the lighting such that the viewer can see your face. Basically, what you are doing is setting up what the picture of you and your environment is, so that it tells as accurate as possible a story about you.

Some tips about using the video or Skype are helpful. First, with each use, test your connections ahead of time, to be sure you have a solid internet connection, and that you know how the sound and video displays can be accessed or muted. You should also have a wired connection to maximize the speed; with slow connections, you may end up with a freeze-frame effect, something that is quite disruptive to the flow of the discussion or interview. Second, you should be present with the technology early, to address any potential technical issues. Third, make sure that you have a back-up plan; this could be contact numbers for those with whom you will be talking or meeting, alternative equipment, technical assistance that can be accessed with limited notice and other support that might become necessary. This technology and its widespread utilization is still relatively new, and is unlikely to be relatively flawless all of the time (as a telephone line is now, but certainly wasn't in its earliest days). Fourth, from a technology perspective, you may find that it is helpful to have a plug-in microphone (which is not very costly) that you use to provide better sound; some of the built-in microphones are not of good quality.

Surveys and forms

Helpful for your communications efforts is gathering and using information. As described in the evaluation chapter, surveys can be very helpful to document your needs, pilot test your efforts and gather information about what results you achieve. Numerous tools exist that can be helpful. You might consider the use of Wufoo, Survey Monkey and Google Forms as starting points. Other software programs exist, with various levels of cost and sophistication. Plus, over the years, newer and more user-friendly functions will undoubtedly be implemented.

From a basic perspective, you use the software's platform to build the questions. Different protocols and formats exist for accomplishing these; some software allows you to see the form as it is created, and others do not have this simultaneous function as easily accessed. The questions asked may have varied styles: you may find single line questions, with a short answer or a unique answer. You may also have multiple choice responses, where a person can provide one or more responses to specific pre-identified choices. With any type of question, you may decide to offer the opportunity for individuals to respond with a choice of "other," which can also include an option for a short detail of what this was. Your responses can include checkboxes, or also Likert-type scales with a value from, for example, "strongly disagree" to "strongly agree." Some questions may generate additional questions as relevant; for example, a question may have follow-on questions that would be relevant only if a respondent made a specific selection (such as a response of 4 or 5 on a 5-point scale), then generating a follow-on question. You may also include images; for example, you may ask a respondent to assess various posters or logos (this may be helpful with clarifying what imagery works best for what audience, or it can be helpful for your pilot testing of a product or strategy).

With thoughtful survey design, what you want to do is to maximize the responses gathered from respondents. You want to make sure that the survey is clear and not cumbersome. You want to avoid frustrating the respondent which may result in a premature ending of survey participation. You want to have questions that are clear and concise, and that do not confuse the reader. You want basic language that does not have to be interpreted. With questions with choices, it is wise to include as many appropriate options as possible. You also want to have the type of question that maximizes your interpretation later; a simple "yes/no" set of choices may or may not do this for you; also, a "don't know" or "does not apply" response may be viable and appropriate. Further, consider whether you have open-ended responses, such as "Name three challenges that you faced since …"; this elicits very rich data, yet becomes a labor-intensive task for coding and analyzing the data. Clearly, with any data collection process, tradeoffs exist; in this case it is rich data versus the effort for coding and analyzing the data.

With these various software products, you can use the form or data collection tool for any of a variety of aims. You may decide that you want to use the form to get more information; you can ask an important question that may otherwise go unaddressed. You don't need to use this survey as the vehicle to ask everything; you may decide that follow-on questions or queries warrant another survey.

You can also use a survey to educate—this can engage the recipient, whether s/he is a student, an organization member or a community participant. You may build a survey form that walks them through a process, and thus it can have some text. You might ask them about what their choices are (e.g., "first choice," "second choice," "third choice"), and where you can embed links for providing more information based on the choice selected. The form can include some rule building, whereby you hide various fields or choices; if they answer a certain question with a particular response, then the form shows another question that otherwise would not be shown. This can be the case for an entire page, with the rule allowing for a whole page to be shown, or skipped.

Overall, the idea of having a form, or a survey, can be used for various purposes. This can be very helpful for gathering information. Similarly, just as with Prezi, it can guide the user toward an outcome, based on the responses garnered along the way. Different information can be unveiled as needed and as appropriate. This is another tool that can provide information both to you and the respondent, and also provide direction to the respondent.

Blogging

Preparing a blog is a way of sharing your thoughts and perspectives, or those of your organization. A blog, short for a "web log," can be periodic or regular. They can be planned or more spontaneous. They provide an opportunity for you to have a presence in a more in-depth manner. While Twitter limits you to 140 characters, the blog is the opposite, as it allows you to expand on your thoughts in a commentary type of format. Various approaches are used with blogs, whether a diary or random thoughts, whether with photos and images or just words, and whether incorporating links to others or stand-alone. Countless numbers of blogs exist, and linkages for blogs exist within various other software packages and protocols.

How can you get started relatively easily with doing a blog? Consider the use of Wordpress.com; while other programs exist, this provides a fairly easy-to-use starting point for the preparation of a blog. One of the first things to do with this program is to establish a blog address; you can start with your own domain name, or you can use one with the tagline "wordpress.com" at no cost. Make sure the username doesn't exist, and then proceed. You want to make sure that your information is correct, including an email, website and information about you. Again, this helps with you establishing an appropriate digital presence, so someone can find you and follow you.

Once you have yourself established, create a blog title, a tagline, a theme and then the blog! You write this, and then you can share your blog posts. This sharing can be done through other approaches, such as Twitter or Facebook. With creating your blog, you will be adding a new one. You may choose to reuse content that you already have, from some other approach or strategy with which you have been involved. You may insert content, pictures (media) and then publish it. You might add some tags, so that when people do searches by themes, they could come up with your blog that relates to that theme of interest to them.

You typically will have the opportunity to show the "likes" when viewers have that response to your blog; also, others are able to share your blog, so that they can further promote what you have already said. You can have comments posted; that way, people will be likely to visit the blog more often if they feel like they are in a conversation, rather than just seeing information posted.

The intent with the blog is to focus mainly on the content. Your emphasis should be upon good content, and with an aim of engaging the audience. Again, this is a way of getting your content distributed widely, and thus promotes your "brand" or your message more widely than if you relied simply on the traditional approaches of print materials.

Messages from the field

Technology implementation model

Edmund T. Cabellon, Ed.D., Bridgewater State University

A technology implementation model aids professionals leading departments, divisions and associations implementing digital technology tools to build capacity, augment engagement and catalyze change.[6] This six-part model guides organization leaders as they prepare their social media and other technology initiatives, with more detail available at http://edcabellon.com.

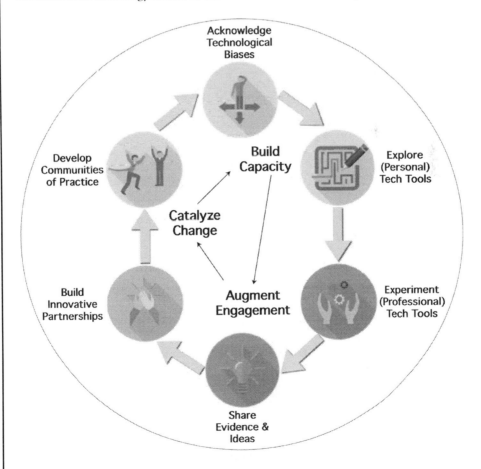

Acknowledge technological biases. Acknowledging and sharing one's technological biases provides a direction and movement. For example, leaders might lead a discussion at a staff meeting or retreat about technology perceptions and attitudes, seeking to gain a mutual understanding. These discussions might uncover why previous technology was not implemented and inspire new energy to take future action.

Explore personal uses of digital technology. Leaders are asked to explore personal uses of various digital technology tools that might have shared meaning in their higher education work. Given digital technology's ubiquity, leaders could create opportunities for their departments and divisions to explore how various digital technology tools might have broader purposes. For example, senior leaders might create a technology committee to regularly explore new technologies, present their value to division leaders and create a general inventory of how professionals are harnessing technology in their work.

Experiment professionally with digital technology tools. Then, leaders are asked to intentionally experiment professionally with digital technology tools. For example, leaders might add a technology marketplace to their annual conferences by inviting a variety of technology vendors and technology minded leaders to share their latest successful technology implementation.

Share digital technology evidence and ideas. Leaders are encouraged to share digital technology use evidence and ideas within departments and across the organizational structure. For example, when multiple departments seek the same hardware or third-party developed software (e.g., iPads, digital duty logs, content management systems), senior leaders should select specific units to initially conduct a pilot test, whose data should drive future investment. Certainly, new technologies should only be brought on with department heads' commitment to publically present and share data annually.

Build cross-divisional, innovative partnerships. This sharing process actualizes the next phase of the design, where leaders are inspired to build cross-organizational partnerships with those in a range of roles: information technology, marketing and communication, program development, and education. For example, executive leaders might request an annual presentation during a senior leadership meeting focused on divisional collaborations with digital technology. Certainly, executive leaders could benefit from the data collected, analyzed and implemented throughout their respective organizations and units, possibly impacting future budget decisions.

Develop communities of practice. Leaders institutionalize their digital technology use through organizational communities of practice. This collaboration allows for intentional overlap among units and highlights the benefits associated with this technology.

Forward!

In summary, the idea of emerging approaches can be seen as a constantly moving target. For you to do your health and safety communications most effectively, it's important to stay up-to-date with the various approaches and know–feel–do strategies that are emerging. Many of the approaches in this chapter could not have been written about, much less envisioned, just a few short years ago. Plus, whenever these words are read, new know–feel–do strategies not now envisioned or conceptualized, much less developed, will exist. The specific software cited will likely have expanded to make it more user-friendly, and demonstrate increased integration of function within its form.

The important thing is to stay current. Just as Chapter 2 on the audience emphasizes knowing what is important and relevant for your audience, and Chapter 3 on aims and goals emphasizes staying current, this chapter focuses on the tools that help you remain increasingly relevant and appropriate with your content and your process. As you step back and look at yourself and your efforts, your aim is to be as effective as possible. These tools are ways of reframing and reorganizing the content which you already know. With some confidence, some boldness, and some flair, you can both make a broader impact and have fun in the process of doing so!

Notes

1 Social media. (n.d.). Retrieved April 28, 2016, from www.merriam-webster.com/dictionary/social media.
2 Toffler, A. (1970). *Future Shock.* New York: Random House, Inc.
3 Twitter Company | About. (2016). Retrieved May 3, 2016, from https://about.twitter.com/company.
4 Facebook Company Info | Facebook. (2016). Retrieved May 3, 2016, from http://newsroom.fb.com/company-info.
5 Qualman, E. (2013). *Socialnomics: How Social Media Transforms the Way We Live and Do Business.* New Jersey: John Wiley and Son, Inc.
6 Cabellon, E. T. (2016). *Redefining Student Affairs Through Digital Technology: A Ten-Year Historiography of Digital Technology Use by Student Affairs Administrators* (Doctoral dissertation). Retrieved from ProQuest Dissertations and Theses. (Accession Order No. 10013238).

13 Pulling it together

Some perspectives

You are a health and safety communicator. Whether based on your motivation, the role you have in your organization, an assignment or a blend of these, you aim to improve the lives of others through messaging on health and safety issues. To do well, you have a model to follow and a range of know-feel-do strategies and approaches designed to assist with your success. Hopefully, this guide helps with your success.

Throughout this guide, you have been introduced to several examples and recommendations from the field that help you use the model. The examples demonstrate ways in which communities and organizations, agencies and individuals, have had an impact.

There is, in fact, no "conclusion" that says "The End." This chapter is not like a movie that has an end; it is more like a beginning, or a new beginning, for you. Implementing health and safety communications is a process. The desired endpoint—increased health and safety—can always be better; our lives can always be improved. It's like the goal line is continuously moving. Further, the effectiveness of your work can always improve.

As you strive to make a difference with a health or safety issue, you have noticed a gap or a need, and you want to do something about it. You want to accomplish your goal and you want to see change. In this process, your aim is to change people's minds. This is no easy task. People have worked for years and years on various health and safety issues, and change is slow. As you work on your issue, you must keep in mind that your task of changing others' minds, through whatever processes and efforts you use, is a daunting one. Remember, throughout the process, that you have an aim, or a mission, and that is to make a difference in their lives.

With this, you must have a strategy. You must be strategic and organized. To summarize, ten tips are offered in this chapter to help remind you about the importance of staying on track. This strategy is not a simple one, such that you will accomplish your goal with, for example, the implementation of a single approach. With your health and safety communications effort, you must be committed to working on the issue—the gaps—for the long haul. Your aim of changing minds, and hearts, must be viewed as a slow, strategic focus. You must be both patient and persistent.

As cited in Chapter 12 on social media and various emerging technologies, as well as Chapter 6 that encompassed evaluation efforts, there's a distinction that exists between your output and your throughput. All too often, your focus may be upon your throughput; after all it is these things and activities upon which you spend your time and energy. What is important is to review your results and modify and update your efforts as needed. Consider the following:

- You conducted two dozen workshops throughout the region on your area of specialization.
- You prepared a monthly poster series, and got this distributed throughout the community.
- Your promotional campaign had packets delivered to thousands of homes.
- Your ad in the magazine had several thousand impressions.
- Your television PSA was seen by thousands of people.
- You personally spoke with five thousand people.

These may all be good. These productions may be necessary to achieve your ultimate aim; and they may be sufficient. But that's not the best measure. The aim was not one of preparing the posters or doing the workshops; the aim was not one of having packets designed, nor of looking good. Your aim was having an impact on individuals; your aim was one of providing information and enhancing motivation so a change in knowledge, attitudes and/or behavior (and ultimately behavior) was achieved.

You needed to do the "throughput" to achieve the end result; however, it's important to keep your attention on the "output" so that, ultimately, it is achieved. Your efforts are, primarily, about impact, results and change. That's what got you started in the first place. And the effort is not one of just "willing" the end result to be achieved; you do have to invest in significant resources and planning to achieve this end result. So paying attention to the results, as well as the effort and quality of effort to achieve these results, are all important. Your effort is all about something of value—it is changing the minds of others, to ultimately result in changes in their behavior. This endpoint is of value to you and to those served by you. You are seeking, ideally, to produce something of value to the world (or to a small portion of it). That's your end goal, that's your aim, and that's your dream.

As such, it is important for you to acknowledge that small steps toward your ultimate goal are valuable and important. Even seemingly insignificant progress is vital toward the ultimate aim you seek. Periodically, it is valuable to step back and review your efforts and any progress, and then celebrate the progress that you make. When changing the minds of others, achieving movement is a big accomplishment and one that deserves to be celebrated. So take the time to step back and reflect on this progress, albeit as small or seemingly minor as it may be, and celebrate it.

Be cautioned, however, that "winning is not won." The small steps that you have made, the intermediate goals you have achieved and the progress that you celebrate do not necessarily translate into "mission accomplished." You do want to give praise—to yourself and to others—for the progress that is made. However, you undoubtedly have a long way to go. If your aim is limited in scope, that's fine; you want to appreciate what you have accomplished. However, if your aim is much broader and more grandiose, you and others working with you are to be thanked, in advance, for your perseverance and dedication to continue with these efforts. You know that small steps are to be counted and celebrated; but you also know that it is not appropriate to sit back and quit your effort, just because you have made progress in the short run. The progress made is important, yet it is important to also attend to sustaining this progress.

A final reflective thought is that you might consider that you are part of a "movement." You have undoubtedly heard about movements that bring about large-scale societal change, such as the women's rights movement, the civil rights movement, the movement to reduce childhood obesity or the movement to eradicate smoking. These are major initiatives and are long-term commitments by a variety of people and organiza-tions. You may have your own movement, or you may be part of a larger movement.

In most cases, health and safety communications work occurs at the local level—you are working on a brochure or media event, a campaign or a workshop, that will have a local and limited audience. Thus, the scope of your effort may be quite limited; and, if it is a larger scope, the "movement" with which you are affiliated may be local or limited in nature. That's fine—as it is still an important undertaking, and one that can have a tremen-dous impact on the health and lives of those affected directly and indirectly by your work. The context of this is that your work, however large or small, is important work. It may seem tedious or lack reward at times; however, it is helpful to step back and look at the larger picture of what you seek to accomplish. Certainly, if things are not moving in the direction you seek, then step back and assess, evaluate and determine what may be lacking or what could be enhanced. That's all part of the process of monitoring and reviewing your work, again within the context of making progress and, ultimately, doing good work.

Ten tips

Throughout this guide, you have been reminded that your preparation for health and safety communications involves a type of "tool box." There are dozens of tools avail-able, with new ones and various permutations and combinations continually emerging. You cannot and need not use them all. As you think about a construction worker's tool box, an artist's palatte and a chef's kitchen, all the tools won't be used; different ones are appropriate for different purposes. With you, various know-feel-do strategies and tools are available; you have workshops and media and print materials and public presence and more; plus, there are tools within the tools, such as testimonials and creative epidemiol-ogy and attending to the data and the qualitative stories. Plus, you are best served when your efforts are grounded on the theory—as well as the audience and their needs—and what is current with you and with them.

Pulling this together, ten summary tips can be helpful to remind you about your work. These may be like a final checklist helpful to guide you, keep you focused, and sustain you throughout your work.

Tip #1: Be clear. Be very specific, in your own mind, with what you want the audi-ence to know, feel or do as a result of your specific efforts. While you have an overall vision in mind, the emphasis here is upon what is most immediate as a direct result of the workshop, PSA, brochure or other effort. The clearer you are at the onset, the greater likelihood you are to have quality results.

Tip #2: Be strategic. Have a design for how you're going to pull together and orches-trate your effort. The best advice is to follow the health and safety communications model (see page 8); this involves the five steps, and involves other people in your effort. It also incorporates thoughts about evaluation from the earliest planning stages; you don't want to just tack on the evaluation at the end.

Tip #3: Be grounded. Not only should your effort have theoretical underpinnings, but it should also be up-to-date with its information, incorporate what you know about your audience and match the approaches to the audience's needs and learning styles. You will want to think about the theory or theories upon which your efforts are based and use those constructs to help frame your thinking.

Tip #4: Be imperfect. While this may sound inappropriate, it's actually an action-oriented tip. Three overarching themes throughout this book help guide this. First, there is no one single best way to accomplish your health and safety communications goal. Second, no health and safety communications effort is 100 percent perfect. Third, you should feel empowered to try, and then learn from that and improve. How often have you seen the process as one of "ready, aim, aim, aim, aim, aim"? This is about having the confidence, and using known approaches as outlined here, to proceed.

Tip #5: Find your stride. Learn what you do well, whether that reflects on your area of emphasis, the approaches used, the look, the style or other factors. With the hundreds of health and safety topics, and the countless and changing tools and approaches, you cannot do it all. You will benefit from finding your niche and the type of approach that you take. It is best to be known for whatever is important for you or your organization and to be known for quality work and for efforts that have value. This may mean that you stand out; positioning yourself for aspects of your work is most helpful for achieving your ultimate aims.

Tip #6: Engage various resources. Your work is stronger when you use appropriate resources throughout the process. You know or will learn where your areas of strength are; similarly, you may have some weaker areas. Engage others to fill in the gaps and to complement your efforts. Garner others' perspectives, obtain critiques and suggestions and collaborate to both share the burden and strengthen the design. The resources you gather may extend beyond other people and include new approaches, cutting edge technologies, planning know–feel–do strategies and concepts previously untested or not used with your audience or issue.

Tip #7: Be bold. To do the same effort as has been done in the past will likely produce the same results as have been found. Since your effort is based on a need or a gap, you want to do something different. Be innovative with your thinking and planning; try something new. Through this, still be grounded and organize your efforts with a reason (and not just do something "because it looks good"). Do seriously consider extending the traditional boundaries. Just having the discussion of being creative or innovative can unlock some potential that you otherwise wouldn't have thought about.

Tip #8: Continue to learn. Health and safety communication is a process, and one that requires you to stay up to date with new science about your areas of interest and importance. Further, your audience's needs and interests will evolve, so you must stay current about them so you can reach them. New technologies will continue to appear; the approaches identified as "cutting edge" in the social media chapter (Chapter 12) will continue to evolve. Similarly, advertising and marketing know–feel–do strategies, as well as what seems to motivate people, will evolve.

Tip #9: Recall your vision. As you get engrossed with the day-to-day minutia of planning and executing quality communications efforts, remember the "big picture." Recall often the impact that you are trying to have; then, in your own mind, incorporate the specific know–feel–do strategies or efforts into that context. This helps keep you on target and motivated, to help sustain your commitment to your mission. You can think about various analogies, such as moving the football toward the goal line one yard (or ten) at a time. Or, the classic starfish story ending with "For this one, it makes a difference."

Tip #10: Have fun! Health and safety communication is a journey, with an endpoint or a series of midway points in mind. Some of the preparation will be arduous or tedious, and other parts may be confusing or elusive. Hopefully the overall experience is a good one. Yes, you might be quite stressed out over a television appearance or speech, and yes, your workshop or campaign may not have been as well received as you would have liked. But throughout these processes and efforts, you are finding some rewards and, hopefully, enjoyment that makes it all worth your while.

Forward!

This guide has been designed to provide you with tools, large and small, concrete and more conceptual, to help you succeed. Your efforts are important to change the status quo around a range of health and safety issues. Your vision is helping to move beyond coping or survival and emphasizing thriving. This resource is designed to help maximize others' hopes and dreams, through you doing even better with your hopes and dreams vis-à-vis health and safety communications.

It is important that you have *competence*—the skills and resources that are appropriate for achieving your goals. It is important that you have *confidence*—the belief in yourself that you can make a difference. And it is important that you have *commitment*—staying with this and persevering for the long run, as change is different and is best viewed with small steps toward the larger goal. With these three elements, and all three of them, you are better equipped and sustained for having an impact.

Use the planning model, draw upon the tool kit and reflect on the ten tips. This is a journey for impact and results. There's not a clear endpoint nor a magic answer. There can be a better tomorrow, healthier and safer, through the good works of dedicated people such as yourself. So continue to grow and learn, and spread the word. And, strive to do well while you are doing good ... all the while moving Forward!

Appendix

Calendar of health and safety events

This calendar serves as a starting point for scheduling a health or safety initiative, whether that is a campaign or other event.

Each month includes examples of established events at the national level:
* Events for the entire month are identified at the top of the monthly calendar
* Events for a week are illustrated for a particular week
* Events for a day are identified by that date

The examples here are from 2014; specific dates and weeks may vary from year to year; some day- or week-focused events are based on the specific date (e.g., the 3rd), and others are based on a specific day of the week and month (e.g., the first Thursday of the month).

Other health and safety examples exist at the national level; further more initiatives are found at the state level, which may or may not coincide with this national listing.

JANUARY

Birth Defects Prevention Awareness · Stalking Awareness · Radon Action
Cervical Cancer Screening · Daffodil Days (through March) · Blood Donor
Thyroid Awareness · Winter Sports TBI Awareness · Cervical Health Awareness
Slavery, Human Trafficking Prevention · Glaucoma Awareness

	MONDAY	TUESDAY	WEDNESDAY	THURSDAY	FRIDAY	SATURDAY	SUNDAY
WEEK 1			New Year's Day 1	2	3	4	5
WEEK 2	National Folic Acid Awareness Week (6–12) 6	7	8	9	10	11	12
WEEK 3	13	14	15	16	17	18	19
WEEK 4	Martin Luther King, Jr. Day 20	Healthy Weight Week (20–26) (Nat) Medical Group Practice Week (21–25) 21	22	National Nuclear Science Week (Jan 28–Feb 1) 23	24	25	26
WEEK 5	National Drug Facts Week (Jan 27–Feb 2) 27	28	29	30	31		

Women's Healthy Weight Day

Find a Dentist Day and IV Nurse Day

FEBRUARY

Age-Related Macular Degeneration/ Low Vision Awareness — Heart Month
Condom Month — Children's Dental Health — Therapeutic Recreation
Prenatal Infection Prevention — Kids ENT Health — Wise Health Care Consumer
Gall Bladder and Bile Duct Cancer Awareness — Teen Dating Violence Awareness
Cancer Prevention

	MONDAY	TUESDAY	WEDNESDAY	THURSDAY	FRIDAY	SATURDAY	SUNDAY
WEEK 1	Establishing and Repairing Healthy Relationships, Feb 7–14th	National Burn Awareness Week (2–8)				National Freedom Day **1**	Groundhog Day **2**
WEEK 2	African Heritage and Health Week (1–7) **3**	PeriAnesthesia Nurse Awareness Week (4–10) **4**	**5**	National Black HIV/AIDS Awareness Day, 7th **6**	Natl Wear Red Day and Give Kids a Smile Day, 7th **7**	Nuclear Science Drug Facts Week / African Heritage and Health Week (1–7) **8**	Burn Awareness RA Awareness **9**
WEEK 3	PA Nurse Week **10**	Cardiac Rehabilitation Week and Cardiovascular Professionals Week (10–16) / National Condom Week (11–15) / World Day of the Sick **11**	Congenital Heart Defect Awareness Week (7–14) **12**	Natl Donor Day and Valentine's **13** / **14**	**14**	**15**	Congenital Heart Defect Awareness Week (7–14) **16**
WEEK 4	President's Day **17**	National Eating Disorders Awareness Week (Feb 24–Mar 2) **18**	**19**	**20**	**21**	**22**	**23**
WEEK 5	**24**	**25**	**26**	**27**	**28**		

MARCH

	MONDAY	TUESDAY	WEDNESDAY	THURSDAY	FRIDAY	SATURDAY	SUNDAY
WEEK 1	Spring Break Safety, March 1–10th					Eating Disorders Awareness / Self-Harm Awareness Day **1**	Sleep Awareness / Patient Safety **2**
WEEK 2	Youth Violence Prevention **3**	**4**	**5**	**6**	**7**	**8**	**9**
WEEK 3	Natl Women and Girls HIV/AIDS Awareness Day **10**	**11**	**12**	**13**	World Kidney Day **14**	**15**	Poison Prevention **16**
WEEK 4	World Tuberculosis Day **17**	**18**	Kick Butts Day **19**	Native American HIV/AIDS Awareness Day **20**	**21**	World Water Day **22**	Tsunami Prep **23**
WEEK 5	**24**	American Diabetes Alert Day **25**	**26**	**27**	**28**	**29**	**30**
WEEK 6	**31**						

National Sleep Awareness Week (2–9)
Patient Safety Awareness Week (2–8)
National School Breakfast Week (3–7)
Brain Awareness Week (10–16)
National Youth Violence Prevention Week (7–11)
National Inhalants Awareness and Poison Prevention Week (16–22)
Flood Safety Awareness Week (17–21)
National Tsunami Preparedness Week (23–29)
National Work Zone Awareness Week (March 31–April 4)

APRIL

Awareness themes:
Alcohol Awareness · Child Abuse Prevention · IBS Awareness · Autism Awareness · Sarcoidosis Awareness · Facial Protection · Distracted Driving Awareness · Occupational Therapy · Donate Life · Sexual Assault Awareness and Prevention · Minority Health · Sports Eye Safety Awareness · STI Awareness · Earth Month · Cancer Control · Injury Prevention · Women's Eye Health · Youth Sports Safety · Esophageal Cancer · Head and Neck Cancer · Stress Awareness · Testicular Cancer

	MONDAY	TUESDAY	WEDNESDAY	THURSDAY	FRIDAY	SATURDAY	SUNDAY
WEEK 1	National Work Zone Awareness Week (March 31–April 4)		Medication Safety Week (1–7)				
		Sexual Assault Awareness Day of Action **1**	**2**	Natl Alcohol Screening and Youth HIV/AIDS Awareness Day **3**	**4**	Alcohol Free Weekend (4–6) **5**	Window Safety **6**
WEEK 2	Medication Safety National Public Health Week (7–13) National Window Safety Week (6–12) World Health Day **7**	**8**	Natl Youth Violence Prevention Week (7–11) **9**	**10**	**11**	**12**	**13**
WEEK 3	**14**	National Infertility Awareness Week (20–26) Every Kid Healthy Week (21–25) **15**	**16**	**17**	**18**	**19**	Infertility Awareness Easter Sunday **20**
WEEK 4	National Infant Immunization Week (April 26–May 3) World Immunization Week (23–30) **21**	National Playground Safety Week (22–26) Earth Day **22**	World Immunization Week (22–26) **23**	World Immunization Week (23–30) **24**	Infant Immunization **25**	**26**	**27**
WEEK 5	Air Quality Awareness Week (April 28–May 2) Workers' Memorial Day **28**	**29**	**30**				

World Meningitis and Meningitis to Bring Child to Work Day, 24th

National Children's Flag Memorial Day, 25th

MAY

Monthly observances: Arthritis Awareness · Better Hearing and Speech · Global Employee Health and Fitness · Global Youth Traffic Safety · Hepatitis Awareness · Mental Health · Melanoma/Skin Cancer Detection and Prevention · Asthma and Allergy Awareness · Celiac Disease Awareness · Clean Air · Mediterranean Diet · Physical Fitness and Sports · Healthy Vision · Better Sleep · Osteoporosis Awareness and Prevention · Teen Pregnancy Prevention · UV Safety · Ultraviolet Awareness · Preeclampsia Awareness · Motorcycle Safety Awareness · Foster Care · Bicycle Safety · Older Americans · Electrical Safety · Brain Cancer · Lupus

Click It or Ticket Mobilization (May 19–Jun 1) · 101 Critical Days of Summer (May 25–Sep 4)

	MONDAY	TUESDAY	WEDNESDAY	THURSDAY	FRIDAY	SATURDAY	SUNDAY
WEEK 1				**1** Keep Kids Alive—Drive 25 Day; Kids' Mental Health [4–10]	**2**	**3** Cornelia de Lange Syndrome Awareness	**4** Kid's Mental… Occupational…
WEEK 2	**5**	**6**	**7** Bike to School Day 7	**8**	**9**	**10** Food Allergy	**11** Mother's Day; Women's Health
WEEK 3	**12**	**13**	**14**	**15**	**16**	**16**	**17**
WEEK 4	**19**	**20**	**21**	**22** Heat Safety Awareness	**23**	**24**	**25** Hurricane
WEEK 5	Memorial Day **26**	**27**	Natl Senior Health and Fitness Day **28**	**29**	**30**	World No Tobacco Day **31**	

Week-long observances:
- National Infant Immunization Week (April 26–May 3)
- Air Quality Awareness Week
- National Physical Education and Sports Week (1–7)
- International Building Safety Week
- International Building Safety Week (2–8)
- North American Occupational Safety and Health Week (4–10) and Children's Mental Health Awareness Week (4–10)
- Anxiety and Depression Awareness Week (4–10)
- National Neuropathy awareness Week (12–16)
- Natl Women's Health Week (11–17)
- Food Allergy Awareness Week (11–17)
- Stuttering Awareness Week (12–18)
- Natl Alcohol and Other Drug-Related Birth Defects Week (12–16)
- National Safe Boating Week (17–23), Recreational Water Illness, EMS Week (18–24)
- Safe Boating Week
- EMS Week
- Injury Prevention Week (19–25)
- Natl Dog Bite Prevention Week (19–25)
- National Hurricane Preparedness Week (25–31)

Marked days:
- Hand Hygiene Day, 5th
- Childhood Depression Awareness Day, 6th
- Occupational Safety and Health professionals Day, 7th
- Natl Employee Health and Fitness Day, 15th
- Natl Bike to Work Day, 16th
- Women's and Check-up and Fibromyalgia Awareness Day
- Asian and Pacific Islander HIV/AIDS Awareness Day, 19th
- World Autoimmune Arthritis Day
- HIV Vaccine Awareness Day 18

JUNE

101 Critical Days of Summer (May 25–Sep 4) — *Click it or Ticket Mobilization (May 19–Jun 1)*

Aphasia Awareness | Myasthenia Gravis Awareness | Men's Health | Home Safety

Scleroderma Awareness | Cataract Awareness | Congenital Cytomeglovirus Awareness

PTSD Awareness | Safety

	MONDAY	TUESDAY	WEDNESDAY	THURSDAY	FRIDAY	SATURDAY	SUNDAY
WEEK 1							Stand for Children Day 1
WEEK 2	2	3	4	5	6	7	8
WEEK 3	Ride to Work Day 9	10		11	12	13	14
WEEK 4	Ride to Work Day 16	17	18	World Sickle Cell Day 19	20	21	Father's Day 15
WEEK 5	23	24	25	26	Natl PTSD Awareness Day 27	28	Lightning 22
WEEK 6	30						29

National CPR/AED Awareness Week (1–7)
National Rip Current Awareness Week (1–7)
Sun Safety Week (1–7)
Tire Safety Week (2–8)
Men's Health Week (9–15)
National Lightning Safety Awareness Week (22–28)

CPR/AED
Rip Currents
Sun Safety

Natl Cancer Survivors Day, 1st

JULY

101 Critical Days of Summer (May 25–Sep 4)

- Cord Blood Awareness
- Group B Strep Awareness
- Fireworks Safety
- Cleft and Craniofacial Awareness and Prevention
- UV Safety
- Bladder Cancer Awareness
- Sarcoma Awareness
- Juvenile Arthritis Awareness

	MONDAY	TUESDAY	WEDNESDAY	THURSDAY	FRIDAY	SATURDAY	SUNDAY
WEEK 1			1	2	3	Independence Day 4	5	6
WEEK 2	7	8	9	10	11	12	13
WEEK 3	14	15	16	17	18	19	20
WEEK 4	21	22	23	24	25	26	27
WEEK 5	World Hepatitis Day 28	29	30	31			

AUGUST

Psoriasis Awareness
101 Critical Days of Summer (May 25–Sep 4)
Drive Sober or Get Pulled Over (Aug 15–Sep 1)
Back to School Month (Aug 15–Sep 15) Immunization Awareness
Breastfeeding Children's Eye Health and Safety

	MONDAY	TUESDAY	WEDNESDAY	THURSDAY	FRIDAY	SATURDAY	SUNDAY
							Stop on Red
					World Breastfeeding Week (1–7)		
WEEK 1					1	2	3
	World Breastfeeding Week (1–7) National Stop on Red Week (3–9)						
WEEK 2	4	5	6	7	8	9	10
	National Health Center Week (11–17)						
WEEK 3	11	12	13	14	15	16	17
WEEK 4	18	19	20	21	22	23	24
WEEK 5	25	26	27	28	29	30	31

SEPTEMBER

101 Critical Days of Summer (May 25–Sep 4)	Childhood Cancer	Healthy Aging
Recovery	*Drive Sober or Get Pulled Over (Aug 15–Sep 1)*	Alcohol Recovery
Preparedness	Back to School Month (Aug 15–Sep 15)	Leukemia and Lymphoma
TBI	Fruit and Veggies—More Matters	Gynecologic Cancer	Campus Fire Safety
Sickle Cell	ITP Awareness	Food and Safety Education	Atrial Fibrillation
Alzheimer's	Screening	Leukemia and Lymphoma	Head Lice Prevention
Whole Grains	Thyroid Cancer	Prostate Cancer	Yoga	Ovarian Cancer

	MONDAY	TUESDAY	WEDNESDAY	THURSDAY	FRIDAY	SATURDAY	SUNDAY
	National Childhood Injury Prevention Week (1–7)						
WEEK 1	Labor Day 1	2	3	4	5	6	7 Suicide Prevention
	National Suicide Prevention Week (7–13)						
WEEK 2	8	9	World Suicide Prevention Day 10	11	12	Natl Celiac Disease Awareness Day 13	14 Child Passenger
	Child Passenger Safety Week (14–20)						
WEEK 3	15	Get Ready Day 16	Natl School Backpack Awareness Day 17	Natl HIV/AIDS and Aging Awareness Day 18	Intl Talk Like a Pirate Day 19	Natl Seat Check Saturday 20	Farm Safety 21
	National Farm Safety and Health Week (21–27)						
WEEK 4	22	23	Natl Women's Health and Fitness Day 24	25	Sport Purple for Platelets Day 26	Family Health and Fitness Day, RAINN Day 27	World Rabies Day 28
WEEK 5	World Heart Day 29	30					

OCTOBER

Awareness Categories
- ADHD Awareness
- Domestic Violence Awareness and Prevention
- Liver Cancer
- Eye Injury Prevention
- Health Literacy
- Home Eye Safety
- Breast Cancer
- Intl Walk to School
- Learning Disabilities Awareness
- Bullying Prevention
- Crime Prevention
- Down Syndrome Awareness
- Medical Librarians
- Physical Therapy
- Save Your Vision

	MONDAY	TUESDAY	WEDNESDAY	THURSDAY	FRIDAY	SATURDAY	SUNDAY
WEEK 1			1	Natl Depression Screening Day, 9th — 2	3	4	Fire Prevention — 5
WEEK 2	Metastatic Breast Cancer Awareness Day, 13th — 6 National Fire Prevention Week (5–11) Mental Illness Awareness Week (6–10)	7 Drive Safely Work Week (7–11)	8	Intl Walk to School Day — 9	10	11	Bone and Joint — 5/11 World Pediatric Bone and Joint Day, 19th
WEEK 3	Bone and Joint Health National Awareness Week (13–17) National Health Education Week (13–17)	MBCA and Columbus Day 13	14	Natl Latino AIDS Awareness Day 15	World Food Day 16	Natl Mammography Day 17	Infection / Teen Driver / Respiratory Care — 19
WEEK 4	Bone and Joint International Infection Prevention Week (19–25) National Teen Driver Safety Week (19–25) Respiratory Care Week (19–25)	20	21 National School Bus Safety Week (20–24)	Intl Stuttering Awareness Day, 22nd — 22	International Red Ribbon Week (23–31) — 23	24	25
WEEK 5	International Red Ribbon Week (23–31) — 27	28	World Psoriasis Day 29	30	Halloween 31		26

NOVEMBER

Awareness banners:
- American Diabetes
- Carcinoid Cancer
- COPD Awareness
- Adoption Awareness
- Alzheimer's Disease Awareness
- Lung Cancer
- Diabetic Eye Disease
- Stomach Cancer
- Family Caregiver's
- Healthy Skin
- Hospice Palliative Care
- Pancreatic Cancer
- Tie One On For Safety (MADD), (Nov 21–Jan 1)

	MONDAY	TUESDAY	WEDNESDAY	THURSDAY	FRIDAY	SATURDAY	SUNDAY
WEEK 1						1	2 Daylight Saving Time Ends
WEEK 2	3	4	5	6	7	8	9
WEEK 3	10	11 Veterans Day	12	13	14	15	16
WEEK 4	17	18	19	20 Great American Smokeout	21	22	23
WEEK 5	24	25	26	27 Thanksgiving Day	28	29	30

Drowsy Driving Prevention Week (3–7)

National Hunger and Homelessness Awareness Week (16–22)

Get Smart About Antibiotics Week (17–23)

National Teens Don't Text and Drive Week (17–23)

Gastroesophageal Reflux Disease Awareness Week (23–29)

Gastroesophageal

Hunger and Homeless

Day of Homelessness Awareness, 21st

Intl Survivors of Suicide Day, 22nd

Natl Family Health History Day, 27th

DECEMBER

	MONDAY	TUESDAY	WEDNESDAY	THURSDAY	FRIDAY	SATURDAY	SUNDAY
WEEK 1	World AIDS Day 1	2	3	4	5	6	7
WEEK 2	8	9	10	11	12	13	14
WEEK 3	15	16	17	18	19	20	21
WEEK 4	22	23	Christmas Eve 24	Christmas Day 25	26	27	28
WEEK 5	29	30	New Year's Eve 31				

National Handwashing Awareness Week (7–13)
National Influenza Vaccination Week (7–13)

Handwashing Influenza

Tie One On For Safety (MADD), (Nov 21–Jan 1)
Drunk and Drugged Driving (3D) Prevention
Drive Sober or Get Pulled Over, (Dec 12–Jan 1)
Safe Toys and Gifts Month

Glossary

Advisory group   A group making recommendations on the course of action.

Aim   A purpose or intention. In health and safety communications the aim is to influence or persuade the intended audience to promote their health and reduce their safety risk.

Approach   A delivery medium for conveying a message. In health and safety communications, the preparation of an approach is called a production and the implementation of the approach is called channeling.

Approval agent   Person playing an active role in a process and from whom permission is needed to proceed with a process.

Assessment   Determination of the status of something.

Audience   The receiver and decoder of the message.

Billboards   Large outdoor boards for displaying advertisements.

Brochure   A single-page, folded leaflet.

Campaign   An organized course of action to achieve a particular goal.

Channel   The route of delivery, the medium, or the approach used to transmit the message.

Channeling   Implementing an approach through the route of delivery. In health and safety communications an approach (public service announcement, newsletter, flier, etc.) is produced and then implemented by delivering it to the intended audience.

Concept review   Assessment of the design and implementation of a project. Concept reviews can be conducted throughout the development of a project or product, to assess the content, design, messaging, reach and appropriateness to ensure it is on track for meeting specified needs.

Creative epidemiology   The reformulation or restating of data and numbers in a way that is succinct, memorable, visual and compelling. This may be based on equivalents such as time, money, numbers or other factors that would have meaning to the target audience.

Cultural competence   The ability to interact effectively with people of different cultures and socio-economic backgrounds.

Evaluation   Processes to determine the effectiveness of strategies used and review of approaches incorporated for achieving results. Evaluation often involves instrumentation, protocols, staffing, data analysis and reporting. Quantitative and qualitative evaluation are the primary efforts.

Expert opinions   Statements by or reference to an expert or specialized organization.

Flash lecture   A brief and spontaneous lecture, typcially advertised shortly before the event using social media and offered in a public location where passersby can stop and listen.

Flier   A single-page printed production usually posted on bulletin boards.

Focus group   A qualitative research technique in which an experienced moderator guides about eight to ten participants through a discussion of a selected topic, allowing them to talk freely and spontaneously. Focus groups are often used to identify previously unknown issues or concerns or to explore reactions to potential actions, benefits or concepts during the planning and development stages.

Formative evaluation   Evaluative research conducted during program development. May include state-of-the art reviews, pretesting messages and materials, and pilot testing a program on a small scale before full implementation.

Gatekeeper   An organization or individual you must work with before you can reach an intended audience (e.g., an organization, a schoolteacher, a television public service director).

Goal   A desired state.

Health and safety   A dynamic state of living that involves degrees of risk, functionality and life satisfaction.

Health belief model   A conceptual framework of health behavior stating that health behavior is a function of both knowledge and motivation. Specifically, the model emphasizes the role of perceived vulnerability to a condition, perceived severity of the condition, perceived benefits of the recommended action, perceived barriers to the advised action, cues to action and self-efficacy in terms of one's ability to take action.

Health and safety communications   Conveying messages that raise awareness about health and safety topics and issues for the purpose of changing audience behavior.

Health and safety communications model   A five-step explanation of developing and delivering health and safety communications.

Impact   The degree of influence or persuasion experienced by the receiving audience.

Impact evaluation   A type of summative evaluation used to determine short-term effects of the program.

In-kind donations   Something given for free.

Intermediaries   People acting as a link between others to bring about an agreement or reconciliation.

Interpersonal communication   Messages are conveyed between persons to inform, instruct or persuade, with the audience usually not exceeding 20 persons.

Issues   Important topics for discussion or debate.

Linking and pairing   Building upon the audience's existing thoughts or perceptions to reframe a current message or approach. Linking and pairing extends existing messages and approaches and incorporates similarities.

Mass communication   Media are used to disseminate messages widely, rapidly and continuously to arouse intended meanings in large and diverse audiences and to influence them in a variety of ways.

Mass media   Approaches designed to reach large audiences. These include, but are not limited to, television, radio, newspapers, magazines, and the internet.

Measurement   Assigning scores to data or categorizing data.

Media (the)   Main means of mass communication (i.e., television, radio, newspapers and the internet).

Media advocacy   Having a strategic engagement with the media for the purpose of advancing a social initiative or policy effort.

Media literacy   Having the skills to deconstruct media messages to identify the sponsor's motives and to construct or compose media messages representing the intended audience's point of view. This is often taught to youth so they can evaluate the media messages directed toward them.

Media relations   Working with the media to inform the public of your organization's important communications in a positive, consistent and credible manner.

Message   Sent information from a source to an audience. In health and safety communications it is based on a relevant topic or issue.

Need   Something necessary in given circumstances or a situation requiring a course of action.

Objectives   Statements of what that audience has to accomplish in order to reach a goal. In health and safety communication objectives are organized around what the audience is expected to know, feel and do in order to reach the desired state of promoted health and reduced safety risk.

Op-ed   Short for "opposite the editorial page" in a newspaper, this is a section that includes columns, commentaries, specialized articles, and essays. Op-ed contributions can be found in a newspaper or magazine.

Optimism bias   Perceived invulnerability.

Outcome evaluation   Type of summative evaluation used to determine if goals were reached (long-term effects of the program).

Pamphlet (or booklet)   A multiple-page publication compiled and put together with a booklet stapler or binding machine with the content usually focused on a single topic or issue.

Paradigm   A pattern or template of thought.

Pilot testing   Testing the effort before and during its implementation.

Positioning Using strategies designed to gain the attention and prioritization within the mind of the audience. With so many messages competing for the audience's attention, positioning can emphasize factors such as first, largest, only, lowest cost, most effective or fastest.

Poster Printed production similar to flier yet larger in format.

Press release A communication directed at the news media to announce something of newsworthy importance.

Process evaluation Evaluation directed at individual steps in the health and safety communications model.

Production Preparing the communication approach, including determination of approaches, graphic design and layout, assembly of materials and artwork, editing, pilot testing and review.

Public presence Setting involving a health communicator's active engagement as an individual.

Public service announcement (PSA) A mass media advertisement distributed or broadcasted without charge to the sponsoring organization.

Reasoned action and planned behavior Theory assumes a person makes reasonable and systematic use of information when deciding how to behave. His/her intention to act is the immediate determinant of the health or safety behavior. However, intention is shaped by personal attitude toward the behavior as well as perception of the social pressure to perform the behavior (subjective norm). Perceived behavioral control over the behavior is also an important part.

Research A disciplined effort to answer a question.

Resource A supply of assets to draw upon while designing and implementing health and safety communications messages (e.g., referenced material, data sources, etc.).

Salient health beliefs Immediate, important or conspicuous beliefs.

Selective exposure When a conveyed message reaches a receptive audience who is not the intended target audience.

Social (cognitive) learning theory A theory of human behavior that stresses the dynamic interrelationships among people, their behavior and their environment.

Social marketing A process for influencing human behavior on a large scale, using marketing principles for the purpose of societal benefit rather than commercial profit.

Social norms marketing (social norming) A process that builds upon the social marketing know-feel-do strategies, takes the concept of "misperceptions" and strives both to correct these and to promote positive or healthy and safe behavior.

Source Agent, aide or advisory committee tasked with developing and delivering a message.

Spokespersons Recruited speakers based on credibility.

Stages of change (transtheoretical) model A theoretical framework that explains behavior change as a process rather than as an event. The model identifies individuals at various stages of readiness to attempt, to make and to sustain a behavior change. The stages are precontemplation, contemplation, decision/determination, action and maintenance.

Statistics The use of numerical information or data. Statistics are quantitative in nature, and are used to provide specific documentation on factors such as incidence and prevalence of a behavior; they also are used to test a hypothesis and summarize levels of significance.

Strategy A plan of action to create change.

Summative evaluation Evaluation taking place after program implementation and involved impact and outcome evaluation.

Tailoring Designing a communication so that the message is appropriately designed for the readiness of the target audience to make a change.

Testimonial Formal storytelling on an issue that has affected the lives of individuals and groups.

Theory A set of ideas explaining a situation or justifying a course of action.

Tools Devices to draw upon while designing and implementing health and safety communications messages (e.g., data, expert opinions).

Topic A matter or subject for discussion or presented in text.

Triangulation A technique used to blend evaluation results that emanate from different sources.

Workshop A communication approach that is a time-limited opportunity that prepares participants with a specified set of knowledge, attitudes and/or skills.

Index